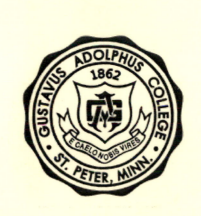

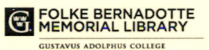
FOLKE BERNADOTTE
MEMORIAL LIBRARY

GUSTAVUS ADOLPHUS COLLEGE

GUSTAVUS LIBRARY
ASSOCIATES

EX LIBRIS 2015-2016

Psychology of Physical Activity

The positive benefits of physical activity for physical and mental health are now widely acknowledged, yet levels of physical inactivity continue to increase throughout the developed world. Understanding the psychology of physical activity has therefore become an important concern for scientists, health professionals and policy-makers alike. *Psychology of Physical Activity* is a comprehensive and in-depth introduction to the fundamentals of exercise psychology, from theories of motivation and adherence to the design of successful interventions for increasing participation.

Now in a fully revised, updated and expanded third edition, *Psychology of Physical Activity* is still the only textbook to offer a full survey of the evidence base for theory and practice in exercise psychology, and the only textbook that explains how to interpret the quality of the research evidence. With international cases, examples and data included throughout, the book also provides a thoroughly detailed examination of the relationship between physical activity and mental health. A full companion website (www.routledge.com/cw/biddle) offers useful features to help students and lecturers get the most out of the book during their course, including multiple-choice revision questions, PowerPoint slides and supplementary learning activities.

Psychology of Physical Activity is the most authoritative, engaging and up-to-date introduction to exercise psychology currently available. It is essential reading for all students working in exercise and health sciences.

Stuart Biddle is Professor of Active Living and Public Health in the Institute of Sport, Exercise & Active Living at Victoria University, Melbourne, Australia. He was previously Professor at Loughborough University where he was Head of the School of Sport & Exercise Sciences, 2001–2007. He was the inaugural Editor-In-Chief of the journal *Psychology of Sport & Exercise* and is a Past-President of both the International Society of Behavioral Nutrition and Physical Activity and the European Federation for the Psychology of Sport and Physical Activity (FEPSAC). In 2010 he received the Distinguished Contribution to Sport & Exercise Psychology Award from the British Psychological Society. Stuart has published over 250 research papers and sits on editorial boards of several leading peer-reviewed scientific journals, including *Preventive Medicine*, *International Journal of Behavioral Nutrition and Physical Activity*, and *Psychology of Sport and Exercise*.

Nanette Mutrie is Chair of Physical Activity for Health at the University of Edinburgh, Scotland, and she directs the Physical Activity for Health Research Centre there. She is also a visiting Professor at the MRC Social and Public Health Sciences Unit at the University of Glasgow and at the University of Ulster. Nanette is a Chartered Psychologist with the British

Psychological Society and has extensive experience of conducting interventions aimed at increasing physical activity. She is also an Honorary Fellow of BASES. She has contributed to policy, for example, 'Let's make Scotland more active', and the National Institute of Health and Clinical Excellence (NICE) programmes on physical activity and the environment and the promotion of walking and cycling (www.nice.org.uk). Nanette was awarded an MBE in the UK New Year's Honours list 2015 for services to physical activity for health. She gets her own exercise by commuter cycling, dog walking and playing golf (badly, so a lot more walking involved!).

Trish Gorely is a Senior Lecturer in Physical Activity and Health in the School of Sport at the University of Stirling, UK. Her research interests are in the psychology of physical activity and health, and understanding physical activity and sedentary behaviour in young people and adults. Trish is an Associate Editor for the *International Review of Sport and Exercise Psychology*.

Psychology of Physical Activity

Determinants, well-being
and interventions

Third edition

**Stuart J.H. Biddle, Nanette Mutrie
and Trish Gorely**

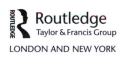

Routledge
Taylor & Francis Group

LONDON AND NEW YORK

First published 2001
by Routledge
2 Park Square, Milton Park, Abingdon, Oxon OX14 4RN

Second edition published 2007
by Routledge
2 Park Square, Milton Park, Abingdon, Oxon OX14 4RN

This edition published 2015
by Routledge
2 Park Square, Milton Park, Abingdon, Oxon OX14 4RN

and by Routledge
711 Third Avenue, New York, NY 10017

Routledge is an imprint of the Taylor & Francis Group, an informa business

British Library Cataloguing-in-Publication Data
A catalogue record for this book is available from the British Library

Library of Congress Cataloging in Publication Data
Biddle, Stuart.
Psychology of physical activity : determinants, well-being and interventions /
Stuart J. H. Biddle, Professor Nanette Mutrie and Trish Gorely. -- Third edition.
pages cm
Includes bibliographical references and index.
1. Exercise--Psychological aspects. 2. Clinical health psychology. 3. Health promotion.
I. Mutrie, Nanette, 1953- II. Mutrie, Professor Nanette. III. Gorely, Trish. IV. Title.
RA781.B486 2015
613.7--dc23
2014029401

ISBN: 978-0-415-51817-8 (hbk)
ISBN: 978-0-415-51818-5 (pbk)
ISBN: 978-0-203-12349-2 (ebk)

Typeset in Perpetua
by Fakenham Prepress Solutions, Fakenham, Norfolk NR21 8NN

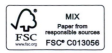

Printed and bound in Great Britain by
TJ International Ltd, Padstow, Cornwall

Contents

List of figures

List of tables

Preface

The psychology of physical activity for health is a field that has grown very rapidly since our first text in 1991 (Biddle and Mutrie, 1991). Indeed, we said this in the Preface to the 2008 edition of the current book. However, it seems even more obvious to make this statement today. To reflect this, we have made many changes to the current edition.

In writing this book, not only did Stuart and Nanette recruit an extra pair of able hands in Trish Gorely, but they reorganised a great deal of material from the 2nd edition (see Biddle and Mutrie, 2008). This meant that new chapters were written while some old chapters were discarded. What was clear in doing this was that a great deal has developed in recent years. This includes the continued growth in physical activity and mental health, an increase in the number of physical activity interventions being conducted and reported, and a significant expansion in research synthesis through systematic reviews and meta-analyses. We have expanded on some of these issues in Chapter 17.

At the same time, although not a central focus of this book, there has been a great deal of expansion – and recognition – of physical activity in national and international policy (see Chapter 1). This means that the material covered in this book is becoming increasingly recognised as a vitally important aspect of public health.

We have reorganised the order of the book to make it what we see as more logical. It also follows the behavioural epidemiological framework (Sallis and Owen, 1999). After the Introduction, we introduce topics on health outcomes that are most germane to psychology – mental health. Here we expand into five chapters from the three in the 2nd edition. We have added new chapters on cognitive functioning and self-esteem.

In Part III we address the correlates and theories of physical activity through five chapters. We felt that this rather dominated previous editions of the book and so have tried to keep a balance between historical context of theory (e.g. Health Belief Model) and contemporary research findings. We have also tried to summarise trends through reviews and exemplar studies.

In Part IV we expand on previous editions by considering physical activity interventions across different age and clinical groups, as well as considering planning and design issues. All chapters in this section are completely new. In addition, in Part V (Chapter 16) we introduce for the first time in a book on 'exercise psychology' the topic of sedentary behaviour. Moreover, new learning and teaching support materials are now available with this book.

Stuart acknowledges Loughborough University for granting a study leave during his period of writing this book. It is often claimed that Loughborough is in Stuart's blood, and that is true. However, towards the end of the writing of the book, he moved to Victoria University in Melbourne, Australia, where he hopes to have an equally enjoyable and productive time.

Nanette had to have her arm twisted into participating in this revision but after successful physiotherapy for that she has enjoyed the way the rewrite was approached. Three memorable writing retreats in Inverness, Stirling and Glasgow made the work more enjoyable. The University of Edinburgh provided some of the time required for this in the workload model, and colleagues in Edinburgh were encouraging about the revision and promised to use it! At home Kay, and Ellie (the border terrier) provided support, often involving walking, and I very much appreciated that. The support often started with the phrase 'walk away from that computer!' – sage advice to all authors.

Trish has enjoyed joining the writing team and has learned much in the process. Thanks guys. She acknowledges the support of the University of Stirling in writing this book and the encouragement she received from friends and colleagues to keep bashing away at it. Finally, we thank the staff at Routledge for their support and encouragement.

Stuart Biddle
Loughborough University

Nanette Mutrie
University of Edinburgh

Trish Gorely
University of Stirling

June 2014

References

Biddle, S.J.H. and Mutrie, N. (1991) *Psychology of Physical Activity and Exercise: A health-related perspective.* London: Springer-Verlag.

Biddle, S.J.H. and Mutrie, N. (2008) *Psychology of Physical Activity: Determinants, well-being and interventions* (2nd edn). London: Routledge.

Sallis, J.F. and Owen, N. (1999) *Physical Activity and Behavioral Medicine.* Thousand Oaks, CA: Sage.

List of abbreviations

ACSM	American College of Sports Medicine
BCT	behaviour change technique
BCW	Behaviour change wheel
BDI	Beck Depression Inventory
BMI	body mass index
CVD	Cardiovascular disease
DSM	*Diagnostic and Statistical Manual of Mental Disorders*
ES	effect size
FFIT	Football Fans in Training
GAPA	Global Advocacy for Physical Activity
HAPA	Health Action Process Approach
HRQL	health-related quality of life
MAACL	Multiple Affect Adjective Checklist
MI	myocardial infarction *or* motivational interviewing
MRC	Medical Research Council
MVPA	moderate to vigorous structured physical activity
NCD	Non-communicable Disease
NHANES	National Health and Nutrition Examination Survey
NICE	National Institute for Health and Care Excellence; *formerly* National Institute for Health and Clinical Excellence
PACE	Physician-based Assessment and Counselling for Exercise
PHC	primary health care
POMS	Profile of Mood States
PPI	positive psychological intervention *or* Patient and Public involvement
PWB	psychological well-being
QALY	quality adjusted life year
RR	relative risk
SES	socio-economic status
TTM	Transtheoretical Model

Part I

Introduction and rationale

1 Introduction and rationale

Why you should take your dog for a walk even if you don't have one!

Purpose of the chapter

This chapter introduces key concepts in the study of physical activity, exercise and health as a prelude to a more extensive discussion in subsequent chapters on the psychology of physical activity. Specifically, in this chapter we aim to:

- introduce the concept of physical activity psychology;
- explain the behavioural epidemiological and ecological frameworks;
- provide a brief synopsis of human evolution and history that is relevant to current physical activity and health behaviours in contemporary society;
- define key terms;
- highlight recent policy and position statements and guidelines on physical activity;
- summarise the evidence linking physical activity with various health outcomes and risks;
- review the prevalence and trends in physical activity and sedentary behaviour.

Many forms of physical activity are healthy! As a result we have been interested in the promotion of physical activity for some time and our first text on the subject was published in the early 1990s (Biddle and Mutrie, 1991). It is pleasing to see that physical activity for health is now a very high priority for governments and other agencies. The Toronto Charter for physical activity, which was launched in 2010 by the Global Advocacy Council for Physical Activity, has provided a landmark moment in our field (Global Advocacy Council for Physical Activity International Society for Physical Activity and Health, 2010). The Charter establishes the case for the promotion of physical activity for health and calls for global action from governments to create policies and opportunities for everyone to lead physically active lives. The rationale for this call to action from the Toronto Charter is shown in Figure 1.1.

This is now a very different context than the early years of investigation of the relationship between physical activity and health. Previously, a great deal of time was spent in identifying the biological mechanisms of the health effects of activity and inactivity – indeed an essential aspect of our knowledge – but rather less attention was devoted to the issues of why people are or are not physically active, what the psychological benefits might be, or the best ways of promoting physical activity. But we are glad to report a significant increase in interest, over the past decade or so, in 'exercise or physical activity psychology', behavioural interventions, and how being active influences how people feel.

This shift in our field from needing to show that physical activity has plausible biological mechanisms that promote health, to realising that we need to provide interventions that will

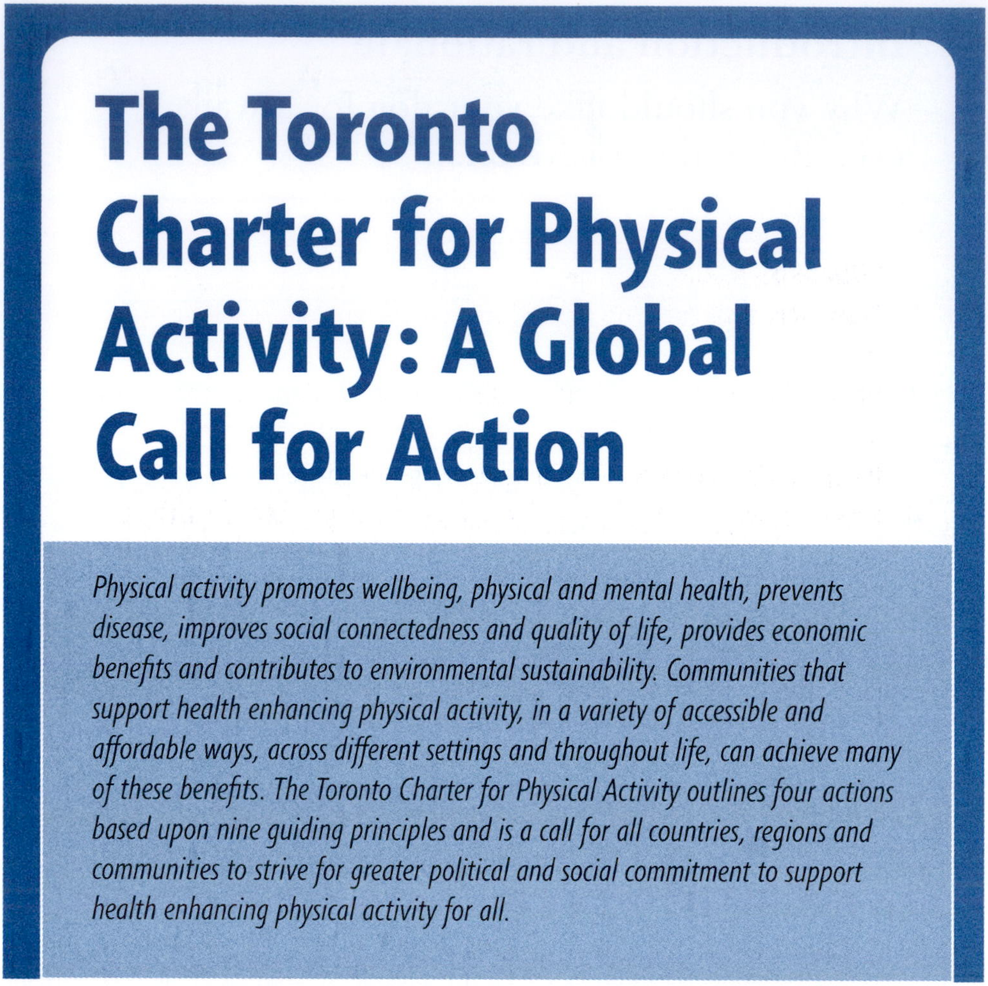

The Toronto Charter for Physical Activity: A Global Call for Action

Physical activity promotes wellbeing, physical and mental health, prevents disease, improves social connectedness and quality of life, provides economic benefits and contributes to environmental sustainability. Communities that support health enhancing physical activity, in a variety of accessible and affordable ways, across different settings and throughout life, can achieve many of these benefits. The Toronto Charter for Physical Activity outlines four actions based upon nine guiding principles and is a call for all countries, regions and communities to strive for greater political and social commitment to support health enhancing physical activity for all.

Figure 1.1   The Toronto Charter for Physical Activity

help people become more active, is emphasised in the Toronto Charter. Experts from around the world reviewed the evidence for interventions that were effective in increasing physical activity levels. This review led to the production of a companion document to the Toronto Charter, entitled 'Seven investments that work' (Global Advocacy for Physical Activity, 2012). These seven investments are shown in Figure 1.2.

When writing our book in 1991 there were few textbooks giving more than cursory attention to how we might help people become more active. Today, however, nearly all works in the field address at least some aspect of psychology, behaviour change or behavioural interventions. This challenge has been noted by England's Chief Medical Officer at the time, Sir Liam Donaldson, who said in his 2009 annual report:

> The benefits of regular physical activity to health, longevity, well being and protection from serious illness have long been established. They easily surpass the effectiveness of

7 Investments that work for physical activity

1. **'Whole-of-school'** programs
2. **Transport policies** and systems that prioritise walking, cycling and public transport
3. **Urban design** regulations and infrastructure that provides for equitable and safe access for recreational physical activity, and recreational and transport-related walking and cycling across the life course
4. Physical activity and NCD prevention integrated into **primary health care** systems
5. **Public education**, including mass media to raise awareness and change social norms on physical activity
6. **Community-wide programs** involving multiple settings and sectors & that mobilize and integrate community engagement and resources
7. Sports systems and programs that promote '**sport for all**' and encourage participation across the life span

GAPA
GLOBAL ADVOCACY
FOR PHYSICAL ACTIVITY
Advocacy Council of ISPAH

Figure 1.2 Seven investments that work for physical activity

any drugs or other medical treatment. The challenge for everyone, young and old alike, is to build these benefits into their daily lives.

(Department of Health, 2009, p. 21)

Even within the field of physical activity psychology there has been a greater recognition of physical activity and exercise for health, whereas in the past the vast majority of the literature focused on competitive sport. For example, one of the key research journals, *Journal of Sport Psychology*, became the *Journal of Sport and Exercise Psychology* (*JSEP*) in 1988 to better reflect the field, and now nearly all such journals have the word 'exercise' in their title.

Medical journals have also increased their interest in the topic of physical activity and in the behavioural challenges of increasing the population level of physical activity. For example, *The Lancet* is one of the world's leading medical journals with almost 200 years of publication history. In that time and up until July 2012 only 62 articles with the words 'physical activity' in the title had been published. Perhaps the most notable *Lancet* article relating to physical activity was that written by Jeremy Morris in 1953 in which he pointed out that active London bus conductors were at lower risk of cardiovascular disease than their much less active (seated) colleagues – the drivers of the buses (Morris *et al.*, 1953). That article was the foundation of the following half-century of work that has now resulted in a *Lancet* series relating to physical activity for health, which was published to coincide with the hosting of the Olympic and Paralympic Games in London in 2012. This series is already a major point of reference for everyone teaching and researching in this area or those making the case to government, local authorities, schools or hospitals about the role of physical activity for health. The editor of *The Lancet* series has been bold enough to call the lack of physical activity a 'pandemic' health concern and this quote appears on the front cover of the journal (Das and Horton, 2012):

> In view of the prevalence, global reach, and health effect of physical inactivity, the issue should be appropriately described as pandemic, with far-reaching health, economic, environmental, and social consequences.

The series includes editorial commentary and research articles with new global evidence on the risks of inactivity, reviews of interventions, the uses of technology and issues relating to surveillance. The series calls for us to rethink our approach to physical activity (Das and Horton, 2012). This quote from the editors supports the approach we have taken in this book. We have approached physical activity from the broadest definition and the following quote demonstrates that narrowly defined 'sport' and 'exercise' alone cannot solve the pandemic of physical inactivity that exists across the world:

> This Series on physical activity is not about sport and it is about more than just exercise. It is about the relationship between human beings and their environment, and about improving human wellbeing by strengthening that relationship. It is not about running on a treadmill, whilst staring at a mirror and listening to your iPod. It is about using the body that we have in the way it was designed, which is to walk often, run sometimes, and move in ways where we physically exert ourselves regularly whether that is at work, at home, in transport to and from places, or during leisure time in our daily lives.
>
> (Das and Horton, 2012, p. 1)

This book provides a review of contemporary psychological knowledge about physical activity. We will *focus exclusively on physical activity for health rather than on sport performance.* Although usually referred to as 'exercise psychology', we feel that this may reflect only structured bouts of physical activity, as we discuss in the definitions section shortly. We therefore prefer to broaden the discussion to 'physical activity' in its widest sense, at least as far as health is concerned. However, as you will see, a great deal of the literature does actually refer to exercise, as this is often a behaviour that is easier to quantify and study. We think it may be time to reconsider the name of the field of 'sport and exercise' psychology – is it time to re-brand to the overarching term 'physical activity psychology'? Interestingly, Division 47 (Exercise and Sport Psychology) of the American Psychology Association has also been debating this issue (see http://www.apadivisions.org/division-47/about/resources/index.aspx and http://www.apadivisions.org/division-47/about/resources/defining.pdf) and have concluded that 'performance psychology' is a more accurate reflection of practice than sport psychology, and that exercise psychology might be better aligned with health psychology. Perhaps this debate is also needed in the UK.

The behavioural epidemiological and ecological frameworks

We adopt a 'behavioural epidemiological' framework advocated by Sallis and Owen (1999). Applying this to physical activity, the framework proposes a five-stage model in which correlates of physical activity build on an understanding of the relationship between physical activity and health and the measurement of physical activity. Correlates then inform the development of interventions, the results of which are translated into action. The framework is illustrated in Figure 1.3.

The five-phase behavioural epidemiology framework is a useful way of viewing various processes in the understanding of physical activity and health. Behavioural epidemiology considers the link between behaviours and health and disease, such as why some people are physically active and others are not. The five main phases are as follows:

1. *To establish the link between physical activity and health.* This is now well documented for many diverse conditions as well as well-being (Dishman *et al.*, 2013; Lee *et al.*, 2012). Many of these conditions are described in this chapter. Psychological outcomes of physical activity are dealt with in the next section of this book.
2. *To develop methods for the accurate assessment of physical activity.* Large-scale surveillance of population trends often relies on self-reported levels of physical activity, a method that is fraught with validity and reliability problems. Recent 'objective' methods, such as movement sensors, heart rate monitors or pedometers are very important and useful, although they do not necessarily give all the information required, such as type of activity or the setting in which activity took place. We must continue to develop better measures of the behaviour itself – physical activity – for the field to progress.
3. *To identify factors that are associated with different levels of physical activity.* Given the evidence supporting the beneficial effects of physical activity on health, it is important to identify factors that might be associated with the adoption and maintenance of the behaviour. This area is referred to as the study of 'correlates' or 'determinants' of physical activity. This is the main theme in Section 3 of the book.
4. *To evaluate interventions designed to promote physical activity.* Once a variable is identified as a correlate of physical activity (e.g. self-efficacy), then interventions can manipulate this variable to test if it is, in fact, a determinant. The number of intervention studies in physical activity is increasing (Foster *et al.*, 2005; Heath *et al.*, 2012). We discuss interventions in Section 4.

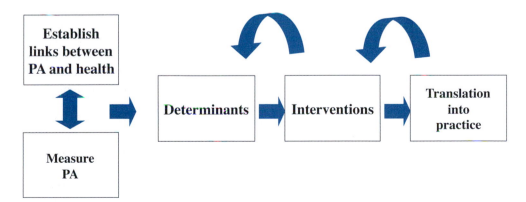

Figure 1.3   Behavioural epidemiological framework

5.   *To translate findings from research into practice.* If interventions work, it is appropriate to translate such findings into ecologically valid settings outside of the research environment.

It is important to realise that the above sequence is not linear. For example, measures of physical activity are developed and refined alongside tests of outcomes, and community projects are often established prior to convincing evidence, but may include a monitoring and evaluation element to test the efficacy of such an intervention before refining future interventions (see Figure 1.3). The whole process then becomes iterative.

Although this book is focused on psychological and behavioural factors, we also advocate the adoption of an *ecological framework* because it highlights the multiple influences on physical activity and sedentary behaviour. Essentially, the ecological framework suggests that behaviour may be the product of multiple influences, such as individual psychology, social circumstances, the surrounding physical environment, and wider socio-political influences (e.g. policy). This is important to highlight in a book that emphasises a psychological approach because such an approach can only be viewed properly in the wider context of an ecological framework. That is, how we think and feel will be important, but they are not the only influences on behaviour – we need to look at the 'bigger picture' too. For example, interventions might target individual motivation when people do not adopt the target behaviour of physical activity yet operate in a favourable environment. On the other hand, motivated people might struggle to be as active as they wish if environmental constraints are severe. At the level of public (population) health, typically we need to address both, as neither will be at optimal levels. That is to say, we need to create supportive environments in which people can operate, yet provide individuals with the psychological tools to change and regulate their own behaviour.

This approach recognises that individual approaches take us only so far and that behaviour is also affected by wider social and environmental influences. An ecological framework recognises *intra*personal (individual), *inter*personal (social), physical environmental, and societal/legislative influences on behaviour. Although we do address environmental, policy and social issues, we can only give these issues brief coverage. However, we fully acknowledge that psychological factors are but one set of influences, or potential influences, on physical activity (see Figure 1.4).

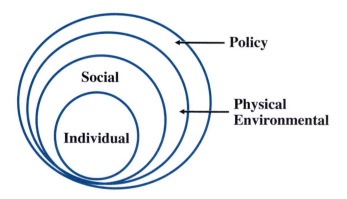

Figure 1.4   Ecological framework

Key point: Physical activity may be influenced by many factors. Psychological influences coexist with social, environmental, and wider policy/legislative influences.

In this introductory chapter, we present a rationale for the study of physical activity, outline briefly some of the health benefits of physical activity, and summarise initiatives and statements from key organisations that illustrate the importance of the topic. Finally, we give an overview of the evidence on how active, or inactive, people are. The chapter provides a background on which to judge and assess the role of behavioural and psychological factors in physical activity. Following this introductory chapter we then divide the book into the following three main parts:

- **Part II Physical activity and mental health**
- **Part III Physical activity correlates and theories**
- **Part IV Physical activity behaviour change**

Physical activity, evolution and history

In the wonderful animated 'Wallace & Grommit' film *The Wrong Trousers*, Wallace buys his dog, Grommit, a pair of 'techno-trousers' – automatic walking trousers that allow Wallace to sit at home while the techno-trousers take Grommit for a walk. Is this the shape of things to come, namely seeking ways of allowing our pets to exercise without moving ourselves? As Wallace said, 'I think you will find these a valuable addition to our modern lifestyle.' It is ironic that we wouldn't dream of depriving our dogs of their walk!

From Grommit to Astrand: 'There is virtually no way of reverting to our "natural" way of life, but with insight into our biological heritage we may be able to modify the current, self-destructive, elements of our modern lifestyle' (Astrand, 1994, p. 103). Astrand's fascinating analysis of evolutionary history in relation to current lifestyles highlights the central issue: we are now living our lives, at least in developed countries, and increasingly in developing ones too, in ways that are largely unhealthy and different from what we have done for most of our past. As some have expressed it, we are living twenty-first-century lifestyles with hunter-gatherer genes. Indeed, Astrand's (1994) analysis of lifestyles of humans since we first appeared on Earth some four million years ago led him to conclude: 'during more than 99% of our existence we were hunters and food gatherers. Now we are exposed to an enormous experiment – without control groups' (p. 101).

From Astrand to Grommit: Professor Astrand often finishes his eloquent lectures with the statement 'you should always take your dog for a walk – even if you don't have one!'

Blair (1988), for example, suggested that four evolutionary periods are important in understanding the relationship between physical activity and health. The pre-agricultural period (up until about 10,000 years ago) was characterised by hunting-and-gathering activities. Physical activity was high and diet was low in fat. The agricultural period (from 10,000 years ago until about the beginning of the nineteenth century) was characterised again by reasonably high physical activity levels and relatively low-fat diets, although the fat content probably increased during this time.

The industrial period (1800–1945) saw the development of the 'industrialised society' with the accompanying problems of overcrowding, poor diet, poor public health measures, and inadequate medical facilities and care. Infectious diseases were responsible for a high proportion of premature deaths. However, this trend was reversed in the 'nuclear/techno-logical' period, which Blair (1988) identified as from 1945 up until the present. The major improvement in public health measures and medical advances meant that infectious diseases were becoming less common in developed societies. However, health problems were merely shifted in terms of causes and outcomes. The major causes of premature mortality have now become 'lifestyle related', such as coronary heart disease and cancers, with risk factors such as cigarette smoking, poor diet and lack of physical activity (Katzmarzyk and Mason, 2009). As Paffenbarger *et al.* (1994) put it, 'both energy intake and energy output are determined primarily by individual behavior' (p. 119).

This is well illustrated by a study from Bassett and colleagues in which they provide a fascinating view on what physical activity levels might have been some 100 to 150 years ago by studying a community of Amish people in Ontario, Canada, in 2002 (Tudor-Locke and Bassett, 2004). The Amish – known to many through Harrison Ford's film *Witness* – shun modern 'conveniences' and motorised transport, and essentially live rural, farming-based lives.

Although not all women in the study led highly active lives, often due to the traditional roles of women in Amish communities centred on the house and cooking, they still had greater physical activity than one might expect today. The men, however, showed excep-tionally high levels of physical activity by today's standards. For example, as Figure 1.5 shows, the average number of steps per day for men and women easily exceeded the 12,500 considered 'highly active' for contemporary Western societies (Tudor-Locke and Bassett, 2004). Overweight and obesity levels were also much lower than in traditional Western communities. If the Amish community studied here is similar to that of many communities in the UK and other Western countries 150 years ago, it suggests that physical activity levels have declined markedly.

Such a change across generations has been referred to as the 'physical activity transition' (Katzmarzyk and Mason, 2009). This is where we have 'transitioned' from active occupations and transport to a period where humans have door-to-door motorised transport, inactive jobs, and more leisure time filled with sedentary pursuits.

In short, humans have now adopted lifestyles in industrialised countries that were quite unknown until very recently in terms of human evolution. This is not to say, of course, that

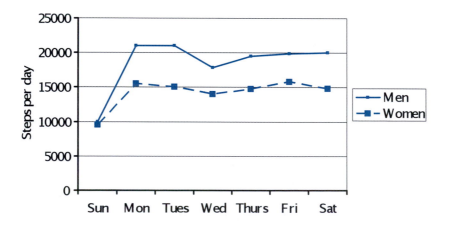

Figure 1.5   Average number of steps a day: Amish community

'health' has necessarily deteriorated; far from it in some cases, although this depends on the definition and measurement of health. Life span itself has increased dramatically. In 1960 the average life expectancy was 68 years in OECD countries but is now 80 years (http://www.compareyourcountry.org/health?lg=en).

> Key point: For 99 per cent of human existence being physically active was needed for survival. We are now living our lives in totally different ways in which activity is no longer needed for survival. Inactivity has become a major new health challenge.

Defining key terms

The terminology adopted in the study of health and physical activity has not always been consistent. This section will give operational definitions and clarifications to key words and terms. In practical terms we see physical activity as an umbrella term that covers all kinds of movement. We see sport and exercise and subdivisions of general physical activity with their own definitions. Specific definitions now follow, including the 'new kid on the block', sedentary behaviour (see Chapter 16).

Physical activity

Caspersen and colleagues (1985) define physical activity in terms of the three following elements:

- Movement of the body produced by the skeletal muscles.
- Resulting energy expenditure which varies from low to high.
- A positive correlation with physical fitness.

This definition of physical activity has been cited many times now and is well accepted. An alternative perspective has also been presented (Winter and Fowler, 2009).

As far as health outcomes are concerned, the energy expenditure is usually required to be well above resting levels and the physical activity is usually referred to as 'moderate-to-vigorous' (MVPA). For example, while I could be classified as being physically active while writing this book (fingers are moving fairly rapidly across the keyboard), this type of physical activity is less than MVPA and has largely been ignored in the study of 'physical activity for health'. However, recently scientists have shown a great deal of interest in the potential health benefits of 'light physical activity', such as standing and more gentle movement. This has been studied primarily from the point of view of reducing excessive sitting time (Wilmot *et al.*, 2012) (see Chapter 16).

Given the decline in the amount of physical activity that most people have to perform in work duties (as illustrated by the example of the Amish community), and the increase in motorised transport, a great deal of the physical activity that is necessary for health must be freely chosen in leisure time or consciously integrated into one's normal daily routine. This, in itself, justifies the increasing importance of studying psychological processes, such as motivation and decision-making, in physical activity, alongside other influences such as social and environmental factors. This is not to say that behaviour change cannot be achieved by other, less conscious means, such as 'nudging', or by 'stealth' (Marteau *et al.*, 2011). Indeed, these may prove to be highly useful.

Sedentary behaviour

High levels of sitting are ubiquitous. With increasing evidence showing deleterious health effects of sitting (Bauman *et al.*, 2013; Wilmot *et al.*, 2012), 'sedentary behaviour' is an important topic. It has been defined as sitting or lying during waking hours (hence does not include sleep), with low levels of energy expenditure (Sedentary Behaviour Research Network, 2012). From a practical point of view, it is 'sitting time'. It is not the same as low levels of physical activity or lack of exercise. This is 'inactivity'.

Exercise

Given that physical activity includes all movement, it is helpful also to recognise sub-components, or elements, of physical activity. Caspersen *et al.* (1985) defined exercise with reference to the following factors:

- body movement produced by skeletal muscles;
- resulting energy expenditure varying from low to high (so far, these points are the same as for physical activity);
- 'very positively correlated with physical fitness';
- 'planned, structured and repetitive bodily movement' (p. 127);
- the objective is to maintain or improve physical fitness.

Exercise may also have the objective of health enhancement or improving performance; for example, improving 10k running time. However, the distinction between physical activity and exercise is not always easy and one should recognise an overlap between the two constructs. In this book, exercise will usually refer to more structured leisure-time physical activity, such as participation in jogging, swimming, 'keep-fit' activities, and recreational sports, which are often supervised and require special facilities or equipment.

It has been recognised that, for many, exercise is perceived as being hard work, vigorous, and possibly unpleasant (see Chapter 2). Consequently, the need to promote 'active living', which may be defined as taking everyday opportunities to be active such as choosing to walk up the stairs rather than taking the lift (elevator), or walking the kids to school rather than driving them, has been recognised in an effort to produce a more acceptable or palatable message and may be more cost-effective.

Sport

Sport is a sub-component of physical activity, and often exercise too, whereby the activity is rule governed, structured, competitive, and involves gross motor movement characterised by physical strategy, prowess and chance (Rejeski and Brawley, 1988). The competitive nature of sport has sometimes been difficult to clarify. Indeed, the Sports Councils in the UK (e.g. 'sportscotland') have jurisdiction over activities that are non-competitive (e.g. keep-fit and yoga), and 'Sport for All' campaigns have often included a wider range of activities than 'traditional' competitive sports. Moreover, not all sports will necessarily be 'health-related' in the sense we adopt in this book. For example, playing darts or pool may be enjoyable and require great skill, but it provides minimal physical activity. But they are sports. We must also recognise that training for sport is not automatically health-enhancing because injuries and overtraining may result.

Health and well-being

Health is multi-factorial in nature and includes dimensions of the physical, mental and social, and, some might argue, the 'spiritual'. It involves enhancement of well-being as well as absence of disease. High positive health is sometimes referred to as 'wellness' or high-level well-being. This is positive physical and emotional well-being with a high capacity for enjoying life and its challenges, and possessing adequate coping strategies in the face of difficulties. Negative health is characterised by disease, morbidity and possibly premature death.

Physical fitness

Physical fitness refers to the ability of the individual to perform muscular work. Caspersen *et al.* (1985) defined it as 'a set of attributes that people have or achieve that relates to the ability to perform physical activity' (p. 129). This suggests that physical fitness is partly related to current physical activity levels ('attributes that people *achieve*') and partly a function of heredity ('attributes that people *have*').

The health-related components of physical fitness have traditionally been identified as cardiovascular fitness, muscular strength and endurance, muscle flexibility, and body composition (fatness) (Caspersen *et al.*, 1985). The development of these components of health-related fitness (HRF) has been related to specific 'health' or disease outcomes. Indeed, Pate (1988) has argued that 'physical fitness' should be defined solely in terms of the health-related aspects by stating that the following criteria should be met in such a definition:

- fitness should refer to the functional capacities required for comfortable and productive involvement in day-to-day activities;
- it should 'encompass manifestation of the health-related outcomes of high levels of habitual activity' (p. 177).

Bouchard and Stephens (1994), however, broaden the definition of HRF by referring to morphological, muscular, motor, cardiovascular and metabolic components. Given the public health perspective adopted in this book, the types and forms of exercise and physical activity that have been reviewed in relation to psychological principles and research are generally health-related. Competitive sport, except where it sheds some light on the wider public health aspects of exercise and physical activity, is not covered.

Correlates and determinants

We have used the word 'correlates' to reflect the factors that affect, or are thought to affect, participation in exercise and physical activity. Sometimes the word 'determinants' is also used. 'Correlates' has now become the standard term to use for this in the literature, mainly because it is recognised that many of the factors discussed are not, or may not be, true determinants. In other words, data may show associations but causality cannot always be demonstrated or inferred. The word 'correlates', therefore, seems more appropriate. Buckworth and Dishman (2002) refer to correlates as 'reproducible associations that are potentially causal' (p. 191).

Policy and position statements on physical activity

A number of organisations have produced position statements and policy documents on health-related behaviours, including physical activity. This reflects the increasing concern regarding the changes in morbidity and premature mortality that face many contemporary societies. One of the most important statements about physical activity for health comes from the World Health Organization (WHO).

The World Health Organization

At the public policy level, the initiation, coordination and implementation of policies that promote physical activity, enhance opportunities for whole populations to be active, and develop environments that promote active choices are necessary (Bull *et al.*, 2004). This policy-based approach has been endorsed by the World Health Assembly (in 2004, and again in 2008) in Resolution WHA57.17: Global Strategy on Diet, Physical Activity and Health http://apps.who.int/gb/ebwha/pdf_files/WHA57/A57_R17-en.pdf, and Resolution WHA61.14: Prevention and Control of Non-communicable Diseases (NCD) http://www.who.int/nmh/publications/ncd_action_plan_en.pdf, and most recently in the High-level Meeting of the United Nations General Assembly on the prevention and control of NCD (World Health Organization, 2004, 2008; United Nations General Assembly, 2011 http://www.un.org/en/ga/president/65/issues/ncdiseases.shtml). The resolutions urged member states and governments to develop national physical activity action plans and policies, with the ultimate aim of increasing physical activity levels in their populations. At this global level physical activity now features in the WHO action plan for the prevention and control of non-communicable diseases 2013 to 2020 [http://www.who.int/nmh/events/ncd_action_plan/en/]. The action plan is a set of voluntary global targets to be achieved by 2025. Physical inactivity is one of nine goals in the plan. The exact goal is '10% relative reduction in prevalence of insufficient physical activity'.

Academics and practitioners in the field of physical activity for health have now created worldwide organisations since we wrote the first edition of our book. The International Society for Behavioral Nutrition and Physical Activity was established in 2002 and has the mission to 'stimulate, promote and advocate innovative research and policy in the area of behavioral nutrition and physical activity toward the betterment of human health worldwide' (see https://www.isbnpa.org).

In 2006 the first congress of the International Society for Physical Activity and Health (ISPAH) took place in Atlanta, USA. Global Advocacy for Physical Activity (GAPA) is the newly created Council of ISPAH. The key principles of GAPA include the following:

- the development of actions based on evidence of effectiveness;
- the application of advocacy actions aimed at multiple levels (for example, political, media, professional);
- the involvement of a wide range of organisations with direct and indirect interests in the promotion of physical activity across all regions of the world.

> Key point: The World Health Organization has a goal to achieve a 10 per cent relative reduction in the prevalence of physical inactivity by 2025.

The Toronto Charter for Physical Activity

As mentioned earlier in the chapter, a landmark moment in the field of physical activity for health was the launching of The Toronto Charter for Physical Activity in May 2010 by the GAPA (see http://64.26.159.200/icpaph/en/toronto_charter.php). This document is a call for action and an advocacy tool; its aim is to create sustainable opportunities for physically active lifestyles for everyone. Within the Toronto Charter there are nine guiding principles listed for a population-based approach to physical activity. These guiding principles identify the importance of evidence-based approaches, of embracing equity by reducing social and health inequalities or removing disparities in access to physical activity. Importantly, the principles acknowledge the need to move beyond the individual to include environmental and social determinants of physical inactivity.

Other principles identify sustainability, a life-course approach to promoting activity and the need to garner political support and resource commitment at the highest level. Four key action areas are identified; each area makes a unique contribution but also builds on and is shaped by the other areas. Each area requires action in partnership, and the actors are listed as government, civil society, academic institutions, professional associations, the private sector, other organisations as well as the communities themselves. The four key areas are as follows:

- *Area 1: Implement a national policy and action plan.* The Toronto Charter outlines how the presence of such a policy or plan will unify the many different sectors in working together to achieve a common goal. It also states how it would help clarify political and financial commitment to the promotion of physical activity. Key components of such a policy or plan include: engaging relevant stakeholders, identifying clear leadership, knowing the roles and actions of all stakeholders, having an implementation plan that identifies timelines, funding and accountability. Ensuring that evidence-based guidelines on physical activity and health are adopted and having a repertoire of different strategies that are evidence-informed and inclusive of different social, cultural and economic backgrounds is also recommended. Even though the Toronto Charter stresses the importance of this area as a key population-based approach, it suggests that the absence of such a policy or plan should not prevent or delay regional, state or local efforts to increase physical activity or to develop relevant policy at their levels.
- *Area 2: Introduce policies that support physical activity.* This area highlights supportive policy and the regulatory environment in which this is placed. It cites examples such as urban planning and design to support sustainable transport options, fiscal policies to subsidise physical activity participation or educational policies to ensure quality opportunities are provided to all children both within and outside the curriculum timetable at the school setting.
- *Area 3: Reorient services and funding to prioritise physical activity.* This area explains how different government sectors can still deliver their core business, but change their priorities to focus on health-enhancing physical activity goals. This would allow for multiple benefits to be achieved, but these would need to be recognised as important and given adequate priority (for example, in 'Sport, Parks and Recreation', changing the focus away from elite or competitive sport participation to include a mass participation, an inactive or a disabilities focus and consequently provide staff training to build capacity in these areas). In 'Health' this would involve giving greater priority to primary prevention and health promotion, as opposed to secondary or tertiary prevention.

- *Area 4: Develop partnerships for action.* Programmes that focus on changing the health behaviour of individuals within one sector can be labour, time and money intensive. Rather, partnership that links programmes across sectors (e.g. education; transport; sports, parks and recreation; and other sectors) could create efficiencies, enhance the use of community-based physical activity programmes and increase physical activity (Mowen and Baker, 2009). Examples of different partnerships and collaborations across national, regional and local levels are given within the Toronto Charter (see http://64.26.159.200/icpaph/en/toronto_charter.php).

Initiatives in the UK

In the UK, ambitious targets for increasing the percentage of the population who are regularly active have been set. For example, in Scotland the goal is to have 50 per cent of the adult population regularly active (using the goal of achieving 30 minutes of moderate activity five times per week) by the year 2022 (Scottish Executive, 2003) and in England the suggested target was 70 per cent by 2020 with an interim target of 50 per cent by 2011 (Department for Culture, Media and Sport, 2002). These targets represented an approximate 20 per cent increase for Scotland and a 40 per cent increase for England in the number of people achieving the recommended minimum activity levels. To put this another way, in Scotland there was an expectation that a year-on-year increase of 1 per cent of the population reaching the recommended minimal levels can be achieved, whereas the English target aimed for a 2 per cent year-on-year increase. In the 2008 revision of the current book (Biddle and Mutrie, 2008) we wrote that there were several reasons to consider that these targets were highly ambitious. We note our concerns of 2008 in italics below and then comment on whether or not these concerns remain. The 2008 concerns were as follows:

1. *It is not yet clear exactly how we should intervene to achieve these increases.* As we write the revision in 2014 it remains unclear exactly how to intervene but the companion document to the Toronto Charter ('seven investments that work') provides the clearest statement to date of how to intervene to increase the level of physical activity in a nation. In Scotland, a ten-year implementation plan has been developed that uses the seven investments advocated by GAPA. This plan for a more active Scotland may be found here: http://www.scotland.gov.uk/Topics/ArtsCultureSport/Sport/MajorEvents/Glasgow-2014/Commonwealth-games/Indicators/PAIP.
2. *There is little evidence that this rate of increase is achievable.* It now seems by 2013 that even the 1 per cent increase year on year which Scotland targeted may not be achievable since the most recent Scottish Health Survey results from 2012 show that the overall percentage of the Scottish population achieving the message of accumulating 30 minutes of activity on five days of the week has plateaued at just under 40 per cent for the past five years (see Figure 1.6). The 2 per cent increase year on year – the aspiration target set for England – has certainly not been achieved and the most recent English survey notes a similar plateau, and comments that for the data collected in 2012 there was no evidence of any Olympic legacy effect (Scholes and Mindell, 2013).
3. *There is no clear resourcing model in either country for ensuring that money will be made available to enable the target to be met.* In our view this problem remains partly because physical activity cuts across several government department budgets and because the costs of inactivity are not well documented. However, the economic burden of inactivity is now being quantified and this will become a powerful driver of provision of resources to

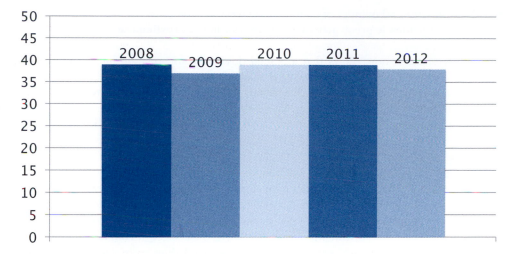

Figure 1.6   Percentage of Scottish adults achieving the 5 x 30 minutes a week recommendation
Source: Bradshaw et al. (2012).

reduce these costs. For example, a review of the cost-effectiveness of physical activity interventions in primary care concluded that 'most interventions … were cost-effective, especially where direct supervision or instruction was not required. … Many physical activity interventions had similar cost-utility estimates to funded pharmaceutical inter-ventions and should be considered for funding at a similar level' (Garrett *et al.*, 2011). It has been estimated that, using 2011 economic values, inactivity costs £18 per person in Scotland (Foster and Allender, on behalf of the Scottish Physical Activity Research Collaboration, 2012). This estimate is very conservative because it does not include some of the major costs, such as mental health, as these are not recorded in routine data.

4. *Increasing physical activity is a task that does not fall easily to one agency such as schools, sport organisations, health boards or transport planners.* We conclude that this challenge remains in the present era.

Position statements

Adults

A number of position statements have emerged that address how much physical activity people need to do to gain health benefits. One of the first statements addressed adults and had a particular focus on achieving physical fitness. Over 30 years ago the American College of Sports Medicine (ACSM) (1978) produced standard guidelines for the development of cardiovascular fitness in healthy adults. This was then revised and extended into a new position paper concerning cardiovascular fitness, as well as muscular strength and endurance and body composition (American College of Sports Medicine, 1990). The recommended amount of activity needed for cardiovascular fitness was noted as follows:

- frequency: three to five days per week;
- intensity: 60 to 90 per cent of maximum heart rate, or 50 to 85 per cent $VO_{2 \, max}$ or heart rate reserve;

- duration: 20 to 60 minutes of continuous aerobic activity;
- mode: large muscle group activities that are continuous, rhythmic and aerobic.

Subsequent research now shows that a graded dose–response relationship exists between physical activity and health; consequently it makes better sense not to 'prescribe' exercise only for the development of cardiovascular fitness but for other health outcomes as well (Lee, 2009). This may be done through more moderate levels of physical activity and that epidemiological knowledge led to the landmark statement by Pate *et al.* (1995) for the Centres for Disease Control and Prevention and ACSM which stated that adults should accumulate 30 minutes or more of moderate intensity physical activity on most, and preferably all, days of the week. This recommendation was adopted in other countries too, such as the UK (Department of Health, 2004), but they have all now been superseded by new messages that were first introduced in the USA (http://www.health.gov/paguidelines/guidelines/default. aspx#toc) and then became the WHO global recommendation on physical activity for health in 2010 (see http://www.who.int/dietphysicalactivity/factsheet_recommendations/en/). After further review by world experts similar recommendations were adopted in the UK (Department of Health, 2011). These new recommendations were established after careful review of emerging evidence and concluded that the volume of activity was more important than the frequency, and thus the core message for adults around the world is now to achieve a minimum of 150 minutes of at least moderate intensity physical activity a week in bouts of at least 10 minutes. Table 1.1 shows the main types and amounts of activity from these universally agreed recommendations.

Young people

The ACSM also made initial statements about the physical fitness and activity for children and youth shortly after they addressed the issue for adults (American College of Sports Medicine, 1988). They made eight specific recommendations, including the development of

Table 1.1   Recommendations from WHO for the amount and type of physical activity that adults aged 18–64 should do to gain health benefits

(http://www.who.int/dietphysicalactivity/factsheet_adults/en/index.html)

Type of activity	Amount of activity
Aerobic activity performed in bouts of at least 10 minutes' duration	At least 150 minutes of moderate intensity throughout the week; or at least 75 minutes of vigorous intensity throughout the week; or an equivalent combination of moderate and vigorous intensity activity.
Higher levels of activity	For additional health benefits, adults should increase their moderate intensity aerobic physical activity to 300 minutes per week, or engage in 150 minutes of vigorous intensity aerobic physical activity per week, or an equivalent combination of moderate and vigorous intensity activity.
Muscle strengthening	Muscle-strengthening activities should be done involving major muscle groups on two or more days a week.

appropriate school physical education programmes that emphasised lifetime exercise habits, enhanced knowledge about exercise, and behaviour change; the encouragement of a greater role in the development of children's activity levels from parents, community organisations and health care professionals; the adoption of a scientifically sound approach to fitness testing in schools whereby the emphasis is placed on health-related aspects assessed in relation to acceptable criteria rather than normative comparison; and finally award schemes for fitness should encourage individual exercise behaviour and achievement rather than superior athletic ability. In 1998, the then Health Education Authority (HEA) in England convened a meeting of experts. Reviews of evidence were written, discussed and revised, and recommendations made for research and policy (Biddle *et al.*, 1998). These were updated in 2011, and a new recommendation was added on sedentary behaviour, giving the following guidelines for young people:

1. All children and young people should engage in moderate to vigorous intensity physical activity for at least 60 minutes and up to several hours every day.
2. Vigorous intensity activities, including those that strengthen muscle and bone, should be incorporated at least three days a week.
3. All children and young people should minimise the amount of time spent being sedentary (sitting) for extended periods.

UK Chief Medical Officers' reports

In 2004, the Chief Medical Officer (CMO) in England published a position paper about physical activity titled 'At least 5 a week' (Department of Health, 2004). The aim of this publication was to provide information on the evidence of the relationship between physical activity and health. The report was compiled from comprehensive reviews of various aspects of the physical activity and health relationship and provided a substantial evidence base to inform practice and policy. In many ways this report replaced and updated the US Surgeon General's Report (US Department of Health and Human Services, 1996) which, for several years, was cited as the most comprehensive evidence base that the world should use as a reference point for the relationship between physical activity and health, and the importance of this topic for public health.

'Start Active, Stay Active', published in 2011, is the first physical activity document that has agreed guidelines for physical activity across all four home countries of the UK (England, Northern Ireland, Scotland and Wales) and updated the evidence from the 2004 CMO report. All four Chief Medical Officers endorsed this report and agreed the guidelines. Broadly speaking, the guidance suggests that adults should accumulate a minimum of 150 minutes of physical activity over the course of the week and that they should undertake strengthening and balance activities and minimise sedentary (sitting) time. The guidelines for adults state the following:

1. Adults should aim to be active daily. Over a week, activity should add up to at least 150 minutes (2.5 hours) of moderate intensity activity in bouts of ten minutes or more – one way to approach this is to do 30 minutes on at least five days a week.
2. Alternatively, comparable benefits can be achieved through 75 minutes of vigorous intensity activity spread across the week or a combination of moderate and vigorous intensity activity.

3.   Adults should also undertake physical activity to improve muscle strength on at least two days a week.
4.   All adults should minimise the amount of time spent being sedentary (sitting) for extended periods.

For the first time, guidelines for older adults were also stated as follows:

1.   Older adults who participate in any amount of physical activity gain some health benefits, including maintenance of good physical and cognitive function. Some physical activity is better than none, and more physical activity provides greater health benefits.
2.   Older adults should aim to be active daily. Over a week, activity should add up to at least 150 minutes (2.5 hours) of moderate intensity activity in bouts of ten minutes or more – one way to approach this is to do 30 minutes on at least five days a week.
3.   For those who are already regularly active at moderate intensity, comparable benefits can be achieved through 75 minutes of vigorous intensity activity spread across the week or a combination of moderate and vigorous activity.
4.   Older adults should also undertake physical activity to improve muscle strength on at least two days a week.
5.   Older adults at risk of falls should incorporate physical activity to improve balance and coordination on at least two days a week.
6.   All older adults should minimise the amount of time spent being sedentary (sitting) for extended periods.

Key point: The importance of physical activity for health is now recognised globally and is supported by international and national guidelines across the life span.

Health-related outcomes of physical activity

To understand behavioural aspects of physical activity, it is important to know the health benefits that accrue from being active. We now believe that there is strong evidence for this. *The Lancet* series of 2012 on physical activity provides some of the very best evidence in this area. In that series, Lee *et al.* (2012) reviewed the global data available and concluded that, in addition to all-cause mortality, there are ten non-communicable diseases that have up to a 30 per cent reduction in risk for people who engage in regular activity at recommended levels. These diseases are listed in Table 1.2. The amazing thing about physical activity is that even when people have these diseases it can still confer benefits. Very few lifestyle issues can both prevent and help in the treatment of so many diseases.

Key point: The benefits of physical activity are numerous and affect multiple health outcomes and conditions. The evidence is now well documented and convincing.

In providing an estimate of the global burden of disease caused by inactivity, Lee *et al.* (2012) note that almost 10 per cent of the burden of colon cancer and diabetes is caused by lack of sufficient activity. Figure 1.7 displays the analysis. One way of demonstrating the public health

Table 1.2   Diseases for which there is strong evidence of protective and beneficial effects from regular physical activity (Lee *et al.*, 2012)

Strong evidence of reduced risk	Strong evidence of benefits of activity to adult
All-cause mortality	Increased cardiorespiratory and muscular fitness
Coronary heart disease	Healthier body mass and composition
High blood pressure	Improved bone health
Stroke	Increased functional health
Falling	Improved cognitive function
Metabolic syndrome	
Type 2 diabetes	
Breast cancer	
Colon cancer	
Depression	

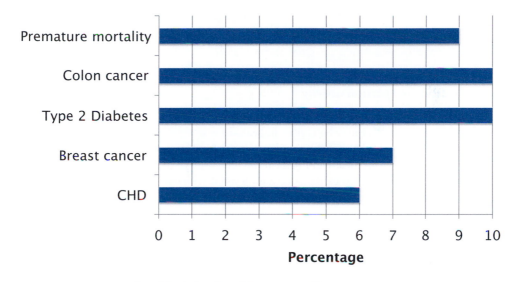

Figure 1.7   Percentage of worldwide burden of disease caused by inactivity

Source: Lee *et al.* (2012).

importance of the global lack of sufficient activity is to make a comparison with the risks associated with smoking. Most people are now aware that smoking is a highly risky activity, but do they also know that lack of sufficient physical activity is equally risky? As part of their review of the global burden of disease, Lee *et al.* made a comparison of the population attributable fraction (PAF) and the number of deaths per year caused by inactivity and smoking. Figure 1.8 shows the results of this comparison. To help in understanding this figure, the PAF is defined as the reduction in population mortality that would occur if the level of smoking or inactivity was reduced to zero. This is usually expressed as a percentage. You will see in the figure that both the PAF and deaths caused in millions across the world are almost identical for smoking and inactivity. This is an important piece of information for advocacy of the high risk of inactivity.

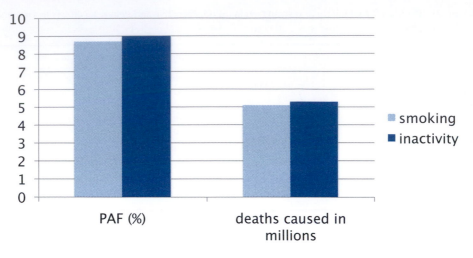

Figure 1.8   Comparison of population attributable fraction and deaths caused in millions by smoking and physical inactivity

Source: Drawn from data in Lee *et al.* (2012).

Risks of exercise and physical activity

Although the evidence supports quite clearly the beneficial health effects of physical activity, there are some aspects that may be contra-indicated for some groups, or situations in which a particular health risk is elevated during physical activity. The most commonly cited risks of exercise are sudden cardiac death and musculoskeletal injury.

Although the risk of sudden cardiac death is elevated with exercise, the balance of cardiac benefit and risk as a result of being a physically active individual is positive (Hardman and Stensel, 2009). Siscovick and colleagues (1984) reported that men who exercised vigorously for more than 20 minutes each week had an overall risk of primary cardiac arrest only 40 per cent of that of their inactive counterparts. It appears, therefore, that despite a temporary rise in risk during exercise, this is outweighed by the long-term effects of exercise on cardiac risk.

Knowledge on the musculoskeletal risks of exercise is not extensive, although clinical studies have been conducted on swimming, running, cycling, callisthenics and racket sports and have identified a number of injuries (Koplan *et al.*, 1985; Pate and Macera, 1994). It is difficult to find prevalence data on these kinds of injuries across the population and it is also difficult to reach a consensus on the meaning of an injury. For example, a feeling of tightness in the hamstring may be considered an injury by some people that would stop them taking part in their weekly tennis game. For other people that same feeling of tightness just means that they need to warm up more before their weekly tennis game. A recent study has shown that for women who achieve the 150 minutes per week threshold of moderate intensity activity there is an increased risk of musculoskeletal injury (Morrow *et al.*, 2012). However, the authors conclude that this modest increased risk of injury is far outweighed by the substantial health benefits that can be gained.

Some mental health problems have been identified with exercise, such as eating disorders or dependence on exercise. Such problems are likely to be unhealthy due to increased risk of injury, fatigue, illness and psychological ill health. However, the prevalence of exercise dependence is not known and is likely to be very small (Szabo, 2000), and eating disorders are likely to be a primary health concern in which over-exercising is a secondary symptom. The issue of negative psychological outcomes from physical activity is discussed more fully in Chapter 2.

Patterns of physical activity across the world

The wide array of positive health outcomes from physical activity suggests that considerable public health benefits could be achieved through increasing the population levels of physical activity, although some risks are also evident (see Hardman and Stensel (2014) for a detailed analysis). The identification of patterns of physical activity and sedentary living is important in any effort to plan public health initiatives in this field.

Measurement and surveillance of physical activity and sedentary behaviours

We believe it is important to assess both physically active and sedentary behaviours in order to better understand population prevalence of these behaviours. The problems in determining the activity levels of the population should not be underestimated. The measurement of physical activity becomes less reliable as techniques more suited to large-scale surveys – often self-report methods – are used (Sallis and Saelens, 2000). In a review of physical activity assessment in epidemiological research, LaPorte *et al.* (1985) identified over 30 different techniques, and a study of self-report measures in physical activity surveillance for young people located 89 instruments (Biddle *et al.*, 2011). For large-scale population-based research, however, the use of some variation on survey recall of activity is almost inevitable. However, 'objective' measures, such as heart rate monitors or movement sensors, are possible and are now being used in large samples (Mattocks *et al.*, 2008; Riddoch *et al.*, 2007). The instrument of choice for such measures is the Actigraph accelerometer, although inconsistency on data collection and analysis protocols can be a problem (Ridgers and Fairclough, 2011).

In an effort to obtain greater standardisation of self-reported physical activity levels across countries, a group of researchers developed the International Physical Activity Questionnaire (IPAQ) for both the monitoring of international surveillance trends and more focused research projects (Craig *et al.*, 2003). Several forms of the IPAQ were developed. These include long and short forms, self-administered and those administered by telephone, and those that refer to the 'last seven days' and a 'usual week'. The long form of IPAQ allows for assessment of different types of activity, including occupational, transport, yard/garden, household, leisure and sitting.

Satisfactory reliability and validity, at least comparable with other self-report measures, were reported and it was recommended that the short form (seven-day version) be used for national physical activity monitoring purposes. In addition, it was proposed that the long form be used for research purposes where more detailed assessing is required (Craig *et al.*, 2003). Further details are available at http://www.ipaq.ki.se.

Sedentary behaviour can also be assessed using self-report and objective methods (Atkin *et al.*, 2012). Objective methods, such as looking at low levels of activity with the Actigraph or thigh angle as a marker of sitting in the ActivPal, are increasingly used in the assessment of sedentary behaviour. To measure different types of sedentary behaviour, such as TV time or computer use, self-report instruments are required (Marshall *et al.*, 2010).

Prevalence of physical activity and sedentary behaviour

The estimates of activity levels of a population will be partly dependent on the method used. The more stringent the criteria adopted for classifying people as 'active', the fewer people will be classified as active, as shown in current estimates (Riddoch *et al.*, 2007). In an effort to provide a more global picture of the prevalence of physical activity, Hallal and colleagues synthesised data from 122 countries (Hallal *et al.*, 2012). They set out three criteria that would allow comparisons between datasets of adult levels of sufficient activity for health. These criteria were: achieving a minimum of 30 minutes of moderate intensity activity on five days of the week or achieving a minimum of 20 minutes of vigorous activity on three days of the week, or a combination of moderate and vigorous that would equate to 600 MET minutes per week (1 MET is energy expenditure at rest). The findings suggest that around one-third of the world's population is not sufficiently active. The percentage of those classified as inactive varies by area, with South East Asia having low levels of inactivity (17%) while the Americas and Eastern Mediterranean have higher levels of inactivity (43%). There were also three very important findings in term of issues of equality:

1.   universally, women are less active than men;
2.   across the globe, activity levels decrease dramatically with age;
3.   inactivity is increasing in high-income countries.

These authors also analysed the same datasets to make a global comparison of activity levels for children. Here the criteria were set as a minimum of 60 minutes of moderate intensity physical activity each day. The findings suggest that only 20 per cent of the world's adolescents aged 13 to 15 years achieve this recommended level of activity. Hallal *et al.* (2012) point out that the history of this level of surveillance of physical activity levels around the world is very short in comparison to other health behaviours such as smoking. However, we need this surveillance to understand the temporal patterns of activity. Many suspect that activity levels are decreasing over time but we have few datasets to draw firm conclusions about this. However, one systematic review of these temporal trends did find over 40 articles with sufficient quality to be included (Knuth and Hallal, 2009). The authors concluded that there was evidence that while adult leisure-time physical activity levels had *increased* over time, occupational levels of activity had decreased. This is confirmed by an elegant analysis by Church and colleagues (2011). A worrying finding from this review was the conclusion that levels of activity in youth are declining over time.

Sedentary behaviours

Key sedentary behaviours include TV viewing, leisure-time computer use, overall 'screen time', sitting in a car or other forms of motorised transport, sitting at work, sitting to socialise, sitting to read and sitting to do homework. Essentially, sedentary behaviour takes place in all contexts – leisure, work/school, travel. Objective estimates of total sedentary time during the waking day from the large 2004 National Health and Nutrition Examination Survey for over 6,000 US children and adults showed that participants spent 55 per cent of their monitored time in sedentary behaviour. This is just over 7.5 hours per day, and excludes sleep. The amount of sedentary time varied by subgroups, with the most sedentary being older adolescents and adults aged over 60 years. Estimates from self-reported single sedentary behaviours, such as TV viewing, are less precise, but typically people watch about two hours of TV per day, and more at weekends. The 2010 Kaiser Foundation Report (Rideout *et al.*, 2010) produced higher values, but this often includes sitting in front of the TV doing other tasks – multi-tasking, for example, with a laptop or smartphone. Levels of recreational 'screen time' include TV and computer use and, given the developments in computer technology, prevalence of screen time is on the increase.

Conclusion

Many adults across the world appear not to be active enough for optimal health benefits. In addition, those identified as inactive are more likely to be female, older, and to come from higher income countries. Current data are not sufficient to give us a clear picture of trends over time but there is an indication that gains in leisure-time activity levels across the world may be offset by losses in occupational activity. Moreover, increasing leisure-time sedentary behaviour is likely to be increasing from previous generations, and probably substantially (Katzmarzyk and Mason, 2009). In addition, there is some evidence that a small percentage of youth achieve the current recommendations of activity and that youth activity levels may be declining over time. Overall, and in line with recommendations in the Toronto Charter, there is a need for investment in national surveillance of physical activity, particularly for low- and middle-income countries. Over the next decade we will certainly know more about the pattern of physical activity levels around the world from these data. More information is also needed on the physical activity levels of those with disabilities (Shields *et al.*, 2012).

> Key point: Despite the difficulties in assessing physical activity and sedentary behaviour accurately at population levels, there seems little doubt that many people are not active enough for health benefits and are too sedentary.

Chapter summary

Evidence supports the view that appropriate physical activity can have significant health benefits for all sectors of the population. This book, therefore, will consider psychological and wider behavioural factors likely to influence the participation of individuals in physical activity, as well as the likely psychological outcomes of such involvement. Through a better understanding of these outcomes, including mental health, as well as determinants (corre-lates) and interventions, we should be able to increase participation rates, decrease sedentary behaviour, and bring about significant public health benefits.

In summary, therefore, we conclude the following:

- Human beings in developed Western societies have lifestyles quite dissimilar to those for which our evolution has prepared us and that this is likely to be a major factor in modern non-communicable disease patterns.
- A number of national and international organisations have supported the promotion of physical activity as an important health behaviour through the publication of policy and position statements.
- Physical activity has been shown to be beneficial for many important health outcomes.
- Physical activity in the form of vigorous exercise does have risks, such as injury and

occasional sudden cardiac death, but the evidence shows clearly that people are at greater risk if they are physically inactive.

• Data from around the world show that the adult and youth population is not active enough for health benefits, although trends suggest that leisure-time physical activity may have increased. This has been more than offset by declines in occupational physical activity.

• Sedentary behaviours are highly prevalent and associated with negative health outcomes.

References

American College of Sports Medicine. (1978). Position statement on the recommended quantity and quality of exercise for developing and maintaining fitness in healthy adults. *Medicine and Science in Sports, 10*, vii–x.

——. (1988). Opinion statement on physical fitness in children and youth. *Medicine and Science in Sports and Exercise, 20*, 422–423.

——. (1990). Position stand: The recommended quantity and quality of exercise for developing and maintaining cardiorespiratory and muscular fitness in healthy adults. *Medicine and Science in Sports and Exercise, 22*, 265–274.

Astrand, P-O. (1994). Physical activity and fitness: Evolutionary perspective and trends for the future. In C. Bouchard, R.J. Shephard and T. Stephens (eds), *Physical Activity, Fitness, and Health* (pp. 98–105). Champaign, IL: Human Kinetics.

Atkin, A.J., Gorely, T., Clemes, S.A., Yates, T., Edwardson, C., Brage, S. and Biddle, S.J.H. (2012). Methods of measurement in epidemiology: Sedentary behaviour. *International Journal of Epidemiology, 41*, 1460–1471.

Bauman, A.E., Chau, J.Y., Ding, D. and Bennie, J. (2013). Too much sitting and cardio-metabolic risk: An update of epidemiological evidence. *Current Cardiovascular Risk Reports*. doi: 10.1007/s12170-013-0316-y.

Biddle, S.J.H. and Mutrie, N. (1991). *Psychology of Physical Activity and Exercise: A health-related perspective*. London: Springer-Verlag.

——. (2008). *Psychology of Physical Activity: Determinants, well-being and interventions* (2nd edn). London: Routledge.

Biddle, S.J.H., Sallis, J.F. and Cavill, N. (eds). (1998). *Young and Active? Young people and health-enhancing physical activity: Evidence and implications*. London: Health Education Authority.

Biddle, S.J.H., Gorely, T., Pearson, N. and Bull, F.C. (2011). An assessment of self-reported physical activity instruments in young people for population surveillance: Project ALPHA. *International Journal of Behavioral Nutrition and Physical Activity, 8*(1), doi: 10.1186/1479-5868-1188-1181.

Blair, S.N. (1988). Exercise within a healthy lifestyle. In R.K. Dishman (ed.), *Exercise Adherence: Its impact on public health* (pp. 75–89). Champaign, IL: Human Kinetics.

Bouchard, C., and Shephard, R.J. (1994). Physical activity, fitness, and health: The model and key concepts. In C. Bouchard, R.J. Shephard and T. Stephens (eds), *Physical activity, fitness, and health* (pp. 77–88). Champaign, IL: Human Kinetics.

Bradshaw, P., Bromley, C., Corbett, J., *et al.* (2012). The Scottish health survey. (Vol. 1 adults). Edinburgh.

Buckworth, J. and Dishman, R.K. (2002). *Exercise Psychology*. Champaign, IL: Human Kinetics.

Bull, F.C., Bellew, B., Schoppe, S. and Bauman, A.E. (2004). Developments in national physical activity policy: An international review and recommendations towards better practice. *Journal of Science and Medicine in Sport, 7*(1, Supplement), 93–104.

Caspersen, C.J., Powell, K.E. and Christenson, G.M. (1985). Physical activity, exercise and physical fitness: Definitions and distinctions for health-related research. *Public Health Reports, 100*, 126–131.

Church, T.S., Thomas, D.M., Tudor-Locke, C., Katzmarzyk, P.T., Earnest, C.P., Rodarte, R.Q. and

Bouchard, C. (2011). Trends over 5 decades in U.S. occupation-related physical activity and their associations with obesity. *PLoS ONE, 6*(5), e19657. doi: 10.1371/journal.pone.0019657.

Craig, C.L., Marshall, A.L., Sjostrom, M., Bauman, A.E., Booth, M.L., Ainsworth, B.E. and Oja, P. (2003). International physical activity questionnaire: 12-country reliability and validity. *Medicine and Science in Sports and Exercise, 35*(8), 1381–1395.

Das, P. and Horton, R. (2012). Rethinking our approach to physical activity. *The Lancet, 380*(9838), 189–190.

Department for Culture, Media and Sport. (2002). *Game Plan: A strategy for delivering government's sport and physical activity objectives*. London: Cabinet Office.

Department of Health. (2004). *At Least Five a Week: Evidence on the impact of physical activity and its relationship to health. A report from the Chief Medical Officer*. London: Author.

——. (2011). *Start Active, Stay Active: A report on physical activity for health from the four home countries' Chief Medical Officers*. London: Author.

Department of Health. (2009). *On the state of public health: Annual report of the Chief Medical Officer*. London: Crown.

Dishman, R.K., Heath, G.W. and Lee, I-M. (2013). *Physical Activity Epidemiology* (2nd edn). Champaign, IL: Human Kinetics.

Foster, C. and Allender, S., on behalf of the Scottish Physical Activity Research Collaboration. (2012). Costing the burden of ill health related to physical inactivity for Scotland. Edinburgh: NHS Health Scotland.

Foster, C., Hillsdon, M. and Thorogood, M. (2005). Interventions for physical activity. *Cochrane Database of Systematic Reviews,* Issue 1. Art. No.: CD003180. doi: 10.1002/14651858.CD003180.pub2.

Garrett, S., Elley, C., Raina, R., Sally, B., O'Dea, D., Lawton, B.A. and Dowell, A.C. (2011). Are physical activity interventions in primary care and the community cost-effective? A systematic review of the evidence. *British Journal of General Practice, 61*, 125–133. doi: 10.3399/bjgp11X561249.

Global Advocacy Council for Physical Activity International Society for Physical Activity and Health. (2010). The Toronto Charter for Physical Activity: A Global Call to Action.

Global Advocacy for Physical Activity (GAPA) the Advocacy Council of the International Society for Physical Activity and Health (ISPAH). NCD Prevention: Investments that Work for Physical Activity. Br J Sports Med 2012; 46: 709–712.

Hallal, P.C., Andersen, L.B., Bull, F.C., Guthold, R., Haskell, W., Ekelund, U. and Lancet Physical Activity Series Working Group. (2012). Global physical activity levels: Surveillance progress, pitfalls, and prospects. *Lancet, 380*(9838), 247–257. doi: 10.1016/S0140-6736(12)60646-1.

Hardman, A.E. and Stensel, D.J. (2009). *Physical Activity and Health: The evidence explained* (2nd edn). London: Routledge.

Heath, G.W., Parra, D.C., Sarmiento, O.L., Andersen, L.B., Owen, N. and Goenka, S. for the Lancet Physical Activity Series Working Group. (2012). Evidence-based intervention in physical activity: Lessons from around the world. *The Lancet, July*, 45–54.

Katzmarzyk, P.T. and Mason, C. (2009). The physical activity transition. *Journal of Physical Activity and Health, 6*, 269–280.

Knuth, A.G. and Hallal, P.C. (2009). Temporal trends in physical activity: A systematic review. *Journal of Physical Activity and Health, 6*(5), 548–559.

Koplan, J.P., Siscovick, D.S. and Goldbaum, G.M. (1985). The risks of exercise: A public health view of injuries and hazards. *Public Health Reports, 100*, 189–195.

LaPorte, R.E., Montoye, H.J. and Caspersen, C.J. (1985). Assessment of physical activity in epidemiological research: Problems and prospects. *Public Health Reports, 100*, 131–146.

Lee, I-M. (ed.). (2009). *Epidemiological Methods in Physical Activity Studies*. New York: Oxford University Press.

Lee, I-M., Shiroma, E.J., Lobelo, F., Puska, P., Blair, S.N., Katzmarzyk, P.T. and Lancet Physical Activity Series Working Group. (2012). Effect of physical inactivity on major non-communicable diseases worldwide: An analysis of burden of disease and life expectancy. *The Lancet, 380*(9838), 219–229. doi: 10.1016/S0140-6736(12)61031-9.

Malina, R.M. (1988). Physical activity in early and modern populations: An evolutionary view. In R.M. Malina and H.M. Eckert (eds), *Physical Activity in Early and Modern Populations* (pp. 1–12). Champaign, IL: Human Kinetics and the American Academy of Physical Education.

Marshall, A.L., Miller, Y.D., Burton, N.W. and Brown, W.J. (2010). Measuring total and domain-specific sitting: A study of reliability and validity. *Medicine and Science in Sports and Exercise, 42*(6), 1094–1102.

Marteau, T.M., Ogilvie, D., Roland, M., Suhrcke, M. and Kelly, M.P. (2011). Judging nudging: Can nudging improve population health? *British Medical Journal, 342*, d228.

Mattocks, C., Ness, A., Leary, S., Tilling, K., Blair, S.N., Shield, J. and Riddoch, C. (2008). Use of accelerometers in a large field-based study of children: Protocols, design issues, and effects on precision. *Journal of Physical Activity and Health, 5*(Suppl. 1), S98–S111.

Morris, J.N, Heady, J.A., Raffle, P.A.B., Roberts, C.G. and Parks, J.W. (1953). Coronary heart disease and physical activity of work. *The Lancet, ii*, 1053–1057; 1111–1120.

Morrow, J.R., Jr., Defina, L.F., Leonard, D., Trudelle-Jackson, E. and Custodio, M.A. (2012). Meeting physical activity guidelines and musculoskeletal injury: The WIN study. *Medical Science and Sports Exercise, 44*(10), 1986–1992. doi: 10.1249/MSS.0b013e31825a36c6.

Mowen, A.J., and Baker, B.L. (2009). Park, Recreation, Fitness and Sport Sector Recommendations for a more physically active America: A white paper for the United States National Physical Activity Plan. *Journal of Physical Activity and Health, 6*(S2), S236–S244.

Paffenbarger, R.S., Hyde, R.T., Wing, A.L., Lee, I-M. and Kampert, J.B. (1994). Some interrelations of physical activity, physiological fitness, health and longevity. In C. Bouchard, R.J. Shephard and T. Stephens (eds), *Physical Activity, Fitness, and Health* (pp. 119–133). Champaign, IL: Human Kinetics.

Pate, R.R. (1988). The evolving definition of physical fitness. *Quest, 40*, 174–179.

Pate, R.R. and Macera, C.A. (1994). Risks of exercising: Musculoskeletal injuries. In C. Bouchard, R.J. Shephard and T. Stephens (eds), *Physical Activity, Fitness, and Health* (pp. 1008–1018). Champaign, IL: Human Kinetics.

Pate, R.R., Pratt, M., Blair, S.N., Haskel, W.L., Macera, C.A., Bouchard, C. and Wilmore, J.H. (1995). Physical activity and public health: A recommendation from the Centers for Disease Control and Prevention and the American College of Sports Medicine. *Journal of the American Medical Association, 273*, 402–407.

Rejeski, W.J. and Brawley, L.R. (1988). Defining the boundaries of sport psychology. *The Sport Psychologist, 2*, 231–242.

Riddoch, C.J., Mattocks, C., Deere, K., Saunders, J., Kirkby, J., Tilling, K. and Ness, A.R. (2007). Objective measurement of levels and patterns of physical activity. *Archives of Disease in Childhood, 92*, 963–969.

Rideout, V.J., Foehr, U.G. and Roberts, D.F. (2010). *Generation M2: Media in the lives of 8 to 18 year olds.* The Henry J. Kaiser Family Foundation.

Ridgers, N.D. and Fairclough, S.J. (2011). Assessing free-living physical activity using acceler-ometry: Practical issues for researchers and practitioners. *European Journal of Sport Science, 11*(3), 205–213.

Sallis, J.F. and Owen, N. (1999). *Physical Activity and Behavioral Medicine.* Thousand Oaks, CA: Sage.

Sallis, J.F. and Saelens, B.E. (2000). Assessment of physical activity by self-report: Status, limitations, and future directions. *Research Quarterly for Exercise and Sport, 71*, 1–14.

Scholes, S. and Mindell, J. (2013). Physical activity in adults. *Health Survey England 2012 Volume 1* (pp. 1–49). London: The Health and Social Care Information Centre.

Scottish Executive. (2003). *Let's Make Scotland More Active: A strategy for physical activity.* Edinburgh: Author.

Sedentary Behaviour Research Network. (2012). Letter to the Editor: Standardized use of the terms 'sedentary' and 'sedentary behaviours'. *Applied Physiology, Nutrition and Metabolism, 37*, 540–542.

Shields, N., Synnot, A.J. and Barr, M. (2012). Perceived barriers and facilitators to physical activity for children with disability: A systematic review. *British Journal of Sports Medicine, 46*, 989–997. doi:910.1136/bjsports-2012-090236.

Siscovick, D.S., Weiss, N.S., Fletcher, R.H. and Lasky, T. (1984). The incidence of primary cardiac arrest during vigorous physical exercise. *New England Journal of Medicine, 311*, 874–877.

Szabo, A. (2000). Physical activity as a source of psychological dysfunction. In S.J.H. Biddle, K.R. Fox and S.H. Boutcher (eds), *Physical Activity and Psychological Well-being* (pp. 130–153). London: Routledge.

Tudor-Locke, C. and Bassett, D.R. (2004). How many steps/day are enough? Preliminary pedometer indices for public health. *Sports Medicine, 34*, 1–8.

US Department of Health and Human Services. (1996). Physical Activity and health: A report of the Surgeon General. Atlanta: US Department of Health and Human Services, Centers for Disease Control and Prevention, National Center for Chronic Disease Prevention and Health Promotion.

Wilmot, E.G., Edwardson, C.L., Achana, F.A., Davies, M.J., Gorely, T., Gray, L.J. and Biddle, S.J.H. (2012). Sedentary time in adults and the association with diabetes, cardiovascular disease and death: Systematic review and meta-analysis. *Diabetologia, 55*(11), 2895–2905. doi: 10.1007/s00125-012-2677-z.

Winter, E.M. and Fowler, N. (2009). Exercise defined and quantified according to the Systeme International d'Unites. *Journal of Sports Science, 27*(5), 447–460. doi: 10.1080/02640410802658461.

World Health Organization (2004). Global strategy on diet, physical activity and health. World Health Organization.

Part II

Physical activity and mental health

2 Physical activity and psychological well-being

Does physical activity make us feel good?

Buckworth and Dishman (2002) pointed out that as long ago as 1899 William James said that 'our muscular vigor will … always be needed to furnish the background of sanity, and cheerfulness to life, to give moral elasticity to our dispositions, to round off the wiry edge of our fretfulness, and make us good-humoured' (p. 91). Perhaps now we are ready to listen to this message.

A fundamental question in the psychology of physical activity is 'does physical activity make you feel good?' – healthy mind in a healthy body and all that. In this chapter, therefore, we review the evidence on the relationship between participation in physical activity and psychological well-being (PWB). Specifically, we review the areas of mood and affect, enjoyment, and sleep, as well as psychological well-being for women. In addition, possible mental health outcomes of too much sedentary behaviour (sitting time) are discussed. Specifically, in this chapter we aim to:

- introduce the concept of health-related quality of life and how it is typically measured;
- review the evidence linking physical activity with measures of mood and affect;
- highlight the construct of physical activity enjoyment and present three approaches to understanding this construct;
- comment on the psychological effects of depriving people of physical activity;
- highlight results on the effect of physical activity on sleep;
- appraise the evidence on the association between sedentary behaviour (sitting) and psychological well-being;
- explore the evidence for the existence of 'exercise dependence';
- discuss physical activity and psychological well-being for women.

A case was made in Chapter 1 for the diverse health benefits of a physically active lifestyle. However, although there is plenty of anecdotal support for the view that physical activity has positive effects on psychological well-being, the emphasis is often placed more firmly on the physical outcomes. Yet evidence on psychological well-being is far from just anecdotal; there is a great deal of research evidence linking physical activity to many elements of mental health (Ekkekakis, 2013). Indeed, there is now an academic journal devoted solely to this topic (see http://www.journals.elsevier.com/mental-health-and-physical-activity/).

The publication of health-related documents in England by the government in the 1990s (Department of Health, 1993) marked a significant change in approach in health care and promotion, and placed greater emphasis on aspects of well-being. For example, in the overall aims of the government's Health of the Nation initiative were the desire for 'adding years to life' – to reduce premature mortality and improve life expectancy – and 'adding life to years'; that is, improving the quality of life. Similarly, the influential and seminal Surgeon General's Report on physical activity and health in the United States (US Department of Health and Human Services, 1996) recognised the importance of physical activity for well-being as well as disease prevention. More recently, the report from the four Chief Medical Officers of the UK on physical activity and health recognised the positive effects that physical activity can have on various elements of psychological well-being (Chief Medical Officers of England, Scotland, Wales and Northern Ireland, 2011).

The promotion of health through physical activity, therefore, now incorporates the recognition of the importance of psychological well-being. This chapter reviews the evidence on the links between physical activity and psychological well-being, with a main emphasis on mood and 'core' affect. More discrete forms of mental health, such as depression and self-esteem, are dealt with elsewhere in the book (see Chapters 3 to 6). Specifically in this chapter, we review evidence concerning the following:

- health-related quality of life
- core affect
- mood
- enjoyment
- sleep
- sedentary behaviour (sitting) and psychological well-being
- exercise deprivation and dependence.

Health-related quality of life

Quality of life is typically assessed in health behaviour trials, including those involving physical activity (Focht, 2012). Rejeski and colleagues (1996) suggest that it is typical for health-related quality of life (HRQL) to be defined in terms of participants' perceptions of function. They outline six types of HRQL measures:

- global indices of HRQL: these might include general life satisfaction, or self-esteem;
- physical function: perceptions of function, physical self-perceptions, health-related perceptions;
- physical symptoms: fatigue, energy, sleep;
- emotional function: depression, anxiety, mood, affect;
- social function: social dependency, family/work roles;
- cognitive function: memory, attention, problem-solving.

HRQL measures are usually viewed simply in terms of physical function and this may be considered a narrow view. There are many HRQL instruments and these include affective measures. Some suggest a simple division of HRQL into functional measures and those assessing quality of life (Muldoon *et al.*, 1998). The issue of quality of life has become increasingly important because health economists use measures of quality of life to quantify the benefits of different approaches to treatment. The concept of the quality adjusted life year (QALY) is used to estimate how much it would cost to improve someone's quality of life or extend that person's life with a new treatment.

Key HRQL measures include the SF-36, The Nottingham Health Profile (Hunt *et al.*, 1986) and the EQ-5D (Buxton *et al.*, 1990, 1992) [see http://www.euroqol.org/]. The SF-36 is the best-known measure and is a 36-item questionnaire designed to assess eight health dimensions covering functional status, well-being and overall evaluation of health (Dixon *et al.*, 1994). The SF-36 (also known as the SF-36 Health Survey and the Rand 36-item Health Survey) has an anglicised version for use in the UK as well as a short form (SF-12). The SF-36 assesses the following dimensions of well-being: physical functioning, social functioning, role limitations due to physical problems, mental health, energy/vitality, pain, and general health perception. It also has one item assessing perceptions of recent changes in health (Bowling, 1997).

The EQ-5D is used for quality of life and economic appraisal. It consists of two parts: (1) a 15-item instrument assessing self-description of perceived mobility (e.g. 'I have some problems in walking about'), self-care (e.g. 'I have some problems washing and dressing myself'), usual activities (e.g. 'I am unable to perform my usual activities'), pain/discomfort (e.g. 'I have no pain or discomfort'), and anxiety/depression (e.g. 'I am extremely anxious and depressed'); and (2) a visual analogue scale ranging from 'worst imaginable health state' (score = 0) to 'best imaginable health state' (score = 100).

One global dimension of HRQL is perceptions of life satisfaction. This might be particularly important for older adults if they experience physical and mental decline. McAuley and colleagues have conducted extensive research on HRQL outcomes in older adults involved in physical activity interventions. For example, in a five-year follow-up, Elavsky *et al.* (2005) showed that positive self-efficacy, physical self-worth and affect resulting from enhanced levels of physical activity predicted life satisfaction after one year. Moreover, self-efficacy, physical self-worth and affect showed good stability over four years and again predicted life satisfaction. The authors concluded that enhanced life satisfaction associated with physical activity is mediated by enhanced feelings of self-efficacy, physical self-worth and affect.

Rejeski *et al.* (1996) provide a comprehensive review of HRQL and physical activity, and offer the following conclusions:

- HRQL test batteries should include general and condition- or population-specific measures.
- The degree of change observed in HRQL through physical activity will depend on baseline levels.
- The degree of impact of physical activity on HRQL will depend on both the physiological stimulus as well as social and behavioural characteristics of the treatment or intervention.
- People vary in the extent to which they value certain health-related outcomes from physical activity; hence this will affect HRQL perceptions of those in intervention studies.

Focht (2012) concludes that findings 'clearly demonstrate that exercise consistently results in statistically significant, clinically meaningful improvements in a variety of quality-of-life outcomes' (p. 110).

Affective outcomes of physical activity

The affective reactions associated with physical activity play a potentially important role in physical activity and health promotion. If we believe that physical activity is a positive health behaviour to be encouraged and promoted, how people feel during and after activity may be critical in determining whether they maintain their involvement. This means that issues concerning participation, motivation and adherence cannot be divorced from aspects of psychological well-being. Affect may have motivational properties for important health-related behaviours. In addition, positive affect is an important health outcome in its own right. As stated by Hefferon and Mutrie (2012), 'activity participation is an exceptionally effective strategy for facilitating psychological well-being within individuals and societies' (p. 125).

> Key point: How people feel during and after physical activity will influence whether they maintain their involvement.

Defining terms: affect, emotion and mood

The terms 'affect', 'emotion' and 'mood' are closely related and often perceived to be synonymous concepts. However, this requires careful clarification and definition. These are necessarily difficult concepts to define, and demarcations are not always clear, but an effort to summarise them is given in Table 2.1.

'Affect', sometimes referred to as 'core affect' or 'basic affect', is the generic 'valenced' (good/bad) response that is a broader construct than emotion. It is a basic human response. Russell and Feldman-Barrett (1999) refer to 'core affect' as 'the most elementary consciously accessible affective feelings' (p. 806).

Moods or 'mood states' are commonly targeted in physical activity studies. Mood may be seen as a global set of affective (feeling) states we experience on a day-to-day basis and may last for hours, days, weeks, or even months. Mood may be conceptualised in terms of distinct mood states, such as vigour and depression, but these, as mood states, are not a reaction to a specified event but more likely stem from generic feelings. The origin of mood states is more difficult to specify, such as 'feeling down' for no obvious reason, hence they tend to be 'diffuse' and relatively low in intensity.

Emotion is normally defined in terms of specific feeling states generated in reaction to certain events or appraisals. They are likely to last for minutes or hours, but for no longer, and can be intense. Given that a cognitive appraisal takes place for an emotional reaction to be elicited, physical activity studies do not always assess true emotional outcomes. Most physical activity studies are testing the affective states, or changes, resulting from single or multiple bouts of activity and may not test cognitive appraisals of specific events. However, emotions can sometimes be assessed in physical activity, such as feelings of efficacy following successful negotiation of a new exercise programme. Regrettably, the distinction between mood and emotion in physical activity research studies is often not made clear.

It is important to note that affect can also be a component of moods and emotions. For example, pride will feel pleasant and depression will feel unpleasant. Readers are referred to Ekkekakis and Russell (2013) for further discussion on definitional issues.

> Key point: Defining the key terms of affect, mood and emotion is not easy, but we should provide working definitions in research projects and not assume they are one and the same.

Table 2.1   Defining features of affect, emotion and mood

Construct	Defining features	Intensity and time	Cognitive mediation	Example
Affect (core affect; basic affect)	Basic and generic valenced (pleasant/ unpleasant) responses	Varied	A cognitive appraisal might be involved when affect is a component of emotion or mood, but is not necessary (see text). Affect can occur independently.	Feeling 'good', pleasant
Emotion	Affective states resulting from an appraisal of specific events	Usually high intensity; short duration	Cognitive appraisal of a specific eliciting event	Proud or ashamed
Mood	Diffuse affective states not resulting from specific events but more likely associated with general views at a point in time	Lower intensity; may be prolonged	Cognitive appraisal of larger issues or events in the distant past or future	Irritable or jovial

Measurement issues

In psychology, there is a debate concerning the nature of affective states, including emotion (Ekkekakis and Russell, 2013). Some prefer to define affective states in terms of discrete emotional reactions, such as pleasure and fear, and this is the 'categorical' approach to measurement of affect. Others suggest that affect is best defined in terms of their common properties, or dimensions, such as positive and negative affect (Watson *et al.*, 1988) – the 'dimensional' approach. Lazarus (1991), however, argues that the distinct qualities of emotional reactions are lost, or blurred, when reduced to a few affective dimensions. He argues that each emotion is unique because it is created by a different appraisal of the perceived significance of an event. However, it is also logical to see emotions clustered according to common categories. Watson *et al.* (1988) have derived two major factors from an analysis of emotions: positive affect and negative affect. The former refers to feelings such as alert and active, whereas negative affect refers to unpleasant affective states such as anger.

Russell has also advocated a dimensional approach to the study of affect (Russell, 1980). In his 'circumplex' model, he suggests that emotion may best be defined in terms of the two dimensions of valence (i.e. pleasant–unpleasant) and arousal (i.e. high–low). This gives rise to affective states being classified into four quadrants, as shown in Figure 2.1.

Ekkekakis and Petruzzello (2000) argue that the decision on whether categorical or dimensional approaches should be used depends on the nature of the research question. For studies wishing to test the affective responses to exercise in the context of exercise adherence, dimensional measures of affective valence (good/bad) are likely to be appropriate, particularly when the current state of knowledge is such that hypotheses concerning specific affective states or emotions are not always possible. This is because reinforcement of exercise adherence is likely to be related to generic feelings of 'good' or 'bad'. Nor do we

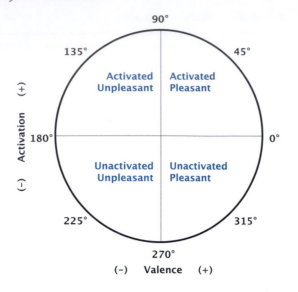

Figure 2.1   The circumplex model of affect proposed by Russell

Source: Russell (1980).

know very much about mediating variables that may be causing the affective responses; hence it is logical to assess along affective dimensions. However, if we wish to test the effects of specific environments (e.g. exercising in classes) or contexts (e.g. trying a new activity), then assessing discrete emotions or feelings may be applicable, such as anxiety or self-efficacy.

Measures of affect, emotion and mood in physical activity

Dimensional measures of affect in physical activity have typically used the circumplex model (Figure 2.1). In addition to the advantages of this approach that have already been discussed, because this method involves simple assessment scales of arousal/activation and valence (good/bad), multiple measures may be taken *during* single exercise bouts. This allows for the assessment of affect before, during and after exercise. Typically, studies have failed to describe the affective states during exercise and may be making erroneous conclusions based on only having measures before and after exercise.

Many studies have used Hardy and Rejeski's (1989) 'Feeling Scale' to assess affective valence. This scale requires the participant to rate their feeling on an 11-point scale anchored by 'Very Good' (+5) and 'Very Bad' (-5). Activation/arousal may be measured using the Felt Arousal Scale (Svebak and Murgatroyd, 1985) – a 6-point scale anchored by 'low arousal' (0) and 'high arousal' (6). Using the circumplex, affective states may be plotted, such as shown in Figure 2.2. This example shows that a 15-minute treadmill walk at a self-chosen pace results in an activated pleasant state during and immediately after its completion. A 10-minute seated recovery period leads to a low-activation pleasant state. A treadmill test, lasting on average just over 11 minutes, during which the speed and grade are gradually increased until the point of volitional exhaustion, leads to an activated *unpleasant* state. A subsequent cool-down and 10-minute seated recovery period bring about a return to a low-activation pleasant state. The ventilatory threshold (indicated by 'VT'), which is a marker of the transition from aerobic to anaerobic metabolism, appears to be the turning point towards displeasure during

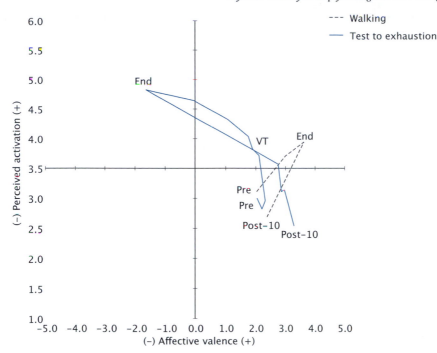

Figure 2.2 Affective responses to two bouts of physical activity, plotted in circumplex space, where the horizontal dimension represents self-rated affective valence, ranging from displeasure to pleasure and the vertical dimension represents perceived activation. 'Pre' indicates the beginning of each activity, 'End' indicates its end and 'Post-10' indicates 10 minutes after the end.

Source: Plotted with data from Ekkekakis *et al.* (2000) and Hall *et al.* (2002).

Note: VT = ventilatory threshold.

the treadmill test. This is discussed in more detail later, but does question the common assumption that exercise is always associated with positive affect or that high-intensity exercise is a sensible public health strategy when considering adherence. There are likely to be situations, possibly related to higher intensity exercise, where affective valence becomes negative and thus may affect motivation and adherence (Ekkekakis, 2003).

The majority of studies in physical activity and affect have adopted the categorical approach to measurement. Where generic measures of mood have been used, typically the Profile of Mood States (POMS) (McNair *et al.*, 1971) has been the instrument of choice. The POMS assesses five negative moods and only one positive mood (vigour), although the bipolar form of the POMS allows the assessment of both positive and negative poles for each construct. The bipolar form has rarely been used in physical activity research. The POMS may also be varied according to the instructions, such as how participants feel 'right now' or 'over the past few weeks', depending on the research question.

In addition to more generic measures of mood and affect, some researchers have developed scales for the assessment of 'exercise-related' affect or 'feeling states'. Both types of measures used in physical activity research are summarised in Table 2.2, showing dimensional and categorical measures.

Table 2.2   Examples of categorical and dimensional measures of mood and affect commonly used in physical activity research

Instrument	Reference	Measures	Comments
Dimensional measures			
PANAS (Positive and Negative Affect Schedule)	Watson *et al.* (1988)	Two 10-item affect scales assessing: • positive affect (e.g. excited, enthusiastic, inspired) • negative affect (e.g. distressed, hostile, irritable)	• good psychometric properties • assesses only two general dimensions • time instructions can be varied • can be a state or trait scale • general scale not specific to physical activity
FS (Feeling Scale)	Hardy and Rejeski (1989)	• single-item scale assessing hedonic tone (pleasure–displeasure)	• developed for exercise research • state scale • 11-point scale ranging from −5 to +5
Categorical measures			
POMS (Profile of Mood States)	McNair *et al.* (1971)	65-item scale assessing: • tension • depression • anger • vigour • fatigue • confusion	• only one positive subscale • used extensively in PA research • short and bipolar forms available • time instructions can be varied • can be a state or trait scale • general scale not specific to physical activity
MAACL (Multiple Affect Adjective Check List)	Zuckerman and Lubin (1965)	• scale comprises 132 adjectives • assesses anxiety, depression and hostility	• time instructions can be varied • can be a state or trait scale • general scale not specific to physical activity • some doubts expressed about psychometric properties (see McDonald and Hodgdon, 1991)
EFI (Exercise Feeling Inventory)	Gauvin and Rejeski (1993)	12-item adjective scale assessing four dimensions: • positive engagement • tranquillity • revitalisation • physical exhaustion	• developed for exercise research • sound psychometric properties • state scale
SEES (Subjective Exercise Experiences Scale)	McAuley and Courneya (1994)	12-item adjective scale assessing three dimensions: • positive well-being • psychological distress • fatigue	• developed for exercise research • sound psychometric properties • state scale

In reaction to their dissatisfaction with global measures, such as the PANAS, Gauvin and Rejeski (1993) developed the Exercise-induced Feeling Inventory (EFI) in an effort to capture four distinct feeling states in exercise: revitalisation, tranquillity, positive engagement and physical exhaustion. The conceptual underpinnings of such 'exercise-specific' measures have been criticised (Ekkekakis and Petruzzello, 2001a, 2001b):

> A measure of affect tailored to tap only those affective states believed to be relevant to exercise leads to some considerable logical problems. An important problem stems from the fact that most studies investigating the exercise–affect relationship involve assessments of affect under non-exercise conditions, such as before exercise … how meaningful would any comparisons be between exercise and all the non-exercise conditions where this measure is likely to be employed?
>
> (Ekkekakis and Petruzzello, 2001a, p. 7)

Key point: How you measure affective responses to physical activity, such as whether you choose a categorical or dimensional approach, will depend on the research question.

Evidence for relationships between physical activity and affect

There are a very large number of studies investigating the relationship between physical activity, usually structured exercise, and affective states. Conclusions are drawn from both acute exercise studies, where the exercise is just a single session, and studies involving a programme of physical activity over time (chronic exercise studies).

Narrative and meta-analytic reviews

From the numerous narrative reviews available, there is cautious support for the proposition that exercise is associated with enhanced affect and mood (Biddle, 2000). The caution comes from the relatively weak research designs utilised. To that end, it is often better to draw conclusions from systematic reviews, including meta-analyses where they exist.

McDonald and Hodgdon (1991) conducted one of the first meta-analyses of exercise and mood research. They delimited their review to aerobic fitness training studies and found that researchers used mainly the unipolar POMS or Multiple Affect Adjective Checklist (MAACL). Results showed a clear relationship between exercise and vigour and a lack of negative mood, and this corresponds to the typical 'iceberg profile' (see Figure 2.3). McDonald and Hodgdon concluded that 'aerobic fitness training produces some positive change in mood – at least on a short-term basis' (p. 98). Whether the POMS is the best measure for testing such effects is another matter and readers are advised to consider whether such a measure captures the responses deemed relevant to physical activity situations. Moreover, it is worth noting that the POMS does not adequately assess the four quadrants of the circumplex model.

A meta-analysis summarising the effects of exercise on positive and negative affect in older adults (Arent *et al.*, 2000) also showed beneficial effects. Selected results are shown in Figure 2.4. Positive effects were found for experimental over control groups for all forms of physical activity, but particularly mixed exercise modes, and greater effects were noted for lower intensities of physical activity, consistent with evidence from other approaches, such as the circumplex model (Ekkekakis, 2003).

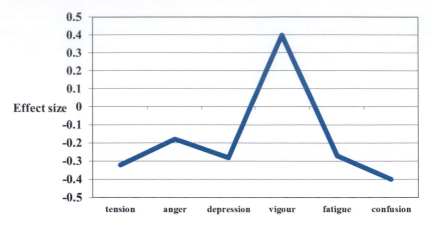
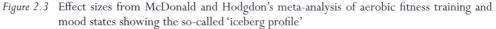

Figure 2.3 Effect sizes from McDonald and Hodgdon's meta-analysis of aerobic fitness training and mood states showing the so-called 'iceberg profile'

Source: McDonald and Hodgdon (1991).

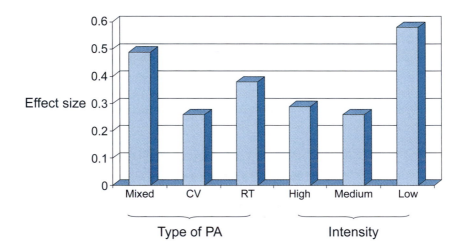

Figure 2.4 Effect sizes for experimental studies investigating exercise and affective ('mood') states in older adults

Source: Arent *et al.* (2000).

The circumplex model shows that the most positive affective state, or at least the one most expected from physical activity, is the quadrant labelled 'positive activated affect' (PAA). This is represented by high affective valence (feeling 'good') and high arousal/activation. Reed and Ones (2006) conducted a comprehensive meta-analysis of 158 studies investigating acute aerobic exercise and measures reflecting PAA. The overall effect size was 0.47 – considered to be just below a 'moderate' effect but clearly meaningful. Effects were consistently positive:

- immediately post-exercise;
- when pre-exercise PAA was lower than average (suggesting that exercise may particularly help those with less positive affect);

- for lower intensity exercise;
- for durations of exercise up to 35 minutes;
- for low to moderate exercise doses (combination of duration and intensity).

The authors also concluded that the effects of aerobic exercise on PAA appear to last for at least 30 minutes after exercise before returning to baseline – the so-called 'rebound' phenomenon.

Reed and Buck (2009) then conducted a meta-analysis of 105 studies investigating participation in regular (chronic) aerobic exercise, rather than the acute studies reported by Reed and Ones. Results showed an overall effect size of 0.57, a moderate effect. Higher levels of PAA were evident with lower initial levels of PAA, and the overall effects were stronger in studies rated as higher quality. Higher PAA was associated with greater exercise frequency whereas higher exercise intensity was associated with lower PAA. Optimal conditions for improving PAA appeared to be low intensity, 30–35 minutes in duration, 3–5 days/week for 10–12 weeks.

These two meta-analyses are informative insofar as they address an important quadrant of the circumplex model. However, weaknesses include the extreme diversity of measures included as 'PAA' alongside weaker research designs. That said, the results are quite consistent across acute and chronic studies, and show that aerobic exercise is associated with positive activated affect and is likely to be more so for those with initially low levels of PAA and for less intense forms of exercise. However, many of the studies included in the meta-analysis were not able to track changes in PAA during exercise, and this is something that researchers need to do more of (Backhouse *et al.*, 2007).

One of the key issues emerging from these reviews is that affective responses to physical activity are likely to be moderated by several factors, including exercise intensity (Ekkekakis, 2013). Ekkekakis' important paper on his 'dual-mode model' in 2003 sums up the state of play regarding affective responses, intensity, and temporal aspects of responses, through five propositions (Ekkekakis, 2003):

- Proposition 1: 'There are positive affective responses during and for a short period following bouts of physical activity of mild intensity and short duration' (p. 217). For example, 15-minute self-paced walks have been shown to produce improved affective valence (Ekkekakis *et al.*, 2000).
- Proposition 2: 'Affective responses during moderately vigorous exercise are characterised by marked intra-individual variability, with some individuals reporting positive and some reporting negative changes' (p. 219). Intra-individual variability has rarely been considered in the literature on exercise and affect, yet the data show that Ekkekakis' proposition is correct (Van Landuyt *et al.*, 2000). For example, Ekkekakis *et al.* (2005) summarise data from five studies showing the variability of responses as a function of exercise intensity. These data are shown in Figure 2.5 and illustrate very clearly that studies 1 and 2 (self-paced 10- and 15-minute walking) produced a highly positive change in affect for over 70 per cent of the participants. Study 3 was 30 minutes of cycling at 60 per cent of maximal oxygen consumption and showed much more variable responses. Conversely, the negative responses in studies 4 and 5 were almost universal. These studies involved exercising to exhaustion.
- Proposition 3: 'Responses immediately following moderately vigorous exercise are almost uniformly positive, regardless of whether the responses during exercise were positive or negative' (p. 221). This is the so-called 'rebound' effect, the robustness of which Ekkekakis (2003) describes as 'remarkable' (p. 221).

- Proposition 4: 'Affective responses during strenuous exercise unify into a negative trend as the intensity of exercise approaches each individual's functional limits' (p. 222). The ventilatory threshold has been suggested as one biological marker for when this shift occurs. As shown in Table 2.3, this level of intensity will mean that the link between affective valence and interoceptive factors will strengthen, often shown by increases in measures such as heart rate, rating of perceived exertion (RPE), and blood lactate.
- Proposition 5: 'There is a homogeneous positive shift in affective valence immediately following strenuous exercise' (p. 224). This is also a rebound effect similar to that observed after moderately vigorous exercise.

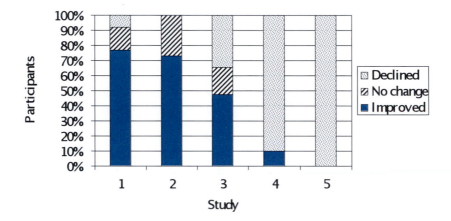

Figure 2.5   Intra-individual variability in affective responses to different exercise stimuli
Source: Data from five studies reported in Ekkekakis *et al.* (2005).
Note: Study 1: 10-minute self-paced walk. Study 2: 15-minute self-paced walk. Study 3: 30 minutes of cycling at 60% of maximal oxygen consumption. Study 4: Incremental treadmill running to exhaustion. Study 5: Cycling to exhaustion under conditions of dehydration.

Table 2.3   Affective responses to varying levels of exercise intensity, proposed by Ekkekakis and colleagues (Ekkekakis, 2003; Ekkekakis *et al.*, 2005)

Intensity range	Affective reaction to exercise	Variability of response	Influencing factors
Moderate – clearly below ventilatory threshold	Pleasure	Homogeneous	Cognitive factors play small role
Heavy – close to the ventilatory threshold	Pleasure or displeasure	Variable	Cognitive factors play a major role
Severe – clearly above ventilatory threshold	Displeasure	Homogeneous	Interoceptive factors play a major role

The role of exercise intensity in affect seems quite clear (Ekkekakis and Dafermos, 2012). High-intensity exercise will yield much less positive, and indeed likely negative, feeling states during participation. Advocating high-intensity exercise as a public health strategy – such as 'HIIT' (high-intensity interval training) protocols currently in vogue with physiologists – is likely to fail due to low rates of adherence. This is probably why exercise has been used as punishment in the past, although we strongly advocate that this practice be discontinued!

> Key point: There are beneficial affective changes with physical activity, but this relationship is influenced by the intensity of physical activity. The 'feel-good' effect is highly unlikely during high-intensity exercise.

Illustrative study: affective responses of obese women to increasing exercise intensity

The propositions stated by Ekkekakis require further testing in diverse groups. To this end, a study was conducted comparing affective responses to increasing exercise intensity for inactive women differing in weight status (Ekkekakis *et al.*, 2010). Normal-weight, overweight and obese women took part in a treadmill protocol of increasing exercise intensity to the point of 'volitional exhaustion'. Different affective measures were taken at various time points. Results at the end of the exercise period showed that ratings of pleasure (using the Feeling Scale) were significantly lower for the obese women than for the other two groups. The same was true for ratings of energy. Of interest was the finding that while ratings of pleasure dropped quite quickly for the obese group, these women reported less pleasure at all levels of exercise intensity. However, even for the normal-weight women, feelings of pleasure dropped markedly at the highest levels of exercise intensity.

Physical activity and feelings of energy and fatigue

Another aspect of psychological well-being that has been studied in the context of physical activity is that of energy and fatigue. Puetz (2006) conducted a meta-analysis of 12 population-based studies that examined the association between physical activity and feelings of energy and fatigue. Results were analysed by comparing active adults with those who were less active. Results showed an association between physical activity and a reduced risk of experiencing feelings of low energy and fatigue with a significant odds ratio of 0.61, thus showing approximately 40 per cent lower scores for inactive people for energy and low fatigue. Studies were supportive of a strong, consistent and temporally appropriate dose–response relationship between physical activity and feelings of energy and fatigue. A similar review was also conducted on energy and fatigue, but this time on the effects of chronic exercise (Puetz *et al.*, 2006). Again, increased feelings were reported of energy and lower fatigue for those active compared with control conditions.

Enjoyment and physical activity

If physical activity is associated with psychological well-being, it seems obvious that an element of enjoyment of physical activity must also be present. Enjoyment is an important part of motivation and participation, and may be particularly crucial when physical effort is required, such as in some structured exercise classes. Despite all of this, enjoyment has remained an elusive concept in research for many years, and the state of knowledge has changed little since our previous edition of this book.

At least three approaches to enjoyment have been identified that are relevant to health-related physical activity:

- Csikszentmihalyi's 'flow' model;
- intrinsic motivational processes;
- exercise-related affective states.

Enjoyment and flow

Csikszentmihalyi (1975) studied why people invest huge amounts of time and energy in tasks appearing to yield limited external rewards. Such activities are described as 'autotelic' (meaning 'self-goal' or 'self-purpose'). In asking people engaged in a range of activities, including rock climbers, composers, chess players, dancers and basketball players, why they enjoyed their chosen activity, 'intrinsic' factors were clearly evident. For example, the highest ranked reasons were 'enjoyment of the experience and use of skills' and 'the activity itself – the pattern, the action, the world it provides'. The least favoured reason was 'prestige/regard/glamour'.

One of Csikszentmihalyi's conclusions was that motivation seemed highest when the difficulty of the task (challenge) was matched by the personal abilities and skills of the individual. This matching led to a state of 'flow', or supreme enjoyment and engagement in the task. A mismatch may lead to either boredom (low challenge relative to skills) or anxiety (high challenge relative to skills), as shown in Figure 2.6.

Enjoyment and intrinsic motivation

The development of intrinsic motivation is a key consideration for many promoting physical activity. High intrinsic motivation includes high effort, feelings of enjoyment, competence and autonomy (self-determination), and low levels of pressure and anxiety (Deci and Ryan,

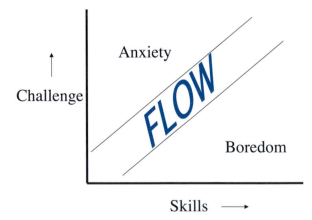

Figure 2.6 Csikzentmihalyi's flow state model, depicting flow as a match of skills and challenge

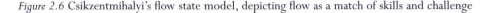

1985). Intrinsic motivation, enjoyment and flow are clearly interrelated. Csikszentmihalyi (1975) spoke of 'autotelic' activities being the ones where flow was most likely, and Deci and Ryan (1985) talked about the 'self-determination' of behaviour through intrinsic motivation. However, 'pure' intrinsic enjoyment is likely to be rare in some forms of physical activity, whereas we may be motivated more by what are called states of 'identified' motivation, such as being physically active for the satisfaction of achieving goals, mastering tasks, etc., rather than just 'fun'. This may account for why there is often a surprisingly low association between physical activity and enjoyment. For example, in a meta-analysis, the association was assessed between 'affective judgement' and physical activity in young people (Nasuti and Rhodes, 2013). Affective judgement was defined as the 'overall pleasure/displeasure, enjoyment, and feeling states expected from enacting an activity or from reflection on past activity' (p. 358). The effect size was small (0.2) but significant. This supports the arguments made above that while enjoyment is important, there will be other factors driving participation.

Future work needs to take into account different motivational elements of intrinsic and extrinsic motivation to better understand 'enjoyment', as well as the role of enjoyment in different forms of physical activity. Studies need to assess enjoyment alongside other motivational constructs, such as perceived value and importance of the activity.

Exercise-related affective states

Earlier, we suggested that a circumplex model of affect can be represented by the activation and evaluation dimensions of affect (see Figure 2.1). Positive feelings, accompanied by high activation, could be associated with enjoyment during physical activity. Similarly, the positive engagement subscale of the Exercise-Induced Feeling Inventory (Gauvin and Rejeski, 1993) is closely associated with enjoyment. However, while enjoyment is a key to motivation, its nature and measurement is still in need of development and refinement. The only specific scale purporting to assess physical activity enjoyment is Kendzierski and DeCarlo's (1991) 18-item Physical Activity Enjoyment Scale (PACES), and this may be overlong for some studies wishing to assess many other constructs. Example items are shown in Table 2.4.

> Key point: Intuition and some empirical evidence tells us that enjoyment is important for exercise motivation. However, the construct of enjoyment has been poorly understood, may only be partially associated with participation, and remains in need of further study.

Table 2.4   Example items from the 20-item Physical Activity Enjoyment Scale (PACES) (Kendzierski and DeCarlo, 1991). All items are rated on a 7-point scale anchored by statements, such as those shown. The instructions state 'please rate how you feel *at the moment* about the physical activity you have been doing'

Item	Anchor 1 (score 1 or 7)	Anchor 2 (score 7 or 1)
1	I enjoy it (score = 7)	I hate it (score = 1)
9	It's very pleasant (score = 7)	It's very unpleasant (score = 1)
15	It's not at all stimulating (score = 1)	It's very stimulating (score = 7)

Exercise deprivation

The literature on exercise deprivation also lends some support to the notion that physical activity is associated with psychological well-being. Exercise deprivation occurs when regular exercisers are forced (often for experimental purposes but sometimes through injuries or illness) to give up their usual pattern of physical activity. Studying the psychological consequences of such deprivation provides an interesting way of looking at the benefits of physical activity and an insight into why some people continue to engage in regular physical activities. It may also assist in our understanding of the mechanisms of psychological benefits from physical activity.

Researchers have asked regular exercisers to stop exercise for a period of days, weeks or months and have found that deprivation caused a 'feel-worse' effect which disappeared once exercise was reinstated. However, despite the appeal of this paradigm, the difficulty of recruiting those who are willing to give up their exercise routines for research purposes has prevented there being a substantial literature in this area. A review by Szabo (1995) showed that interruption to the normal exercise pattern of an habitual exerciser will have a negative impact upon psychological well-being. This negative impact is most frequently expressed as a series of 'withdrawal' symptoms such as guilt, irritability, tension and depression.

This literature provides us with two possible ways of understanding psychological outcomes of physical activity (Pierce, 1994). First, it is suggested that some regular exercisers experience withdrawal on deprivation of their usual exercise because this deprives them of regular enjoyable experiences, such as mood enhancement, social interaction and the joy of movement. Alternatively, and perhaps even simultaneously, some exercisers need the increase in arousal level that exercise brings in order to avoid negative feelings from low sympathetic arousal such as lethargy and sluggishness. Thus, the benefit of physical activity may be seen as a way to maintain good feelings and avoid bad feelings associated with physical inactivity.

Exercise dependence

In this book there is a wealth of evidence concerning the psychological benefits of physical activity or exercise and more so than detrimental effects. Anyone who has had negative experiences of being ridiculed for lack of skill by schoolmates may tell a different story. Novice exercisers who judge themselves failures because they give up their exercise plan may also have trouble accepting that exercise is good for mental health. There is an acknowledged 'dark side' to physical activity in which self-esteem may be damaged or physique anxiety created as a result of poor experiences (Brewer, 1993), but much less literature exists on that topic than on the beneficial effects. Recent evidence has suggested that some people will approach exercise in a way that many would see as mentally unhealthy. Some may become dependent on, or addicted to, exercise and will exhibit very high levels of activity on a daily or twice-daily basis. There is often informal discussion among various professionals about the risk of creating people who are dependent on exercise when using exercise as part of treatment. This is particularly true in working with other dependencies such as alcohol or drug use in which it is easy to suggest that the clients are swapping one dependency for another.

The term 'exercise dependence' was first used by Veale (1987) to describe a state in which exercise has become a compulsive behaviour. Previous literature describing this phenomenon was hampered by lack of an agreed definition. For example, the term 'obligatory exercise' has been used and a questionnaire exists to measure this trait (Thompson and Pasman, 1991).

Davis and colleagues (1993) note that lack of agreement on terminology and measurement has plagued this area of research. Veale (1987) provided a set of diagnostic criteria to help researchers and clinicians describe this kind of exercise behaviour in a consistent manner. Veale used his knowledge of dependence syndrome and developed specific exercise criteria from them (see Table 2.5). In addition, he distinguished between primary exercise dependence and exercise dependence that is secondary to eating disorders.

Exercise dependence is characterised by the following:

- a frequency of at least one exercise session per day;
- a stereotypical daily or weekly pattern of exercise;
- recognition of exercise being compulsive and of withdrawal symptoms if there is an interruption to the normal routine;
- reinstatement of the normal pattern within one or two days of a stoppage.

The problems that exercise dependence can create range from tiredness and chronic injury to relationship problems and eating disorders (Veale and Le Fevre, 1988). However, there is no known prevalence for this problem and no universal agreement on these criteria. Szabo (2000) suggests that it is very rare. Other authors who have reviewed the topic, but used other terms such as obligatory exercise, call for better assessment of the extent of the problem (Draeger *et al.*, 2005).

Hausenblas and Downs (2002a) completed a systematic review of the literature on exercise dependence and found 77 studies on the topic. However, their review could not provide clear conclusions because of the lack of good experimental designs, lack of definition of terms and poor measures.

A textbook on the topic of exercise dependence has now been produced by Kerr and colleagues (2007). Here the issue of dependence receives some appropriate in-depth

Table 2.5   Diagnostic criteria for exercise dependence (Veale, 1987)

Criteria	
A	Narrowing of repertoire leading to a stereotyped pattern of exercise with a regular schedule once or more daily.
B	Salience with the individual giving increasing priority over other activities to maintain the pattern of exercise.
C	Increased tolerance to the amount of exercise performed over the years.
D	Withdrawal symptoms related to a disorder of mood following the cessation of the exercise schedule.
E	Relief or avoidance of withdrawal symptoms by further exercise.
F	Subjective awareness of the compulsion to exercise.
G	Rapid reinstatement of the previous pattern of exercise and withdrawal symptoms after a period of abstinence.

Associated features	
H	Either the individual continues to exercise despite a serious physical disorder known to be caused, aggravated or prolonged by exercise and is advised as such by a health professional, or the individual has arguments or difficulties with his or her partner, family, friends or occupation.
I	Self-inflicted loss of weight by dieting as a means towards improving performance.

examination with chapters on theoretical approaches, achieving the psychological buzz, issues of dependence in relation to being thin and on being thin to win, case studies and possible interventions. The authors themselves introduce their book as follows:

> Exercise dependence has been described as a 'positive addiction', but it can have links with damaging dysfunctional and excessive behaviours, including eating disorders. Clinical and sport psychologists now acknowledge the condition and report that it can be found in both recreational exercisers and competitive athletes.
>
> (Foreword)

Sometimes we are faced with people who do not know the world of physical activity for health very well and who counter our promotional efforts with the comments about risking creating more exercise addicts. We do not believe this is a high risk. Given the real challenges of encouraging the inactive to become regularly active there is a very small risk that some may become dependent on the new exercise opportunities to which they are being introduced. The prevalence is more likely to be involved with what Kerr and colleagues have called 'exercise dependence to be thin or to win'. For us this is the distinction Veale made between primary dependence (people may become dependent on exercise itself) and secondary dependence (dependence may occur for other underlying reasons such at 'to be thin' or 'to win').

> Key point: Dependence is a potentially serious negative consequence of exercise. There is no known prevalence of this problem but it is likely to be very low.

There is clearly a need for a validated questionnaire to measure exercise dependence. Davis *et al.* (1993) have provided some evidence for the validity of the Commitment to Exercise Scale which is related to, but not based on, Veale's concept of exercise dependence. Szabo (2000) has conducted a review of research into this field, but of the 17 studies he cites not one of them is actually measuring exercise dependence. Measures used included questionnaires on commitment to running, self-perceived addiction to running, negative addiction, obligatory running, and in-depth qualitative interviews and case studies. Thus it is difficult to draw conclusions about the extent of the problem. Hausenblas and Downs, who also conducted the systematic review mentioned earlier, have provided preliminary data on an exercise dependence scale which is based on the recognised clinical criteria for dependence (Hausenblas and Downs, 2002b), and this should move the field forward again.

Exercise dependence may well present at a mental health clinic, sports injury clinic or be associated with eating disorders. Given that a very small percentage of the population exercise at a sufficient level to obtain fitness effects, it is likely that only a very small percentage of the overall population could be diagnosed as exercise dependent, and so *it is clearly not a public health problem*. Nevertheless, the media seem interested in this more 'sensational' aspect of exercise and give it greater coverage that it sometimes deserves.

Furthermore, it is difficult to say how harmful exercise dependence really is to an individual. If the person continues to exercise against medical advice then the risk of chronic injury is clear. It may also be economically harmful to neglect work responsibilities in favour of exercise. Damage to personal and social relationships may be psychologically harmful. It is clear in these cases that the exercise-dependent individual needs to regain a balance in terms of their need to exercise and other important life issues. If exercise professionals notice someone who appears to be dependent then some information on seeking appropriate advice or following some self-help strategies should be made available. As with other behaviour change, raising awareness of the issue is a first step. Table 2.6 offers a format for use in creating a poster in gyms and sports injuries clinics to raise awareness and offer avenues of advice.

Exercise dependence secondary to eating disorders

Veale (1995) pointed out that cases of secondary exercise dependence are more frequently encountered than those of primary exercise dependence. Secondary dependence is when a person uses excessive exercise as part of another disorder, such as an eating disorder or a body dysmorphic disorder. He recommended studies that attempt to determine whether or not primary exercise dependence exists independently of eating disorders. Davis *et al.* (1998) suggested that around 80 per cent of patients with anorexia nervosa have exercised extensively, thus indicating the extent of secondary exercise dependence. There is also a suggestion that high levels of exercise may trigger eating disorders, although there is considerable controversy in the literature. For example, Brehm and Steffan (1998) showed in a cross-sectional study that adolescents who were categorised as obligatory exercisers were more likely to have a drive for thinness (a major element in defining eating disorders) compared to adolescents who did exercise but were not classified as obligatory exercisers. The authors concluded that obligatory exercise could trigger eating disorders. Iannos and Tiggeman (1997) showed that for women who exercised for more than 11 hours per week there was a high level of eating-disordered behaviour. This association was not evident for the men in the study who exercised at equally high levels, which suggests that there may be

Table 2.6   Key questions for raising awareness and possible self-help strategies for potential exercise dependents (Veale, 1987; Zaitz, 1989)

	Question
1	Do you think exercise is compulsive for you?
2	Is exercise the most important priority in your life?
3	Is your exercise pattern very routine and rigid? Could people 'set their watches' by your exercise patterns?
4	Are you doing more exercise this year than you did last year to gain that feel-good effect?
5	Do you exercise against medical advice or when injured?
6	Do you get irritable and intolerant when you miss exercise and quickly return to your exercise routine if you are forced to change it?
7	Have you ever considered that you were risking your job, your personal life or your health by overdoing your exercise?
8	Have you ever tried to lose weight just to make your exercise performance better?

If you answered 'yes' to most of these questions, or if you are worried about becoming dependent on exercise, please speak to a member of staff or follow these self-help strategies:
- use cross-training to avoid overuse injuries; remember: aerobic fitness, strength and flexibility are all important aspects of fitness
- schedule a reasonable rest period between two bouts of exercise to prevent physical and mental fatigue
- exercise your mind by getting involved in mental and social activities that can lower anxiety and lift self-esteem
- try to learn a stress management technique such as relaxation, yoga, tai chi or meditation.

different motivations for men and women who are exercise dependent. On the other hand, Szabo (2000) reviewed studies which have explored the association between eating disorders and exercise, and noted that the conclusions are equivocal and that some of the discrepancies in findings related to the definitions of exercise used. This again outlines the need for stand-ardised ways of measuring exercise dependence.

Exercise dependence secondary to muscle dysmorphia

One aspect of secondary exercise dependence relates to the newly named problem of muscle dysmorphia. Pope and colleagues have been the main researchers investigating this topic which was originally named 'reverse anorexia' (Phillips *et al.*, 1997; Pope *et al.*, 1993, 1997). The distinguishing feature of this disorder, which is considered as a special case of body dysmorphic disorder, is the perception of lack of muscularity even when those concerned (mostly men) do have well-developed musculature (Choi *et al.*, 2002). Associated features include fear of public scrutiny of the body, such as in swimming pools or changing rooms, and a lifestyle in which training correctly and eating correctly to enhance muscularity is the most important issue. Having muscle dysmorphic disorder is the primary problem but the secondary issue is the dependence on exercise (typically strength training using weights). It is unclear if this compulsion to eat correctly is perhaps related to eating disorders as well. It is also clear that there may be a degree of social physique anxiety related to this condition and several researchers have shown a high prevalence of steroid and other drug abuse taken with the aim of increasing muscularity (Kanayama *et al.*, 2001). Pope and colleagues have reported levels as high as 46 per cent of steroid use among both males (Olivardia *et al.*, 2000) and females (Pope *et al.*, 1997) identified as having muscle dysmorphic disorder. Pope has also compared quality of life scores for those identified as having body dysmorphic disorder and those with the more specific muscle dysmorphic disorder, and found that the muscle dysmorphic group had lower scores and also reported more suicide attempts. This study also established that the disorder is different to the more general diagnosis of body dysmorphic disorder. Clearly muscle dysmorphia could damage both physical and mental health.

Why does exercise dependence occur?

It is not clear why primary exercise dependence occurs. It has been shown that such extreme exercise behaviour in men is associated with an obsessive-compulsive personality trait (Davis *et al.*, 1993) or that exercise-dependent people are literally 'running away' from other, perhaps undiagnosed, problems. Szabo (2000) suggests that the literature points to self-esteem being negatively related and anxiety positively related to exercise dependence. It has also been proposed that a person who is exercise dependent has become addicted to the feelings associated with increased endorphin or adrenaline production as a result of exercise (Pierce, 1994), but these speculations remain difficult to demonstrate empirically. Another physiologically based explanation has been termed the 'sympathetic arousal hypothesis' (Thompson and Blanton, 1987). Regular exercise may cause decreased sympathetic arousal at rest that feels like lethargy to the individual. Dependence may occur because such an individual seeks out further bouts of activity to help achieve a preferred state of arousal. Beh and colleagues (1996) offered some support for this notion. They measured EEG in dependent and non-dependent exercisers and found that those classified as dependent had higher alpha frequencies than those who were non-dependent. The authors interpreted this as suggesting that dependent exercisers have higher levels of tonic arousal. This runs counter to the idea that sympathetic arousal is depressed as a result of exercise but is consistent with the notion of a preferred arousal level.

Other suggestions about why exercise dependence occurs include the possibility that exercise is an analogue for anorexia nervosa, although this has been heavily criticised and no supportive evidence has been produced. However, Davis *et al.* (1993) did show an association between excessive exercising and weight preoccupation in both men and women and, while this finding may not show an analogue to more serious eating disorders, it certainly suggests a link. Furthermore, we know that exercise dependence is very often present with eating disorders, but what we do not know is whether primary exercise dependence occurs for the same reasons that eating disorders occur.

There is also discussion in the literature on secondary exercise dependence (both in eating disorders and in muscle dysmorphia) being connected to increased pressure from society and the media to have a particular body shape (Leit *et al.*, 2002). The media pressure on women to be thin is one example of this but a more recent example is the media pressure on men to look muscular. In 1999 Pope demonstrated how the notion of the ideal male shape has changed over the years by measuring the features of action toys for boys such as Action Man (Pope *et al.*, 1999). The research showed that current dimensions of chest muscularity exceed those present in the world's largest body builders. These studies show that society may be producing pressures that lead both men and women to be overly concerned about body image and this may result, in extreme cases, in eating disorders or muscle dysmorphic disorder, both of which are associated with excessive amounts of physical activity.

Exercise dependence: conclusions

All health professionals should be aware of the characteristics of exercise dependence. Although the public health risk is negligible, an individual who is exercise dependent may be at risk of mental or physical ill-health. All professionals who are likely to come into contact with such individuals should raise awareness of the issue and offer avenues for seeking help. Those treating eating disorders will be aware of the use of exercise in these conditions but might also consider how exercise could play a positive role in the treatment of eating disorders. Coaches must be aware that there is a risk of triggering eating disorders by demanding a particular body weight or shape. Such issues need to be carefully handled to avoid long-term harm. Finally, further research is required to understand the prevalence and characteristics of those who are exercise dependent. In particular a measurement scale, which could be validated against the diagnostic criteria, is required.

Sitting time: is this associated with poor mental health?

Research is increasing concerning the possible links between sedentary behaviour – essentially 'sitting time' – and indices of psychological well-being. Typically, in addition to depression and cognitive functioning (dealt with in Chapters 3 and 5), these include generic measures of well-being, such as health-related quality of life.

Teychenne and colleagues (2008) conducted a systematic review on depression and sedentary behaviour in adults. Seven observational (five cross-sectional and two longitudinal) and four intervention studies were included. Of the observational studies, six out of seven showed a positive association between sedentary behaviour and depression, showing that higher sedentary behaviour was associated with greater depression. The other study also showed this for time spent surfing the internet, but reported negative associations for depression with hours spent emailing and using chat rooms. This suggests that the type of sedentary behaviour may be an important moderator of any association between sedentary behaviour and depression.

The four intervention studies reviewed by Teychenne *et al.* (2008) showed mixed results: one study showed no effect, and one showed an increase in depression following the introduction of free computer and internet use, while two showed that the risk of depression was reduced during the intervention. One provided extra computer and internet use while the other used extra 'chat' sessions. The latter may have boosted well-being through social interaction.

Since the review by Teychenne and colleagues (2008), there have been several large-scale epidemiological studies published on this topic. Vallance *et al.* (2011) analysed data from nearly 3,000 adults from the American National Health and Nutrition Examination Survey (NHANES). Physical activity and sedentary behaviour were assessed objectively using accelerometers. Depression was assessed using the Patient Health Questionnaire-9. Results showed that in comparison to the least sedentary quartile (the reference group) there was a trend for a greater risk of depression for those with higher levels of sedentary behaviour. This was most clearly shown in the most sedentary quartile.

Hamer and colleagues (2010) analysed data from nearly 4,000 participants from the Scottish Health Survey. Sedentary behaviour in leisure time was the outcome variable of interest and this comprised time spent on television and screen-based entertainment (TVSE). Mental health was assessed using the General Health Questionnaire (GHQ-12) which measures happiness, depression, anxiety and sleep disturbance. The mental health component of the SF-12 was also used. Scores on the GHQ-12 were significantly higher (reflecting worse mental health) with more than four hours per day of TVSE. However, when confounders were included in the analysis, including physical activity and physical function, this was substantially reduced, although the association remained significant.

Another large cross-sectional study, this time from Australia with data from just under 3,500 adults, was reported by Davies *et al.* (2012). Measures were taken of health-related quality of life (HRQL), physical activity and screen time (TV and computer use in leisure time and at work). In men, HRQL was worse for those with no physical activity and high screen time separately. In addition, the risk for having a worse quality of life score was 4.5 times greater for those with no physical activity and high screen time when combined in comparison to those who had 'sufficient' physical activity and low screen time from one measure of HRQL (14 or more 'unhealthy' days in the past 30). However, the trends were not so evident for women.

A study in Spain on over 10,000 university students, with six-year follow-up, was reported by Sanchez-Villegas *et al.* (2008). A sedentary 'index' was computed from self-reported screen time; mental health was assessed through depression, bipolar disorder, anxiety and stress. The group with the highest sedentary index score (>42 hours/week screen time) had increased odds of a mental disorder (Odds Ratio = 1.31) compared with those spending less than 10.5 hours/week.

A prospective cohort study was conducted by Balboa-Castillo *et al.* (2011), also in Spain. Over 1,000 adults aged 62 years and older were assessed in 2003 for leisure-time physical activity (LTPA) and the number of hours they spent sitting each week. Six years later they were assessed for HRQL using the SF-36 (vitality, social functioning, emotional role and mental health). Self-reported weekly hours of sitting predicted HRQL six years later independent of many confounders, including physical activity. All four mental health subscales showed significant linear trends from those with the lowest sitting time to those in the highest quartile for sitting.

Biddle and Asare (2011) conducted a review of reviews concerning physical activity and mental health in children and adolescents. In addition, they summarised associations between sedentary behaviour and mental health for young people. Nine studies were reported and these led the authors to conclude that higher levels of sedentary behaviour (nearly all studies measured this as screen viewing) were associated with poorer mental health. However, only half of the studies analysed physical activity as a confounder, so in these cases we are unable to conclude whether sedentary behaviour has an independent association with poorer mental health in young people.

In summary, therefore, there are cross-sectional associations between sedentary behaviour, and in particular screen viewing, and indicators of poor psychological well-being. Whether these are the product of reverse causality is not known. It is highly likely that those with poor mental health will choose sedentary pursuits. It is also necessary to test diverse sedentary behaviours to see if they differ in their association with mental health. For example, it is plausible that TV viewing, computer game playing and sitting at work or school may be associated with mental health outcomes in different ways.

Exercise and sleep

One important index of 'well-being' is sleep quality. There is anecdotal evidence and a common-sense belief that physical activity can improve quality of sleep. In addition, a number of reviews over many years have shown that sleep can be positively affected by physical activity and exercise (Horne, 1981; O'Connor and Youngstedt, 1995). Kubitz and colleagues (1996) found that acute exercise yielded significant effect sizes for a number of sleep variables. The results showed that individuals who exercised fell asleep faster, and slept longer and deeper than those who did not exercise. The meta-analysis by Youngstedt and colleagues (1997) confirmed these findings, with the exception of sleep onset latency. For chronic exercise, Kubitz et al. (1996) found that fitter individuals fell asleep faster, and slept deeper and longer than less fit individuals. Generally, effects were small to moderate for both acute and chronic exercise.

More recently, a large sample of American adults were analysed to test the association between objectively measured physical activity and sleep (Loprinzi and Cardinal, 2011). Data were from the National Health and Nutrition Examination Survey (NHANES) with over 3,000 adults. Few studies have examined sleep in association with objectively measured physical activity. The relative risk of often feeling overly sleepy during the day compared to never feeling overly sleepy during the day decreased for those meeting physical activity guidelines compared to those not meeting guidelines. Causal links cannot be shown by such a method, but the large population sample and objective measure of activity are strengths to build on for future studies. Another large study, this time with over 11,000 adolescents, also showed an association between meeting physical activity guidelines and having 'sufficient' sleep (Foti et al., 2011).

Physical activity and psychological well-being in women

Our objective in this section is to review the evidence for the role of physical activity psychology on topics relating to women's reproductive functions: menstruation, menopause and pregnancy. Throughout the book we have always tried to include discussion of both men and women whenever data allowed and to point out instances of gender inequality. In this next section we address some particular topics that are specific to women's reproductive function. These topics will relate to how psychology can play a role for these specific times in women's lives either by providing evidence for psychological or physical benefit of physical activity, or by addressing specific issues concerning adherence. First, we discuss what is known about the psychological benefits of physical activity in relation to menstruation. Then we address the topic of psychological responses to exercise during and after pregnancy, including the topic of post-natal depression. Finally, we discuss the growing literature on exercise and menopausal status.

Physical activity and menstruation

Cultural influences passed from mother to daughter may lead to the view for some women that menstruation is a time of incapacity and therefore not a time for participation in physical activity. Every PE teacher will have been faced with notes from parents who want to excuse their daughters from PE 'at that time of the month'. However, the opposite view is that continuing with physical activity and exercise before and during menstruation is normal and could operate to influence feelings of strength rather than incapacity.

One of the areas that has been explored is how the relationship between uncomfortable premenstrual symptoms, such as bloating or pain, could be alleviated by exercise. This idea has been advocated in the lay literature for some time but such recommendations have lacked theoretical rationale and empirical support. The American College of Obstetricians and Gynecologists' website offers a section on frequently asked questions for women's health (http://www.acog.org). In the section regarding premenstrual syndrome (PMS) they suggest that regular exercise may reduce PMS symptoms for many women, and encourage women to take part in regular exercise throughout the menstrual cycle and not just on days when symptoms may be experienced. However, the evidence upon which this advice is based is limited. Daley (2009) completed a comprehensive review of this topic and showed that, from the four studies she identified, there was some evidence that exercise could help reduce PMS. However, she concluded that the evidence was too sparse to make evidenced-based recommendations. We need to see longer term randomised controlled trials to determine the causal relationship but they have not yet appeared in the literature.

> Key point: Physical activity may have a role to play in reducing premenstrual symptoms.

New areas of reproductive health in relation to physical activity and menstruation are now being explored. Polycystic ovary syndrome (PCOS) is a complex condition in which hormone levels are not normal. Ovarian cysts may cause infertility and the condition is often associated with irregular periods. There is also an association with metabolic syndrome and so physical activity should be a possible intervention (see Chapter 15). Some attempts have been made to determine if exercise can help this condition with a systematic review concluding that too few trials are available to make clear conclusions (Harrison *et al.*, 2011). However, the review also suggests that lifestyle modification, such as increasing physical activity, remained a desirable approach to PCOS that should be evaluated in larger well-controlled trials.

Key point: A new area of research relates to the role of physical activity in reducing symptoms and improving quality of life for women with polycystic ovary syndrome.

Exercise and pregnancy

Physical activity and childbirth has engaged the interest of physicians for a very long time. This interest was initially medical with commentary relating to ease of childbirth and health of the baby. For example, in Tudor times in England obstetricians observed that rich women had more difficult births than working-class women and speculated that this was because of sedentary living for the more privileged classes. During the seventeenth and eighteenth centuries pregnant women were encouraged to exercise, with certain limitations and within the acceptable culture of the times, such as use of a spinning wheel and outdoor walking in low-heeled shoes (Rankin *et al.*, 2000). However, during the Victorian era, pregnant women, especially those from the middle and upper classes, were discouraged from activity and pregnancy was seen as 'confinement' with much reduced social interactions. In the early twentieth century, when medical records began to show an association between physical work, typically in lower class women, and lighter birth weight, and therefore easier labour, exercise was advocated as a prerequisite of a healthy pregnancy (Rankin *et al.*, 2000). Nowadays women are encouraged to exercise during pregnancy and the NHS website offers a guide to how to go about this safely (see http://www.nhs.uk/conditions/pregnancy-and-baby/pages/).

An emerging area of importance concerns the role of exercise in psychological well-being during pregnancy. In comparison to the literature available on the physiological issues of exercise during pregnancy (Lokey *et al.*, 1991), there is very little literature on the psychological issues. The transition to parenthood may be seen as a developmental crisis and there are emotional as well as social changes during pregnancy. The pregnant woman may feel that she is perceived only as a 'pregnancy' and that her own identity becomes submerged (Alder, 1994). In addition, a woman's perception of her pregnancy will be influenced by both peer and cultural pressures. Strang and Sullivan (1985) reported that pregnancy resulted in negative changes in body image for many women. In a prospective study, Slavin *et al.* (1988) found that exercise allowed women to feel more in control of their bodies and helped them maintain a positive self-image during pregnancy. These authors suggest that one of the most consistent benefits of exercise during pregnancy is psychological, because it allows women to feel they have control over their bodies at a time when many bodily changes that occur are biologically driven. However, there is a lack of well-designed studies in which exercise 'treatment' was randomly assigned to women and with adequate numbers to allow robust statistical analysis. One study that managed a more controlled design was completed in Scotland by a practising midwife with knowledge of exercise science. Rankin (2002) randomly assigned 157 women to receive either normal antenatal care or normal care plus antenatal exercise. Forty-eight women assigned to the control group and 50 assigned to the exercise intervention completed the three assessments at early pregnancy, late pregnancy and after pregnancy. Many psychological variables were measured alongside variables related to physical health, childbirth and labour. The pattern of results for the psychological variables was remarkably consistent with the control group experiencing a deterioration of positive aspects over the course of the pregnancy and the exercise group showing maintenance of early pregnancy levels of the same variables. An example of one of these variables, namely perceptions of coping assets, is shown in Figure 2.7. Rankin also noted that there were no detrimental effects of the exercise programme on length of labour or on indices of the new-born baby's health. Thus, the conclusion from this study was that adding exercise to routine antenatal care prevented the decline in women's perceptions of well-being that is normally seen through the course of pregnancy. Although more research is needed, this study created changes in the local provision of antenatal exercise classes and training for leaders of such classes; for further details, see Rankin (2002). Despite this promising trial, a systematic review conducted in 2006 found only 14 studies that addressed the question of how exercise might affect pregnancy. The studies involved small numbers and were of poor quality, and so the authors concluded that better, higher quality trials were needed before clear conclusions could be made on the risks or benefits of exercise during pregnancy (Kramer and McDonald, 2006). Since then a new randomised controlled trial with reasonable numbers has shown that women who experience a three-month supervised exercise programme during their pregnancy had reduced depressive symptoms more than the control group who continued normal activities during the pregnancy (Robledo-Colonia *et al.*, 2012).

A further new area of development in terms of exercise psychology and women's reproductive function concerns the topic of post-natal depression. You will see in Chapter 3 that, in our judgement, there is good evidence that exercise can both prevent and treat depression. It would therefore seem obvious that we should study the role of exercise in both the prevention and treatment of post-natal depression (PND). In 2001 we reported that there had been no specific studies in this area but it is pleasing to note that this is changing. In 2009, Daley and colleagues found five studies when they systematically reviewed the literature on this topic (Daley *et al.*, 2009). They found that, when compared with no exercise, exercise reduced symptoms of PND. However, their conclusion has caveats because of the small number of studies, but this group of researchers is currently involved in a large-scale trial which will add to this database.

Physical activity may be very important in PND because standard treatment for depression, that includes either medication or therapy, may be inappropriate at this time owing to issues of feeding the baby. There is also a need for timely intervention since this sort of depression may have a short time course. Physical activity may be particularly good as an alternative

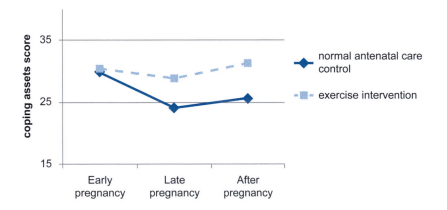

Figure 2.7   Mean scores for perceptions of coping assets over the course of pregnancy
Source: Rankin (2002).

since it is a self-help strategy, could involve socialisation, therefore diminishing isolation as a problem, and literally help women 'get out of the house'. However, it is also clear that physical activity could pose challenges at this time. Sometimes women are still recovering from childbirth and may not feel ready to be active or they may not want to or cannot leave the baby because of feeding or caring needs. One innovative idea has been to introduce exercise for post-partum women in the guise of pram pushing. Armstrong and Edwards (2004), using a randomised controlled design with an exercise and social comparison group, found a significant decrease in depression scores for the pram-pushing group. This is clearly a mode of activity that deserves further attention from exercise psychologists.

> Key point: Physical activity may help pregnant women maintain pre-pregnancy levels of psycho-logical well-being and should be explored as a means to prevent and treat post-natal depression.

Exercise and the menopause

The psychosocial challenges of the transitional years during which women gradually lose their reproductive function (medically termed the climacteric, but more commonly known as the menopause) are many. These include coming to terms with the end of reproductive years, changing roles in the family as children mature and leave home, potential increase in health problems of parents, self and partner, and opportunities for dedicating more time to career and self-development. Many women report that the climacteric is a positive time of change and an opportunity to experience more independence (Musgrave and Menell, 1980). However, some women may experience a certain amount of physical and psychological distress during the climacteric. Vasomotor symptoms, such as nocturnal sweating and hot flushes, are the most commonly reported physical symptoms and are related to hormonal changes (Hunter *et al.*, 1986). There is also evidence of non-clinical psychological symptoms with loss of self-confidence, and increased depression and anxiety being the most frequently reported (Barlow *et al.*, 1989; Hunter and Whitehead, 1989). There are equivocal findings regarding sexual function. It has been suggested that loss of self-esteem is the most general climacteric symptom and several factors combine to reduce a woman's sense of self-esteem during the climacteric. These factors are low socio-economic status, negative attitude towards the menopause and its consequences, limited social network, poor marital relation-ships, and stressful life events.

In the latter part of the twentieth century, Hormone Replacement Therapy (HRT) was heralded as a panacea for women who were suffering from menopausal symptoms with the apparent promise that such therapy might prevent osteoporosis, reduce the risk of cardiovascular disease and make women look and feel younger. Medical opinion now is that HRT should only be prescribed in the smallest dose and for the shortest possible time (UK Committee for Safety and Medicine, 2003). This means that women and clinicians are looking for alternatives to HRT and exercise may come into this frame. Indeed, with substantial evidence for the effectiveness of the role of exercise in the reduction of cardiovascular risk, for prevention and treatment of osteoporosis, for enhanced mood and psychological well-being (Department of Health, 2004), it would certainly seem that exercise has a lot to offer and that women facing the menopause, surrounded by literature of what they should and should not do in terms of supplements, HRT, diet and nutrition, might take our advice – if there is one thing that they should do it is to keep moving!

However, there is still very little experimental research to support the suggestion that women could benefit by increasing activity during the menopause. Daley and colleagues (2011) conducted a systematic review of studies that compared exercise to no treatment and to HRT for vasomotor menopausal symptoms such as hot flushes and night sweats. From six studies, none of the comparisons revealed statistically significant differences. The authors concluded that there was weak evidence in favour of exercise.

It remains feasible that exercise may be a useful self-help and clinical treatment for menopausal symptoms and may be particularly important in promoting positive changes in body image and physical self-perceptions. Future experimental research must establish the effectiveness of such a treatment, and Daley *et al.* (2013) have such a study underway.

Key point: Physical activity may be beneficial for women who are experiencing menopause and our advice is to keep moving!

Is 'fit' a feminist issue?

Although the preceding sections suggest that exercise can be very positive for women facing the various challenges of reproductive function, elsewhere we have noted that the promotion of physical activity for women presents exercise psychologists with certain dilemmas (Mutrie and Choi, 2000). Just as there was a rebellion from feminist thinkers about the constant pressure on women to become thinner, which is best represented in the classic text *Fat is a Feminist Issue* (Orbach, 1978), there is a viewpoint that promoting increased exercise for women represents their 'continued oppression through the sexualisation of physical activity' (Theberge, 1987, p. 389). One dilemma for exercise psychologists is to decide whether or not it matters that one main reason for women to exercise is the pursuit of the 'body beautiful'. If this more 'extrinsic' motivation gets women to initiate activity and that initial experience results in a shift towards more intrinsic motivation, we might expect long-term adherence and thus all the health benefits would follow. That would be ideal. However, we know that it is more likely that women will not achieve body toning and weight-loss goals in the kinds of classes that promise the perfect body, and that their motivation therefore decreases because their unrealistic goals have not been met and they therefore stop exercising.

Our second dilemma relates to perceptions of what some kinds of activity might do to body shape. Anecdotal reports from personal trainers and exercise leaders suggest that many women do not want to do strength training in case they develop 'big muscles'. This is a cultural perception that is difficult to overcome but must always be challenged; otherwise some women will lose out on the benefits of maintaining or gaining strength. Of course, strength training is particularly important for post-menopausal women to help promote bone health and to help prevent falls, and we know also that 'big muscles' would be very difficult for most women to achieve. The reader is referred to the late Precilla Choi's excellent text for further review and discussion of these topics as they relate to women's involvement in physical activity and exercise (Choi, 2000).

Key point: 'Fit' is a feminist issue and exercise psychologists must explore how to promote motivations for exercise that will help women remain active throughout the life course.

Physical activity and psychological well-being: mechanisms

This chapter suggests that physical activity is associated with numerous aspects of psychological well-being. However, we also need to know *why* and *how* such effects occur. This necessitates a brief discussion on the mechanisms of such links, some of which are expanded upon in subsequent chapters.

Mechanisms explaining the effects of physical activity on psychological well-being have not been clearly identified. Several proposed mechanisms are plausible, including biochemical, physiological and social-psychological. Possible mechanisms include the following:

- The effects of exercise on neurotransmitters, such as an increase in endorphins following exercise (Boecker and Dishman, 2013).
- Changes in central serotonergic systems from exercise (Chaouloff *et al.*, 2013).
- The 'feel-better' effect from physical activity may result from changes in physical self-worth and self-esteem from mastering new tasks, having a greater sense of personal control, or from time away and distraction from negative or more stressful aspects of our lives.
- Social interaction, social support and reduced social isolation through physical activity may boost well-being.

In an analysis of possible mechanisms and their interaction with exercise experience, Boutcher (1993) proposes that for those just starting exercise (i.e. in the 'adoption phase'), greater emphasis should be placed on psychological mechanisms, since the exerciser has not yet adapted, physiologically, to the exercise stimulus. In the maintenance phase, Boutcher suggests that both psychological and physiological mechanisms are likely to be important, and in the final habituation phase, he suggests that emphasis should be placed on physiological mechanisms and the influence of behavioural conditioning. These ideas are appealing, since they integrate the context and experience of physical activity with possible mechanisms.

Researchers looking at the psychological outcomes of physical activity are strongly advised to attempt to refine our understanding of mechanisms (Ekkekakis, 2013). Possible explanations for why physical activity may influence psychological well-being are likely to work in a synergistic way in which people may feel better, perceive an increased sense of control, notice less tension in muscles, sleep better, use less effort in daily tasks and have higher levels of circulating mood-enhancing neurotransmitters. Perhaps it is this 'gestalt' which provides the effect rather than one mechanism explaining one outcome.

The link for PWB from physical activity and the field of positive psychology

Seligman has been recognised as the 'father' of the new field of positive psychology. He suggested that the goal of positive psychology is to 'learn how to build the qualities that help individuals and communities not just endure and survive but also flourish' (Seligman, 2002, p. 8). From the range of topics we have reviewed in this chapter we believe that physical activity can help individuals survive and flourish and experience positive emotions. In the following chapters we will also show that physical activity has the capacity to prevent depression, and to buffer individuals against the stresses of life and facilitate thriving after experiencing health-related traumas. At a community level, we suggest that a community in which physical activity is seen as the social norm may be healthier and have greater social capital. Indeed, we would argue that physical activity is a 'stellar' positive psychological intervention (PPI) (Hefferon and Mutrie, 2012, p. 117), as it helps to produce positive emotions, engagement and accomplishment, as well as preventing and reducing more negative experiences and states (e.g. stress, depression). You can explore this connection between the psychological benefits of physical activity and the field of positive psychology in more detail in a chapter in which we claim that physical activity *is* positive psychology in motion (Faulkner *et al.*, in press).

Chapter summary

The relationship between physical activity and psychological well-being is one of the oldest areas of study in philosophy and psychology (Ekkekakis and Dafermos, 2012). It is not surprising, therefore, that evidence is both voluminous and sometimes controversial. Much of the debate stems from weak research designs and low statistical power in studies, thus creating doubt about the true effects of physical activity on psychological well-being. However, nearly all areas studied show positive effects for physical activity across diverse methods of investigation, including meta-analyses, population surveys and experimental trials, and virtually none show negative effects.

From this chapter, we conclude the following:

- Physical activity participation is consistently associated with positive mood and affect, including feelings of 'positive activated affect', energy and lower fatigue.
- Physical activity intensity moderates this relationship, with clearer and more positive results for light to moderate forms of physical activity and negative affect being reported during high-intensity exercise.
- Physically active people who are deprived of exercise report more negative psychological well-being.
- Individuals who exercise fall asleep faster, and sleep longer and deeper than those who do not exercise.
- Exercise can have positive benefits for women's experiences of menstruation, pregnancy and menopause.
- Some people may become dependent on exercise, and exercise leaders should be aware of this and know how to help.
- There are many plausible mechanisms for the 'feel-good' effect from activity and this is a rich area for future research.
- Physical activity is a 'stellar' example of a positive psychology intervention.

References

Alder, B. (1994). Postnatal sexuality. In P.Y.L. Choi and P. Nicolson (eds), *Female Sexuality: Psychology, biology and social context*. London: Harvester Wheatsheaf.

Arent, S.M., Landers, D.M. and Etnier, J.L. (2000). The effects of exercise on mood in older adults: A meta-analytic review. *Journal of Aging and Physical Activity, 8*, 407–430.

Armstrong, K. and Edwards, H. (2004). The effectiveness of a pram-walking exercise programme in reducing depressive symptomatology for postnatal women. *International Journal of Nursing Practice, 10*, 177–194.

Backhouse, S.H., Biddle, S.J.H., Ekkekakis, P., Foskett, A. and Williams, C. (2007). Exercise makes people feel better but people are inactive: Paradox or artefact? *Journal of Sport and Exercise Psychology, 29*, 498–517.

Balboa-Castillo, T., León-Muñoz, L.M, Graciani, A., Rodríguez-Artalejo, F. and Guallar-Castillón, P.

(2011). Longitudinal association of physical activity and sedentary behavior during leisure time with health-related quality of life in community dwelling older adults. *Health and Quality of Life Outcomes, 9*(47). doi: 10.1186/1477-7525-9-47.

Barlow, D.H., Grosset, K.H., Hart, H. and Hart, D.M. (1989). A study of the experience of Glasgow women in the climacteric years. *British Journal of Obstetrics and Gynaecology, 96*, 1192–1197.

Beh, H.C., Mathers, S. and Holden, J. (1996) EEG correlates of exercise dependency. *International Journal of Psychophysiology, 23*, 121–128.

Biddle, S.J.H. (2000). Emotion, mood and physical activity. In S.J.H. Biddle, K.R. Fox and S.H. Boutcher (eds), *Physical Activity and Psychological Well-being* (pp. 63–87). London: Routledge.

Biddle, S.J.H. and Asare, M. (2011). Physical activity and mental health in children and adolescents: A review of reviews. *British Journal of Sports Medicine, 45*, 886–895 doi: 10.1136/bjsports-2011-090185.

Boecker, H. and Dishman, R.K. (2013). Physical activity and reward: The role of endogenous opioids. In P. Ekkekakis (ed.), *Routledge Handbook of Physical Activity and Mental Health*. Abingdon, Oxon: Routledge.

Boutcher, S.H. (1993). Emotion and aerobic exercise. In R.N. Singer, M. Murphey and L.K. Tennant (eds), *Handbook of Research on Sport Psychology* (pp. 799–814). New York: Macmillan.

Bowling, A. (1997). *Measuring Health: A review of quality of life measurement scales* (2nd edn). Buckingham: Open University Press.

Brehm, B.J. and Steffen, J.J. (1998) Relation between obligatory exercise and eating disorders. *American Journal of Health Behavior, 22*(2), 108–119.

Brewer, B.W. (1993) *The dark side of exercise and mental health*. Paper presented at the VIII World Congress of Sport Psychology, Lisbon.

Buckworth, J. and Dishman, R. (2002). *Exercise Psychology*. Champaign, IL: Human Kinetics.

Buxton, M.J., O'Hanlon, M. and Rushby, J. (1990). A new facility for the measurement of health-related quality of life. *Health Policy, 16*, 199–208.

———. (1992). EuroQoL: A reply and reminder. *Health Policy, 20*, 329–332.

Chaouloff, F., Dubreucq, S., Matias, I. and Marsicano, G. (2013). Physical activity feel-good effect: The role of endocannabinoids. In P. Ekkekakis (ed.), *Routledge Handbook of Physical Activity and Mental Health*. Abingdon, Oxon: Routledge.

Chief Medical Officers of England, Scotland, Wales and Northern Ireland. (2011). *Start Active, Stay Active: A report on physical activity from the four home countries' Chief Medical Officers*. London: Department of Health (http://www.dh.gov.uk/en/Publicationsandstatistics/Publications/PublicationsPolicyAndGuidance/DH_128209).

Choi, P.Y.L. (2000). *Femininity and the Physically Active Woman*. London: Routledge.

Choi, P.Y.L., Pope, H.G. and Olivardia, R. (2002). Muscle dysmorphia: A new syndrome in weightlifters. *British Journal of Sports Medicine, 36*(5), 375–376.

Csikszentmihalyi, M. (1975). *Beyond Boredom and Anxiety*. San Francisco, CA: Jossey-Bass.

Daley, A. (2009). Exercise and premenstrual symptomatology: A comprehensive review. *Journal of Women's Health Larchmt, 18*(6), 895–899. doi: 10.1089/jwh.2008.1098.

Daley, A., Jolly, K. and MacArthur, C. (2009). The effectiveness of exercise in the management of post-natal depression: Systematic review and meta-analysis. *Family Practitioner, 26*(2), 154–162. doi: 10.1093/fampra/cmn101.

Daley, A., Stokes-Lampard, H. and Macarthur, C. (2011). Exercise for vasomotor menopausal symptoms. *Cochrane Database System Review* (5), CD006108. doi: 10.1002/14651858.CD006108.pub3.

Daley, A.J., Stokes-Lampard, H., Thomas, A., Rees, M., Coleman, S., Roalfe, A. and Macarthur, C. (2013). Aerobic exercise as a treatment for vasomotor menopausal symptoms: Randomised controlled trial protocol. *Maturitas*. doi: 10.1016/j.maturitas.2013.08.004.

Davies, C.A., Vandelanotte, C., Duncan, M.J. and van Uffelen, J.G.Z. (2012). Associations of physical activity and screen-time on health related quality of life in adults. *Preventive Medicine, 55*(1), 46–49. doi: 10.1016/j.ypmed.2012.05.003.

Davis, C., Brewer, H. and Ratusny, D. (1993). Behavioral frequency and psychological commitment: Necessary concepts in the study of excessive exercising. *Journal of Behavioral Medicine, 16*, 611–628.

Davis, C., Kaptein, S., Kaplan, A.S., Olmsted, M.P., and Woodside, D.B. (1998). Obsessionality in anorexia nervosa: The moderating influence of exercise. *Psychosomatic Medicine, 60*, 192–197.

Deci, E.L. and Ryan, R.M. (1985). *Intrinsic Motivation and Self-determination in Human Behavior*. New York: Plenum Press.

Department of Health. (1993). *The Health of the Nation: A strategy for health for England*. London: HMSO.

——. (2004). *At Least Five a Week: Evidence on the impact of physical activity and its relationship to health. A report from the Chief Medical Officer*. London: Author.

Dixon, P., Heaton, J., Long, A. and Warburton, A. (1994). Reviewing and applying the SF-36. *Outcomes Briefing, 4*, 3–25.

Draeger, J., Yates, A. and Crowell, D. (2005). The obligatory exerciser: Assessing an overcommitment to exercise. *Physician and Sportsmedicine, 33*(6), 13–16; 21–23.

Ekkekakis, P. (2003). Pleasure and displeasure from the body: Perspectives from exercise. *Cognition and Emotion, 17*, 213–239.

——. (ed.). (2013). *Routledge Handbook of Physical Activity and Mental Health*. London: Routledge.

Ekkekakis, P. and Dafermos, M. (2012). Exercise is a many-splendored thing, but for some it does not feel so splendid: Staging a resurgence of hedonistic ideas in the quest to understand exercise behavior. In E.O. Acevedo (ed.), *The Oxford Handbook of Exercise Psychology* (pp. 295–333). New York: Oxford University Press.

Ekkekakis, P. and Petruzzello, S.J. (2000). Analysis of the affect measurement conundrum in exercise psychology: I. Fundamental issues. *Psychology of Sport and Exercise, 1*, 71–88.

——. (2001a). Analysis of the affect measurement conundrum in exercise psychology: II. Conceptual and methodological critique of the Exercise-induced Feeling Inventory. *Psychology of Sport and Exercise, 2*, 1–26.

——. (2001b). Analysis of the affect measurement conundrum in exercise psychology: III. Conceptual and methodological critique of the Subjective Exercise Experiences Scale. *Psychology of Sport and Exercise, 2*, 205–232.

Ekkekakis, P. and Russell, J.A. (2013). *The Measurement of Affect, Mood, and Emotion: A guide for health-behavioral research*. Cambridge: Cambridge University Press.

Ekkekakis, P., Hall, E.E., Van Landuyt, L.M. and Petruzzello, S.J. (2000). Walking in (affective) circles: Can short walks enhance affect? *Journal of Behavioral Medicine, 23*, 245–275.

Ekkekakis, P., Hall, E.E. and Petruzzello, S.J. (2005). Variation and homogeniety in affective responses to physical activity of varying intensities: An alternative perspective on dose-response based on evolutionary considerations. *Journal of Sports Sciences, 23*, 477–500.

Ekkekakis, P., Lind, E. and Vazou, S. (2010). Affective responses to increasing levels of exercise intensity in normal-weight, overweight, and obese middle-aged women. *Obesity, 18*(1), 79–85. doi: 10.1038/oby.2009.204.

Elavsky, S., McAuley, E., Motl, R.W., Konopack, J.F., Marquez, D.X., Hu, L. and Diener, E. (2005). Physical activity enhances long-term quality of life in older adults: Efficacy, esteem, and affective influences. *Annals of Behavioral Medicine, 30*(2), 138–145. doi: 10.1207/s15324796abm3002_6.

Faulkner, G., Hefferon, K. and Mutrie, N. (in press). Physical activity: Positive psychology in motion. In S. Joseph (ed.), *Positive Psychology in Practice* (2nd edn). New Jersey, USA: Wiley.

Focht, B.C. (2012). Exercise and health-related quality of life. In E.O. Acevedo (ed.), *The Oxford Handbook of Exercise Psychology* (pp. 97–116). New York: Oxford University Press.

Foti, K.E., Eaton, D.K., Lowry, R. and McKnight-Ely, L.R. (2011). Sufficient sleep, physical activity, and sedentary behaviors. *American Journal of Preventive Medicine, 41*(6), 596–602. doi: http://dx.doi.org/10.1016/j.amepre.2011.08.009.

Gauvin, L. and Rejeski, W.J. (1993). The Exercise-Induced Feeling Inventory: Development and initial validation. *Journal of Sport and Exercise Psychology, 15*, 403–423.

Hall, E.E., Ekkekakis, P. and Petruzzello, S.J. (2002). The affective beneficence of vigorous exercise revisited. *British Journal of Health Psychology, 7*, 47–66.

Hamer, M., Stamatakis, E. and Mishra, G. (2010). Television- and screen-based activity and mental well-being in adults. *American Journal of Preventive Medicine, 38*(4), 375–380. doi: 10.1016/j. amepre.2009.12.030.

Hardy, C.J. and Rejeski, W.J. (1989). Not what, but how one feels: The measurement of affect during exercise. *Journal of Sport and Exercise Psychology, 11*, 304–317.

Harrison, C.L., Lombard, C.B., Moran, L.J. and Teede, H.J. (2011). Exercise therapy in polycystic ovary syndrome: A systematic review. *Human Reproduction Update, 17*(2), 171–183. doi: 10.1093/humupd/dmq045.

Hausenblas, H.A. and Downs, D.S. (2002a). Exercise dependence: A systematic review. *Psychology of Sport and Exercise, 3*(2), 89–123.

———. (2002b). How much is too much? The development and validation of the exercise dependence scale. *Psychology and Health, 17*(4), 387–404.

Hefferon, K. and Mutrie, N. (2012). Physical activity as 'stellar' positive psychology intervention. In E.O. Acevedo (ed.), *The Oxford Handbook of Exercise Psychology* (pp. 117–128). New York: Oxford University Press.

Horne, J.A. (1981). The effects of exercise upon sleep: A critical review. *Biological Psychology, 12*, 241–290.

Hunt, S.M., McEwan, J. and McKenna, S.P. (1986). *Measuring Health Status*. London: Croom Helm.

Hunter, M. and Whitehead, M. (1989). Psychological experience of the climacteric and post menopause. *Progress in Clinical and Biological Research, 320*, 211–224.

Hunter, M., Battersby, R. and Whitehead, M. (1986). Relationships between psychological symptoms, somatic complaints and menopausal status. *Maturitas, 8*, 217–288.

Iannos, M. and Tiggeman, M. (1997). Personality of the excessive exerciser. *Personality and Individual Differences, 22*, 775–778.

Kanayama, G., Gruber, A.J., Pope, H.G., Borowiecki, J.J. and Hudson, J.I. (2001). Over-the-counter drug use in gymnasiums: An underrecognized substance abuse problem? *Psychotherapy and Psychosomatics, 70*(3), 137–140.

Kendzierski, D. and DeCarlo, K.J. (1991). Physical activity enjoyment scale: Two validation studies. *Journal of Sport and Exercise Psychology, 13*, 50–64.

Kerr, J.H., Lindner, J.K. and Blaydon, M. (2007). *Exercise Dependence*. Abingdon, Oxon: Routledge.

Kramer, M.S. and McDonald, S.W. (2006). Aerobic exercise for women during pregnancy. *Cochrane Database System Review* (3), CD000180. doi: 10.1002/14651858.CD000180.pub2.

Kubitz, K.A., Landers, D.M., Petruzzello, S.J. and Han, M. (1996). The effects of acute and chronic exercise on sleep: A meta-analytic review. *Sports Medicine, 21*, 277–291.

Lazarus, R.S. (1991). *Emotion and Adaptation*. New York: Oxford University Press.

Leit, R.A., Gray, J.J. and Pope, H.G. (2002). The media's representation of the ideal male body: A cause for muscle dysmorphia? *International Journal of Eating Disorders, 31*(3), 334–338.

Lokey, E.A., Tran, Z.V., Wells, C.L., Myers, B.C. and Tran, A.C. (1991). Effects of exercise on pregnancy outcomes: A meta-analytic review. *Medicine and Science in Sports and Exercise, 23*, 1234–1239.

Loprinzi, P.D. and Cardinal, B.J. (2011). Association between objectively-measured physical activity and sleep, NHANES 2005–2006. *Mental Health and Physical Activity, 4*(2), 65–69. doi: 10.1016/j. mhpa.2011.08.001.

McAuley, E. and Courneya, K. (1994). The Subjective Exercise Experiences Scale (SEES): Development and preliminary validation. *Journal of Sport and Exercise Psychology, 16*, 163–177.

McDonald, D.G. and Hodgdon, J.A. (1991). *Psychological Effects of Aerobic Fitness Training: Research and theory*. New York: Springer-Verlag.

McNair, D.M., Lorr, M. and Droppleman, L.F. (1971). *Profile of Mood States Manual*. San Diego, CA: Educational and Industrial Testing Service.

Muldoon, M.F., Barger, S.D., Flory, J.D. and Manuck, S.B. (1998). What are the quality of life measurements measuring? *British Medical Journal, 316*, 542–545.

Musgrave, B. and Menell, Z. (1980). *Change and Choice: Women and middle-age*. London: Peter Owen.

Mutrie, N. and Choi, P.Y.L. (2000). Is 'fit' a feminist issue? Dilemmas for exercise psychology. *Feminism and Psychology, 10*(4), 544–551.

Nasuti, G. and Rhodes, R.E. (2013). Affective judgment and physical activity in youth: Review and meta-analyses. *Annals of Behavioral Medicine, 45*(3), 357–376. doi: 10.1007/s12160-012-9462-6.

O'Connor, P.J. and Youngstedt, S.D. (1995). Influence of exercise on human sleep. *Exercise and Sport Sciences Reviews, 23*, 105–134.

Olivardia, R., Pope, H.G. and Hudson, J. I. (2000). Muscle dysmorphia in male weightlifters: A case-control study. *American Journal of Psychiatry, 157*(8), 1291–1296.

Orbach, S. (1978). *Fat is a Feminist Issue: The anti-diet guide to permanent weight loss.* New York: Paddington Press.

Phillips, K.A., Osullivan, R.L. and Pope, H.G. (1997). Muscle dysmorphia. *Journal of Clinical Psychiatry, 58*(8), 361–361.

Pierce, E. (1994). Exercise dependence syndrome in runners. *Sports Medicine, 18*, 149–155.

Pope, H.G, Katz, D.L. and Hudson, J.I. (1993). Anorexia nervosa and 'reverse anoxeria' among 108 male bodybuilders. *Comprehensive Psychiatry, 34*, 406–409.

Pope, H.G., Gruber, A.J., Choi, P., Olivardia, R. and Phillips, K.A. (1997). Muscle dysmorphia – An underrecognized form of body dysmorphic disorder. *Psychosomatics, 38*(6), 548–557.

Pope, H.G., Olivardia, R., Gruber, A. and Borowiecki, J. (1999). Evolving ideals of male body image as seen through action toys. *International Journal of Eating Disorders, 26*(1), 65–72.

Puetz, T.W. (2006). Physical activity and feelings of energy and fatigue: Epidemiological evidence. *Sports Medicine, 36*, 767–780.

Puetz, T.W., O'Connor, P.J. and Dishman, R.K. (2006). Effects of chronic exercise on feelings of energy and fatigue: A quantitative synthesis. *Psychological Bulletin, 132*, 866–876.

Rankin, J. (2002). *Effects of Antenatal Exercise on Psychological Well-being, Pregnancy and Birth Outcomes.* London: Whurr.

Rankin, J., Hillan, E.M. and Mutrie, N. (2000). An historical overview of physical activity and childbirth. *British Journal of Midwifery, 8*(12), 761–764.

Reed, J. and Buck, S. (2009). The effect of regular aerobic exercise on positive-activated affect: A meta-analysis. *Psychology of Sport and Exercise, 10*(6), 581–594.

Reed, J. Ones, D.S. (2006). The effect of acute aerobic exercise on positive activated affect: A meta-analysis. *Psychology of Sport and Exercise, 7*(5), 477–514.

Rejeski, W.J., Brawley, L.R. and Shumaker, S.A. (1996). Physical activity and health-related quality of life. *Exercise and Sport Sciences Reviews, 24*, 71–108.

Robledo-Colonia, A.F., Sandoval-Restrepo, N., Mosquera-Valderrama, Y.F., Escobar-Hurtado, C. and Ramirez-Velez, R. (2012). Aerobic exercise training during pregnancy reduces depressive symptoms in nulliparous women: A randomised trial. *Journal of Physiotherapy, 58*(1), 9–15. doi: 10.1016/S1836-9553(12)70067-X.

Russell, J.A. (1980). A circumplex model of affect. *Journal of Personality and Social Psychology, 39*, 1161–1178.

Russell, J.A. and Feldman-Barrett, L. (1999). Core affect, prototypical emotional episodes, and other things called emotion: Dissecting the elephant. *Journal of Personality and Social Psychology, 76*, 805–819.

Sanchez-Villegas, A., Ara, I., Guillen-Grima, F., Bes-Rastrollo, M., Varo-Cenarruzabeitia, J.J. and Martinez-Gonzalez, M.A. (2008). Physical activity, sedentary index, and mental disorders in the SUN cohort study. *Medicine and Science in Sports and Exercise, 40*(5), 827–834. doi: 10.1249/MSS0b013e31816348b9.

Seligman, M.E.P. (2002). Positive psychology, positive prevention and positive therapy. In C.R. Snyder and S.J. Lopez (eds), *Handbook of Positive Psychology* (pp. 3–9). New York: Oxford University Press.

Slavin, J.L., Lutter, J.M., Cushman, S. and Lee, V. (1988). Pregnancy and exercise. In J. Puhl, C.H. Brown and R.O. Voy (eds), *Sport Science Perspectives for Women* (pp. 151–160). Champaign, IL: Human Kinetics.

Strang, V.R. and Sullivan, P.L. (1985). Body image attitudes during pregnancy and the postpartum period. *Journal of Obstetric Gynecological Neonatal Nursing, 14*, 332–337.

Svebak, S. and Murgatroyd, S. (1985). Metamotivational dominance: A multimethod validation of reversal theory constructs. *Journal of Personality and Social Psychology, 48*, 107–116.

Szabo, A. (1995). The impact of exercise deprivation on well-being of habitual exercisers. *Australian Journal of Science and Medicine in Sport, 27*(3), 68–75.

———. (2000). Physical activity as a source of psychological dysfunction. In S.J.H. Biddle, K.R. Fox and S.H. Boutcher (eds), *Physical Activity and Psychological Well-being* (pp. 130–153). London: Routledge.

Teychenne, M., Ball, K. and Salmon, J. (2008). Physical activity and likelihood of depression in adults: A review. *Preventive Medicine, 46*(5), 397–411.

Theberge, N. (1987). Sport and women's empowerment. *Women's Studies International Forum, 10*, 387–393.

Thompson, J.K. and Blanton, P. (1987) Energy conservation and exercise dependence: A sympathetic arousal hypothesis. *Medicine and Science in Sports and Exercise, 19*, 91–97.

Thompson, J.K. and Pasman, L. (1991). The obligatory exercise questionnaire. *Behaviour Therapist, 14*, 137.

UK Committee for Safety and Medicine. (2003). HRT: Update on the risk of breast cancer and long-term safety. *Current Problems Pharmacovigil, 29*, 1–3.

US Department of Health and Human Services. (1996). Physical activity and health: A report of the Surgeon General. Atlanta: US Department of Health and Human Services, Centers for Disease Control and Prevention, National Center for Chronic Disease Prevention and Health Promotion.

Vallance, J.K., Winkler, E.A.H., Gardiner, P.A., Healy, G.N., Lynch, B.M. and Owen, N. (2011). Associations of objectively-assessed physical activity and sedentary time with depression: NHANES (2005–2006). *Preventive Medicine, 53*(4–5), 284–288. doi: 10.1016/j.ypmed.2011.07.013.

Van Landuyt, L.M., Ekkekakis, P., Hall, E.E. and Petruzzello, S.J. (2000). Throwing the mountains into the lakes: On the perils of nomothetic conceptions of the exercise–affect relationship. *Journal of Sport and Exercise Psychology, 22*, 208–234.

Veale, D.M.W. (1987). Exercise dependence. *British Journal of Addiction, 82*, 735–740.

———. (1995). Does primary exercise dependence really exist? In J. Annett, B. Cripps and H. Steinberg (eds), *Exercise Addiction: Motivations for participation in sport and exercise* (p. 71). Leicester: The British Psychological Society Sport and Exercise Psychology Section.

Veale, D. and Le Fevre, K. (1988). *A survey of exercise dependence.* Paper presented at the Sport, Health, Psychology and Exercise Symposium, Bisham, Abbey National Sports Centre.

Watson, D., Clark, L.A. and Tellegen, A. (1988). Development and validation of brief measures of positive and negative affect: The PANAS scales. *Journal of Personality and Social Psychology, 54*, 1063–1070.

Youngstedt, S.D., O'Connor, P.J. and Dishman, R.K. (1997). The effects of acute exercise on sleep: A quantitative synthesis. *Sleep, 20*, 203–214.

Zaitz, D. (1989). Are you an exercise addict? *Idea Today, 7*, 44.

Zuckerman, M. and Lubin, B. (1965). *Manual for the Multiple Affect Adjective Checklist.* San Diego, CA: Educational and Industrial Testing Service.

3   Physical activity and clinical depression
Can physical activity beat the blues?

Chapter objectives

Physical activity and depression is one of the most extensively researched areas in 'exercise psychology'. In this chapter, therefore, we focus on how physical activity relates to clinically diagnosed depression in terms of both prevention and treatment.

Specifically, in this chapter we aim to:

- define clinical depression and discuss its prevalence;
- detail prospective epidemiological studies;
- consider an epidemiological study with good design features;
- consider systematic reviews of physical activity and exercise as treatment for clinical depression;
- note the existence of guidelines about the role of physical activity/exercise in the treatment of depression;
- describe a key study concerning exercise as a treatment for depression with good design features;
- critique two studies which have concluded that exercise should not be recommended for depression;
- provide a critique of whether or not the evidence shows a causal relationship between exercise and depression;
- offer directions for future researchers in this area.

Many regular exercisers know that keeping active helps them 'feel good'. It is probably commonly understood that being active has a role to play in positive mental health (see Chapter 2). In the current chapter we deal with poor mental health and ask whether or not regular activity could prevent or treat depression. To begin this exploration we need to define what we mean by depression.

Defining clinical depression

Definitions of depression range from episodes of unhappiness that affect most people from time to time, to recurrent low mood and inability to find enjoyment, and to more extreme dissatisfaction with life that may cause suicide attempts. At one end of the spectrum people may recover relatively quickly from feeling down or blue, but if such feelings persist over time and interfere with our ability to function in work or relationships, they may be classified using standard diagnostic criteria as 'clinical'. In addition, depression may be secondary to other medical conditions, such as alcohol addiction, and is often associated with chronic diseases such as Type 2 diabetes, HIV and cardiac disease. Such feelings may be expected, but to be properly described as depression they will not be transient and will persist over time.

One issue that has plagued our understanding of the relationship between physical activity and depression is the lack of consistency among researchers concerning the criteria for defining depression. Many previous reviews have included cases of 'depression' that would not reach clinically defined criteria and may be better defined as transitory negative affect or minor depression, such as the findings reported in Chapter 2.

> Key point: There is a range of mood states that might be classed as negative but not all of them would classify as 'clinical' depression.

Clinically defined depression will be the main focus of the discussion in this chapter. For clinically defined depression, patients will have sought help for their symptoms and a diagnosis made using standard instruments or interviews. For most people experiencing symptoms of depression, the first point of contact will be primary care and referrals might then be made to more specialist psychological or psychiatric services.

Classifying the various types of mental illness or psychiatric disorders is commonly done with reference to the *Diagnostic and Statistical Manual of Mental Disorders* (DSM), of which version V is current (DSM-5) (American Psychiatric Association, 2013). Another tool is the *International Classification of Diseases-10* (ICD-10) (World Health Organization, 2010) which classifies, and gives a numerical code to, all diseases, including mental and behavioural disorders. These classification systems allow both clinicians and researchers to have a common language concerning the various disorders and a known method of diagnosis, although experience and expert training in psychiatry or psychology is required to undertake any diagnosis. The ICD-10 (1993) chapter on mental and behavioural disorders contains classifications as specified by codes F00-F99 which are shown in Table 3.1.

Table 3.1   ICD-10 codes for mental and behavioural disorders

Numerical code	Description
F00-F09	Organic, including symptomatic, mental disorders
F10-F19	Mental and behavioural disorders due to psychoactive substance use
F20-F29	Schizophrenia, schizotypal and delusion disorders (e.g. paranoid schizophrenia)
F30-F39	Mood (affective) disorders (e.g. depression)
F40-F48	Neurotic, stress-related and somatoform disorders (e.g. phobias)
F50-F59	Behavioural syndromes associated with physiological disturbances and physical factors (e.g. eating disorders)
F60-F69	Disorders of adult personality and behaviour (e.g. kleptomania)
F70-F79	Mental retardation (e.g. mild mental retardation)
F80-F89	Disorders of psychological development (e.g. developmental disorders of speech and language)
F90-F98	Behavioural and emotional disorders with onset usually occurring in childhood and adolescence (e.g. hyperkinetic disorders)
F99	Unspecified mental disorder

The DSM-5 criteria for a major depressive disorder are summarised in Table 3.2 and the symptoms noted by ICD-10 for depression are summarised in Table 3.3.

Key point: *The Diagnostic and Statistical Manual of Mental Disorders* (DSM-5) and the *International Classification of Diseases-10* (ICD-10) (World Health Organization, 2010) are two standard tools which provide clear definitions of depression.

When a clinical interview is used to diagnose depression, the clinical judgement is made using criteria listed in the DSM-5 or the ICD-10. In research studies, the Research Diagnostic Criteria or the Center for Epidemiological Studies depression scale are often used (Radloff, 1977; Spitzer *et al.*, 1978).

Table 3.2   Summary of DSM-5 criteria for major depressive episode

Category	Criteria
A	At least five of the following symptoms have been present during the same two-week period, nearly every day, and represent a change from previous functioning. At least one of the symptoms must be either (1) depressed mood or (2) loss of interest or pleasure
A(1)	Depressed mood (or alternatively can be irritable mood in children and adolescents)
A(2)	Markedly diminished interest or pleasure in all, or almost all, activities
A(3)	Significant weight loss or weight gain when not dieting
A(4)	Insomnia or hypersomnia
A(5)	Psychomotor agitation or retardation
A(6)	Fatigue or loss of energy
A(7)	Feelings of worthlessness or excessive or inappropriate guilt
A(8)	Diminished ability to think or concentrate
A(9)	Recurrent thoughts of death, recurrent suicidal ideation without a specific plan, or a suicidal attempt or a specific plan for committing suicide
B	Symptoms are not better accounted for by a mood disorder due to a general medical condition, a substance-induced mood disorder, or bereavement (normal reaction to death of a loved one)
C	Symptoms are not better accounted for by a psychotic disorder (e.g. Schizo-affective Disorder)

Table 3.3   Summary of ICD-10 symptoms for depression

General criteria	In mild, moderate and severe episodes the individual usually suffers from depressed mood, loss of interest and enjoyment, and reduced energy leading to increased fatiguability and diminished activity. Marked tiredness after only slight effort is common.
Additional symptoms include:	
	reduced concentration and attention
	reduced self-esteem and self-confidence
	ideas of guilt and unworthiness (even in a mild type of episode)
	bleak and pessimistic views of the future
	ideas or acts of self-harm or suicide
	disturbed sleep
	diminished appetite

The most common questionnaire used for assessment, especially in physical activity studies, is the Beck Depression Inventory (BDI) (Beck *et al.*, 1961). This has now been updated to include the DSM-IV criteria and is called the BDI-II (Beck *et al.*, 1996). Moderate depression on the original BDI was defined as a score of 16 or above. The cut-offs used in the Beck-II differ from the original with moderate depression now being defined as a score of 20–28. Thus it is important to note the version of the Beck being used when interpreting intervention effects. In both forms of the questionnaire, the higher the score, the more severe the depression. However, many exercise studies have included people with scores lower than the moderate level at baseline. Such a score would be considered as mild depression and perhaps transitory. The most recent systematic reviews will be alert to this definition but this was probably not the case in the early narrative reviews in this area.

While the failure to differentiate between clinically defined and more minor depression has led to confusion, or perhaps even overestimation of the effect of physical activity on depression, it would be wrong to ignore the more minor levels of depression. In the UK, NICE guidelines for the diagnosis and treatment of depression noted that there has been recent encouragement to identify what has been termed 'sub-threshold' depression. In this case the clinical diagnosis may not be clear for major depression but could be considered as minor depression (National Institute for Health and Clinical Excellence, 2009). There is clearly a potential role for physical activity in helping this sub-threshold level of depression as well and this has been discussed in Chapter 2.

Prevalence of depression

Depression is one of the most common psychiatric problems. Worldwide estimates for the percentage of the population that may suffer from clinically defined depression, also known as major depressive disorder, varies from 4 to 10 per cent (Waraich *et al.*, 2004). In addition, by analysing American employee health insurance data, depression has been noted as the most common complaint in the workplace with a higher prevalence in women than in men (Anspaugh *et al.*, 1996). In 1997 it was estimated from statistical data that by the year 2020 major depression will be the second leading risk factor for disability-adjusted life expectancy after ischaemic heart disease (Murray and Lopez, 1997). In 2006 that estimate was updated and it was then projected that by the year 2030 depression will be the leading risk factor (Mathers and Loncar, 2006).

> Key point: It has been estimated that by the year 2030 depression will be the leading risk factor for life expectancy.

An analysis of the public health impact of chronic disease in 60 countries distributed across the world has concluded that depression produces the greatest decrement of health, ahead of angina, arthritis, asthma and diabetes (Moussavi *et al.*, 2007). The prevalence of mental illness in the UK is 230 per 1,000 referrals to primary care services and data from social trends analysis in the year 2000 showed that 1 in 6 adults living in the UK reported some kind of neurotic disorder such as depression, anxiety or a phobia, in the week prior to the interview. One in four would experience some kind of mental health problem within 12 months (Office for National Statistics, 2001). These prevalence statistics clearly make clinical depression a major public health issue.

Depression is linked to physical health problems

In addition to the importance of mental health in its own right, it has now been recognised that negative emotions, particularly depression, as well as personality and socio-economic status, may have a negative impact on the functioning of various organs and therefore increase the risk of chronic disease, for example, coronary heart disease (Trigo *et al.*, 2005).

Another new and timely area of interest is the idea that childhood depression may increase the risk of adult weight increase and obesity (Hasler *et al.*, 2005). Given that childhood depression is treatable and given the worldwide concern about obesity levels, this association needs further study. These connections between negative emotion and various diseases suggest an increased role for activity, since it may provide a means of improving positive emotions in those who are at risk of disease because of poor mental health.

Prevention

The strongest epidemiological evidence for a causal relationship between inactivity and developing depression comes from prospective studies that have followed cohorts over time. Cross-sectional studies that have only one point in time cannot provide causal information because it remains just as likely that inactivity may cause depression as it does that depression has caused inactivity. One study has clearly shown this bidirectional relationship using the data from the British Whitehall Cohort study over time. Those who were not depressed at baseline but remained regularly active were less likely to become depressed at the eight-year follow-up than those who were not regularly active. Conversely, those who were depressed at baseline were less likely to be regularly active at the eight-year follow-up than those who were not depressed at baseline (Azevedo Da Silva *et al.*, 2012).

The studies on depression where the outcome was clinically defined by questionnaire or interview are listed in Tables 3.4 and 3.5. In all of these studies, statistical adjustments for potential confounding variables, such as age and socio-economic background, were made. Studies that have measured depressive symptoms but do not define a clinical cut-off or category have been excluded.

In Table 3.4, seven prospective studies show that a low level of activity at some preceding date (minimum three years, maximum around 27 years) is associated with an increased risk of clinically defined depression at a later date. Participants were middle- to older-aged adults. Because of the prospective nature of these studies, it is clear that the inactivity preceded the depression, and thus the possibility that the association is simply a result of those who are depressed being inactive may be refuted. In studies that reported relative risk of inactivity for depression the range was from 1.6 to 2. Since people may well be inactive because they are disabled or have other illnesses, it is important to account for physical health status. One study showed that including or excluding those who were unable to walk did not attenuate the relationship (Strawbridge *et al.*, 2002). However, there are other reasons, such as lack of social skills or socio-economic status, which could also predict both inactivity and depression that may not have been fully accounted for.

In comparison to Table 3.4, Table 3.5 contains three prospective studies that did not show a protective effect from physical activity. The reasons for these null results are unclear but, as noted in the table, the measures of activity are not detailed, relying on self-report of defined categories of activity. Such measurements are likely to underestimate the physical activity and depression relationship. It is also possible that publication bias which favours positive significant results over non-significant outcomes has operated and this is why we have more positive than non-significant results. It should also be noted that no published studies have reported statistically significant negative effects of exercise in which depression scores have increased with increasing activity levels.

In summary, epidemiological studies that go beyond cross-sectional data and report depression (with a clear clinical rationale for the definition) and activity levels at two different time points show somewhat equivocal results. However, the weight of the evidence favours a positive and clinically meaningful reduction in risk of depression when people have been active.

A very helpful approach to concluding about the role of physical activity in the prevention of depression has been published by Mammen and Faulkner (2013). The authors systematically reviewed studies with a prospective-based, longitudinal design examining relationships between physical activity and depression over at least two time intervals. A total of 25 of the 30 studies found a significant, inverse relationship between baseline physical activity and follow-up depression, suggesting that physical activity is preventative in the onset of depression. Given the heterogeneity in physical measurement in the reviewed studies, a clear dose–response relationship between physical activity and reduced depression was not readily apparent. However, this study offers promising evidence that any level of physical activity, including low levels, can prevent future depression.

> Key point: There is more evidence in favour of the preventative effect of physical activity on depression than against it.

A key study with good design features

A good example of one of the prospective studies is described in detail below to show the design features. Camacho and colleagues (1991) found an association between inactivity and incidence of depression in a large population from Almeda County in California. Baseline data were collected in 1965 and followed up in 1974 and 1983. Physical activity was categorised as low, medium or high. In the first wave of follow-up (1974), the relative risk (RR) of developing depression was significantly greater for both men and women who were low active in 1965 (RR 1.8 for men, 1.7 for women) compared to those who were high active. There is some evidence for a dose–response relationship with those who were moderately active in 1965 showing lower risk of developing depression than those who were low active (see Figure 3.1).

In the second follow-up in 1983, four categories of activity status were created. These categories are shown in Table 3.6 and are defined as follows:

1. Those who were low active in 1965 and remained low in 1974 (low/low).
2. Those who had been low active in 1965 but had increased activity level in 1974 (low/high).
3. Those who had been high active in 1965 and decreased activity by 1974 (high/low).
4. Those who had been high active at both times points (high/high).

Those who were inactive in 1965 but had increased activity in 1974 were at no greater risk of developing depression in 1983 than those who had been active at both time points (the reference group for computing the odds ratio). This suggests that physical activity may have

Table 3.4 Prospective studies with measures of clinically defined depression showing a protective effect from physical activity

Authors and country	Participants	Design	Measures of depression and physical activity	Results
Farmer *et al.* (1988) USA	1,497 respondents to the National Health and Nutrition Examination Survey follow-up study (NHANES)	Prospective longitudinal eight-year follow-up	Center for Epidemiological Studies Depression Scale (CES-D) using a cut-off point of 16 to indicate depression. Physical activity categorised as did 'little or none' or 'much or moderate' recreational and non-recreational activity.	Women who had engaged in little or no recreational activity were twice as likely to develop depression at follow-up as those who had engaged in 'much' or 'moderate' activity (95% CI = 1.1–3.2). There was no significant association over the same time period for men or for non-recreational activity in a usual day for either women or men. For men who were depressed at baseline, inactivity was a strong predictor of continued depression at the eight-year follow-up.
Camacho *et al.* (1991) USA	8,023 in systematic sample from community	Nine- and 18-year follow-up after baseline in 1965	Depression measured by standard instrument used in Human Population Laboratory studies. Cut-off of 5 used to indicate depression. Frequency of commonly reported physical activity resulting in a physical activity index ranging from 0 [no activity] to 14 high active with strenuous activity.	In the first wave of follow-up (1974), the relative risk (RR) of developing depression was significantly greater for both men and women who were low active in 1965 (RR 1.8 for men, 1.7 for women) compared to those who were high active (although there was a protective effect for moderate levels of activity for women but not for men). Some evidence of dose–response. The second wave of follow-up (1983) suggested that decreasing activity levels over time increases the risk of subsequent depression (OR = 2.02), although the odds ratio was not significant once the model was fully adjusted (OR = 1.61).
Paffenbarger *et al.* (1994) USA	10,201 Harvard Alumni (men only)	23- to 27-year follow-up	Physician diagnosed depression. Rich data on all types and intensities of physical activity – self-reported.	Men who engaged in three or more hours of sport activity per week at baseline had a 27% reduction in the risk of developing depression at follow-up compared to those who played for less than one hour per week. Statistical evidence of dose–response.

Study	Sample	Design	Measure	Results
Strawbridge et al. (2002) USA	1,947 community-dwelling adults (age 50 to 94)	Baseline 1994 and follow-up 1999	Diagnostic and Statistical Manual (DSM) criteria used to define depression. Physical activity measured on an 8-point scale.	Physical activity was protective of incident depression at five-year follow up (OR .83). Excluding disabled participants, who may be depressed but unable to be active, did not attenuate results.
van Gool et al. (2003) Netherlands	1,280 community-dwelling late middle-aged and older people	Six-year follow-up	Dutch version of Center for Epidemiologic Studies Depression scale (CES-D) with a cut-off point of 16 or above (using 20 items) defining depression. Minutes of physical activity per week were self-reported from a variety of possible activities.	155 people became depressed from baseline to follow-up and this was associated with changing from an active to a sedentary lifestyle (RR 1.62) and significantly associated to a decrease in minutes of physical activity.
Bernaards et al. (2006) Netherlands	1,747 workers from 34 companies	Prospective longitudinal with three-year follow-up	Dutch version of CES-D used to measure depression. Those scoring 6 and above (using 11 items from this scale) defined as depressed. Physical activity measured by response to 'How often within the past four months did you participate in strenuous sports activities or strenuous physical activities that lasted long enough to become sweaty?'	For workers with a sedentary job, strenuous leisure-time physical activity (one to two times per week) was significantly associated with a reduced risk of future depression and emotional exhaustion. Higher frequencies (≥ 3 times per week) did not show this relationship
Gallegos-Carrillo et al. (2013) Mexico	1,047 participants in Health Worker Cohort Study, Mexico who were free of depressive symptoms at baseline	Prospective longitudinal six-year follow-up	Center for Epidemiological Studies Depression Scale (CES-D) using a cut-off point of 16 to indicate depression. Physical activity measured by self-report questionnaire of recreational activities over the last year and converted into average MET/hours per week.	Three patterns of physical activity were created: inactive, moderately active and highly active. Those in the inactive category (just over one-third of the sample) had a higher incidence of depression after six years (16.5%) than among those in the other two categories (10.6%).

Table 3.5 Prospective studies with measures of clinically defined depression that do *not* show a protective effect from physical activity

Authors and country	Participants	Design	Measures	Results
Weyerer *et al.* (1992) Germany	1,536 community dwelling adults	Cross-sectional and prospective (5-year follow-up)	All people in this study were interviewed by a research psychiatrist and 8.3% were identified as depressed using a clinical scale. Physical activity was self-reported as regular, occasional or none.	Cross-sectional data showed that those reporting only occasional physical activity were 1.55 times more likely to have depression than those who were regularly physically active, although this was not statistically significant. Low physical activity was not a predictor of depression at five-year follow-up.
Cooper-Patrick *et al.* (1997) USA	973 physicians (men only)	Prospective study. Baseline taken during medical school, and follow-up happens every five years. In this study baseline was 1978 and follow-up 1993.	Self-reported clinical depression. Self-reported physical activity (frequency of exercising 'to a sweat').	There was no evidence for increased risk of depression for those reported exercising 'to a sweat' compared to those who did not or for those who became inactive over the follow-up period (15 years).
Kritz-Silverstein *et al.* (2001) USA	Adults aged 50 to 89 in 1984 to 1987 (932 men, 1,097 women) and followed up 1992 to 1995 (404 men and 540 women)	Cross-sectional and prospective (12-year follow-up)	Modified Beck Depression Inventory (BDI) with scores below 13 being considered as not depressed. Physical activity graded low/ medium/high by yes/no responses to two questions about strenuous physical activity at leisure or work.	Cross-sectional data showed that physical activity was significantly related to lower depression scores. No evidence of predictive effect of low activity on follow-up depression scores.

a protective effect. None of the odds ratios computed for risk of depression in 1983 showed a significant difference between the four activity categories. The largest odds ratio, however, was for those who had relapsed from activity in 1965 to inactivity in 1974. They were 1.6 times more likely to develop depression in 1983 than those who had maintained activity, but

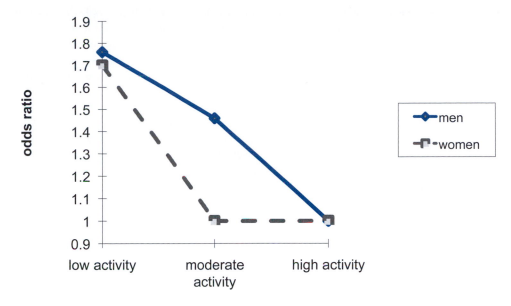

Figure 3.1 1965 physical activity level and 1974 scores for depression

Source: Data from Camacho *et al.* (1991).

Note: Activity level calculated from frequency intensity reports of leisure activities producing a 14-point scale that predicted mortality and morbidity for this sample. Low = 0–4 points; moderate = 5–8; high = 9–14.

Table 3.6 Changes in physical activity status and subsequent depression (Camacho *et al.*, 1991)

Activity status 1965/1974	Odds ratio for developing depression in 1983	Confidence interval for odds ratio
1. low/low	1.22	0.62–2.38
2. low/high	1.11	0.52–2.21
3. high/low	1.61	0.80–3.22
4. high/high	1.00	reference group

it must be remembered that this did not reach significance. The authors note, however, that this odds ratio was relatively unaffected by adjustments for age, sex, physical health, socio-economic status, social support, life events, anomie, smoking status, relative weight, 1965 level of depression and alcohol consumption. This led the authors to believe that it is a robust finding. Given that only 137 people were in this category, it is perhaps not surprising that the odds ratio did not reach significance. However, the 1974 follow-up did provide statistically significant evidence that low activity preceded the reported depression.

Reviewing the evidence base for physical activity as a treatment for depression

Settings for treatment of depression include general practice, hospitals, specialist clinics (or resource centres), private therapy and informal settings. When people do not seek help for feelings of depression they may discuss these feelings informally within family or friendship groups, or they may try to cope with such feelings by themselves. When people do seek out treatment the first port of call may be their GP, in which case some form of medication may be offered. Using data from EU member states from 2000 to 2010 it has been shown that the use of antidepressants increased on average by over 80 per cent in that decade (OECD, 2012). This trend suggests that medication is the first line of treatment and the most frequent.

Some people may be offered counselling-style therapies that include focusing on the way the person is thinking or feeling and acknowledging their social circumstances. Trained professionals who might undertake this therapy include psychiatrists, clinical psychologists, counselling psychologists, hypnotherapists and social workers. Within this area there are many approaches, ranging from psychoanalysis (which is perhaps the layperson's impression of all therapy), to client-centred and cognitive-behavioural approaches. A particular style that has become popular is cognitive behavioural therapy (CBT). Sometimes the whole family may be involved in the therapeutic process. In extreme cases more invasive procedures such as Electro Convulsive Therapy (ECT) or psychosurgery (such as prefrontal lobotomy) may be performed. A good source of reference for understanding these treatments is the Royal College of Physicians in the UK (http://www.rcpsych.ac.uk/default.aspx). Of course, of key interest to us in this chapter is the role of physical activity in the treatment of clinical depression.

Physical activity as a treatment for depression

A BRIEF HISTORY OF REVIEWS ON THE EFFECT OF EXERCISE ON DEPRESSION

We have been interested in the effects of exercise on depression since the first textbook we wrote in 1991 (Biddle and Mutrie, 1991). At that time we described a narrative review that covered an emerging research field with some studies providing randomised designs, some studies reporting on hospitalised designs and some using small-n designs. Not many of these studies would make it into current systematic reviews. We concluded the review by noting that the potential for exercise to decrease depression was clear but that research designs needed to pay more attention to internal validity to enable discussion of causality. Ten years later (Biddle and Mutrie, 2001) we had the benefit of reviewing the new evidence that had emerged from epidemiological studies about the potential for exercise to prevent depression and the first efforts at providing meta-analytic reviews of treatment effects, and so our review was much fuller and reflected a growing field of research. In the 2001 book we concluded that 'the potential benefit of advocating the use of exercise as part of treatment for depression far outweighs the potential risk that no effect will occur' (p. 219). We also concluded that, in our judgement, a causal link existed between exercise and reduction in depression but noted that some people would see this statement as controversial. We therefore advocated the use of exercise as part of the treatment for clinically defined depression and appealed for the next generation of research to focus on the determination of the mechanisms by which exercise could have this effect.

> Key point: Since 2001 we have been suggesting that physical activity should be encouraged for those with clinical depression and we have not changed our minds!

SYSTEMATIC REVIEWS

All of these early reviews and meta-analyses had drawbacks, including the failure to exclude trials in which there was no clinical definition of depression used or to exclude trials that had non-randomised designs, thus leaving results open to bias.

In the second edition of this textbook (Biddle and Mutrie, 2008) we had the advantage of one of the first robust systematic reviews in the area (Lawlor and Hopker, 2001). Systematic reviews have become the gold standard for the synthesis of results in an area where several quality studies are available and are often accompanied by meta-analysis if studies have used the same outcome variables. In Lawlor and Hopker's systematic review and meta-analysis, there was a limited inclusion of studies in the review in two important ways. First, studies had to have defined depression in the clinical range by a recognised method, and second, studies had to be randomised controlled trials. From the 14 studies included, the mean effect size (ES) for exercise compared to no treatment was -1.1 (95% CI -1.5 to -0.6) – a large effect. Cognitive therapy had a similar ES to exercise. There were not sufficient studies to compare exercise to medication. The mean difference between exercise and control groups in BDI score was -7.3 (95% CI -10 to -4.6). Effectiveness has been shown by the ES in this meta-analysis but the clinical significance of this level of change in the BDI was questioned by Lawlor and Hopker, who concluded that 'The effectiveness of exercise in reducing symptoms of depression cannot be determined because of lack of good quality research on clinical populations with adequate follow up' (p. 1).

We were critical of that conclusion in the 2008 edition of the book because the restriction to clinical levels of depression and the inclusion of only randomised controlled trial designs made this a stringent review of the best-quality evidence at the time. The results were similar to other therapies for depression and the effect size was large, and so, while we agreed that there was a need for longer term studies and further research, we could not see why such a negative conclusion had followed on from these results. Such a conclusion in a journal of high impact (*BMJ*) perhaps delayed the acceptance of physical activity as a potential tool for use by mental health practitioners. While we advocated that practitioners should seriously consider the use of physical activity for positive mental health benefits, others would have said that that would be wrong because the evidence remained inconclusive. We could have been accused of taking the 'glass half-full' and optimistic approach to this topic by criticising the overly negative conclusion from that systematic review. We continue to be more optimistic than pessimistic in this area, as the next section shows. Readers will have to make their own judgements from the evidence of whether the glass is half empty or half full.

The science of systematic reviewing has also improved over the past decade and most systematic reviews now follow the guidance of the Cochrane Collaboration. This is an organi-sation of 27,000 contributors from over 120 countries (http://www.cochrane.org). The goal of the Cochrane Collaboration is to make information about the effects of various aspects of health care readily available. The methods adopted involve systematic reviewing of all available literature on the topic in question. The methods handbook that has been produced is seen as the gold standard methodology for systematic reviews (http://www.cochrane.org/training/cochrane-handbook). Guidelines about what kind of evidence will count in a review ensure that the best available evidence is considered. Reviews might cover issues of prevention or treatment. If a review is completed it is published online in the Cochrane Library. The reviews held in the Library help practitioners and policy-makers, and the public, to make decisions about what the evidence suggests about any health intervention.

The most recent review on the topic of exercise as a treatment for depression was published by the Cochrane Library and was conducted by Rimer *et al.* (2012). These authors found 30 studies that met their inclusion criteria. We can clearly see an expansion here from the 14 studies in the Lawlor and Hopker (2001) review in the space of 11 years. The meta-analysis by Rimer *et al.* showed a moderate effect size (-0.67, 95% confidence interval (CI) -0.90 to -0.43) for exercise versus no treatment control conditions.

When studies had potential bias due to lack of allocation concealment or lack of blinding to outcomes, a further meta-analysis of the remaining four trials showed a reduced but still significant effect. Finally, the authors compared the exercise effects to those of cognitive behavioural therapy for the six trials that had these comparisons and found no significant difference. This confirmed the findings of the Lawlor and Hopker review that exercise had a similar effect size to other recognised therapies for depression. However, there were still insufficient studies to compare exercise to drug therapies.

Thus the number of studies has increased and using the Cochrane methodology ensures that there is less chance of bias. The Cochrane Handbook for conducting systematic reviews calls for assessment of the risk of bias, and Rimer *et al.* (2012) provide a graph of their assessments which is shown in Figure 3.2. It may be seen that the main risks to bias are as follows:

- allocation concealment where there is a risk that the person making the allocation to intervention or control knows the sequence and it is therefore not random;
- blinding the outcome assessor where there is a risk that the person assessing physical activity levels or depression levels knows which group the person was in;
- incomplete outcome data where there is a risk that bias occurs because only those completing the intervention have data.

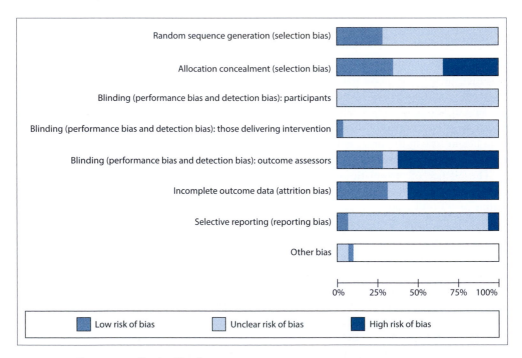

Figure 3.2   Illustration of 'risk of bias'

Source: Rimer *et al.* (2012).

It would still appear that we have not reached the highest standards of design in this area of research because some studies still have some degree of bias, but the risk table provides clear guidance for the next generation of studies. Despite these concerns about bias, the authors of this most recent review are more optimistic and conclude that it is reasonable to recommend exercise as a treatment for depression.

A further update of this review has now been completed and shows a similar effect size for the overall effect (-0.62) for exercise versus no treatment control conditions (Cooney *et al.*, 2013). For the six trials considered to be at low risk of bias (adequate allocation concealment, intention-to-treat analyses and blinded outcome assessment), a further analysis showed a small clinical effect in favour of exercise which did not reach statistical significance. Finally, the authors compared the exercise effects to those of cognitive behavioural therapy for the seven trials that had these comparisons and found no significant difference. Similarly, four trials compared exercise with antidepressant medication and no significant difference was found. One conclusion from the authors of this update is that 'When compared to psychological or pharmacological therapies, exercise appears to be no more effective, though this conclusion is based on a few small trials' (p. 2). This sounds like the glass half-full approach but it could be rewritten with the same underpinning evidence as 'exercise appears to be as effective as other psychological or pharmacological treatments'. Over to you, reader, to decide whether that glass is half full or half empty! However, the authors also note that there are many unanswered questions such as the exact dosage and mode of activity that might work best.

One team of systematic reviewers have taken action on this advice and examined the physical activity mode of walking (Robertson *et al.*, 2012). They found eight trials that met their inclusion criteria and showed a large effect size of 0.86 (CI 1.12, 0.61). The authors concluded that 'Walking has a statistically significant, large effect on the symptoms of depression in some populations but the current evidence base from randomised, controlled trials is limited' (p. 73).

> Key point: A recent systematic review of the studies that have used physical activity or exercise as a treatment for depression concluded that it is reasonable to recommend exercise to people with depressive symptoms.

A KEY STUDY WITH EXCELLENT DESIGN FEATURES

Dunn *et al.* (2005) conducted a very tightly controlled study which aimed to answer some of the questions concerning the relationship between the dose of physical activity provided and the response in terms of decreased depression scores. In particular, this study compared frequency of exercise (three or five days per week) and total energy expenditure per week (7kcal/kg/week 'low dose' versus 17.5kcal/kg/week 'public health dose') in a 12-week protocol. Four aerobic exercise conditions allowed these comparisons; two groups exercised on three days a week – one expended 7kcal/kg/week and the other 17.5kcal/kg/week; two other groups exercise on five days a week but expended the same totals of either 7 or 17.5kcal/kg/week. Participants were randomly assigned to one of these four groups or to a placebo exercise condition which involved stretching exercises on three days of the week. Results showed that the public health dose reduced depression scores more that the lower dose, but that frequency did not matter (see Figure 3.3).

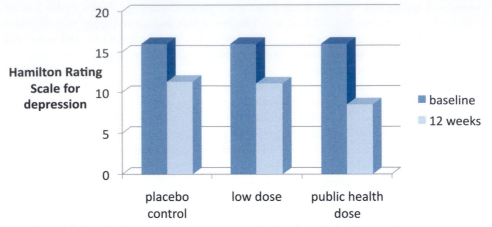

The public health dose of exercise was more effective in reducing depression scores to a clinically acceptable level than the lower dose or the control condition. Frequency of exercise (three or five days/week) was not important.

Figure 3.3 Exercise treatment for depression

Source: Dunn et al. (2005).

All the exercise was completed in sessions which were supervised but in which the participants were isolated from other exercisers. Thus the effect of exercising in a group cannot be one of the possible explanations of these results. This trial has been well enough controlled to rule out a number of previous possible explanations and shows that exercise at a dose recommended for public health (the equivalent of 30 minutes on most days of the week) can be a stand-alone treatment for mild and moderate depression.

It is clearly difficult to conduct studies with good design features in this area. Dunn *et al.*'s study is one of the few that overcomes some of the most common limitations and challenges to researchers in this area.

Limitations and challenges for researchers conducting trials with physical activity or exercise as a treatment for depression

The following bullet points note the challenges that researchers face or the limitations to existing data:

*   Recruiting a large enough sample to ensure statistical power (could the findings of 'no difference' between intervention and control groups in some studies be a type 2 statistical error?).
*   Equalising time in contact with professionals in the different treatment conditions. Control conditions or usual care conditions often have less time in contact with a relevant professional and this could create unintentional bias for the intervention group.
*   Conducting 'double-blind' studies. These are the gold standard within RCTs in which the effect of a drug is being tested. It means that both the researcher and the client/patient are blind to what drug treatment they have been given. In exercise studies this is not possible to achieve because the patient will certainly know that they are exercising, in a way that is different from receiving an unmarked tablet. While every effort should be

made to keep studies at least single blind (that is the researcher taking outcome measures should not know the group assignment), it remains a challenge to achieve this. Clients and patients often reveal their assignment to researchers (who are otherwise blind to assignment) in conversation, such as 'I really enjoyed that weight training'.

- Avoiding resentful demoralisation in a no-treatment group or a group given the 'routine' or placebo condition as opposed to the 'new' treatment. This 'resentful demoralisation' remains a challenge for researchers to overcome because informed consent processes required by ethical procedures mean that the participants are interested in becoming more active. One possible solution is to name the control condition as a waiting list for the intervention so that people assigned to that condition know that they have to wait three or six months, or sometimes 12 months before receiving the intervention.

- In contrast to resentful demoralisation, those assigned to the control group, having been interested in participating in a physical activity study, may find their own motivation or take up local opportunities to become more active. This will diminish the potential contrast between intervention and control conditions in terms of physical activity levels.

- Controlling for the effects of the positive characteristics of an exercise leader or the social effect of a group. The social aspect of group exercise may add further benefits, and group versus individual exercise should now be compared.

- Conducting long-term follow-up. Very few studies have managed to fund adequate follow-up of one or two years.

- Finding adequate measures of the variables of interest, including total energy expenditure. For physical activity measures, objective monitoring should be undertaken because of the acknowledged over-reporting that occurs with self-report measures. For measuring depression a clinical interview may be considered the best option rather than a self-complete questionnaire.

The CONSORT group have considered these inadequacies in trials of a diverse range of medical interventions, and have provided excellent guidance on how to design and report trials that avoid many of these challenges. See the website for further details (http://www.consort-statement.org).

Studies which conclude that exercise cannot be recommended for the treatment of depression

Contrary to the conclusion we have reached above, two recent studies that restricted recruitment to clinical settings and used high-quality research procedures have created new debate in this area because they both conclude that exercise cannot be recommended for depression. However, we contend that their conclusions are erroneous and therefore do not consider that these studies make us more cautious about our conclusion. We offer the following commentary on each study in turn.

The first is a study by Krogh and colleagues (2012), and we commend their attention to detail in terms of compliance with the CONSORT guidelines for conducting randomised controlled trials. The design is a two-arm trial comparing aerobic exercise to an attention control of stretching activity over a three-month programme but there is not a no-treatment or usual care comparison. The results showed no difference between the two groups at three months in terms of depression. The authors conclude that the results do not support referral to aerobic exercise for depression. The design used seems plausible and ethical but we believe there is a potential flaw that could lead to the wrong conclusion. When we look at the results we see that both groups decreased depression scores in the same way over time, and without a no-treatment or usual care comparison we really cannot make conclusions about the effectiveness or lack of effectiveness of aerobic exercise.

In a similar trial design, but with the inclusion of a usual care comparison, we have looked at the effect of aerobic exercise on quality of life for women treated for breast cancer (Daley *et al.*, 2007). In this study the aerobic exercise group improved versus the usual care group but not in relation to the placebo (or attention) control group which was given a light intensity stretching programme of exercise. The placebo group also showed improvements against the usual care group. We concluded that our results showed clinical levels of improvement but we would not have been able to make that conclusion without the usual care comparison. We now believe that even what we may have considered as a placebo or attention control condition involving predominantly stretching activity is probably not an 'inert' treatment. This may be particularly true for people who have not been active for some time for whom even the warming-up activities needed for safe stretching create an increase in activity over resting levels. So even these very low levels of activity may be helping depressed patients with how they feel. We might therefore equally conclude from the Krogh study that both aerobic and stretching activity may be helpful for patients with depression.

International guidelines on how much activity people should do to gain health benefits (including mental health benefits) suggest that while a minimum dose is recommended (typically 150 minutes of moderate intensity activity over the course of the week), we should all be aware that there is a dose–response curve associated with these benefits (Global Advocacy Council for Physical Activity International Society for Physical Activity and Health, 2010). Therefore, even doses of activity such as that achieved via a stretching programme may confer some benefit. Thus we believe that Krogh *et al.* (2012) may have reached an erroneous conclusion.

The second study was completed in the UK and contained the long-awaited results of the TREAD trial (Chalder *et al.*, 2012). This trial had many commendable features, such as large patient numbers, the delivery of the intervention within standard care and a team of experienced researchers, but it did rely on self-reported physical activity. The trial was a two-arm randomised design with both arms receiving usual GP care for depression and the intervention arm also having additional one-to-one sessions with a physical activity counsellor. Both groups decreased depression scores over time but there was no advantage to the facilitated physical activity intervention arm. These results are illustrated in Figure 3.4. The authors noted in the 'what this study adds' section of the paper that 'Clinicians and policy makers should alert people with depression that advice to increase physical activity will not increase their chances of recovery from depression'.

We believe this advice is misguided because, while there are many aspects of this study that are commendable, there are three main flaws that have led to this erroneous conclusion. The first flaw is that most policy-makers and clinicians know that they should not base their decisions on single studies. This is why clinical guidelines, such as those offered by NICE, are based on reviews of all available evidence of high quality. The evidence in the extant literature is supportive of the use of physical activity for the treatment of depression. The second flaw is that there is not a waiting list or a no-treatment control group for comparison. Both intervention and control conditions were receiving standard care which had known efficacy for decreasing depression and both groups improved in the same way. Thus it is not possible to declare that one is less effective than the other. They were both equally effective in reducing depression. In order to test the idea that physical activity could be used to treat depression (and therefore come to their stated conclusion that it cannot do this), the authors would have to have had a study arm with physical activity on its own.

In thinking about this flaw we were reminded of the well-designed study by Blumenthal and colleagues in which exercise was compared to standard drug therapy or a combination of both treatments over a 16-week period. The authors found that all three groups reported significant reductions in depression (see Figure 3.5) (Blumenthal *et al.*, 1999). In a follow-up study of the same participants, Babyack *et al.* (2000) reported some advantages for exercise over a six-month period, including smaller percentages of those in the original exercise group being classified as depressed or using medication. This landmark study was the first to show that exercise by itself had similar outcomes to standard antidepressant medication. However, what if this study had only two arms similar to the TREAD trial? The standard treatment was medication (this would be the usual care arm of the TREAD trial) and the exercise plus medication arm of the Blumenthal trial would have been the intervention arm of the TREAD

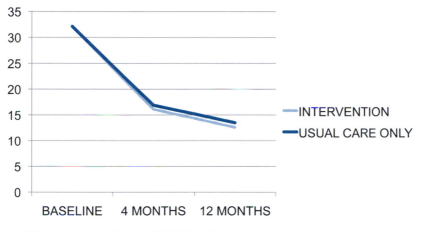

Figure 3.4 BDI scores reported in the TREAD trial

Source: Chalder *et al.* (2012).

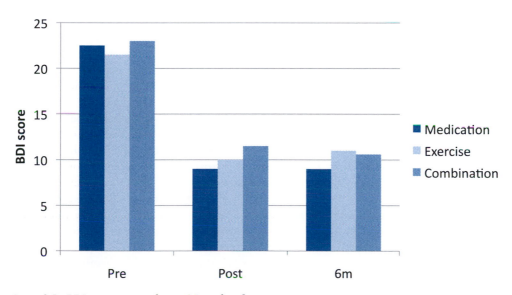

Figure 3.5 BDI scores pre and post 16 weeks of treatment
Source: Data from Blumenthal *et al.* (1999); and six-month follow-up from Babyak *et al.* (2000).

trial. Given that both of these groups improved in the same way would have left Blumenthal unable to conclude about the role of exercise per se, but because there was also an exercise-only arm, then clear conclusions about exercise versus medication were possible. There was also the hypothesis by Blumenthal *et al.* that a combination of two different approaches (exercise and medication) might be superior to either on its own but this was not supported. This is the second flaw of the TREAD trial. Putting increased physical activity alongside an already successful treatment had no added benefit but that does not allow for the conclusion that physical activity would have no benefit on its own.

The third flaw is that 'usual care' included opportunities for increasing physical activity. For participants who provide informed consent for a trial about physical activity, it is likely that many in the usual care arm took up such opportunities to be active. It appears from the results that both groups increased their physical activity levels from baseline. The authors note in relation to the physical activity results that 'there was no evidence that the difference between the groups changed over the duration of the study (time by treatment interaction P = 0.71)' (p. 5). With no significant interaction then, the available evidence is that both groups changed in the same way for physical activity. Thus, because of these three flaws we believe that Chalder *et al.* (2012) have also reached the wrong conclusion in stating that 'The main implication of our results is that advice and encouragement to increase physical activity is not an effective strategy for reducing symptoms of depression' (p. 5).

Key point: We stand by our conclusion that practitioners should encourage patients with depression to become more active.

Further systematic reviews in relation to exercise and depression

In our first overview of this area we noted that there were no studies on young people (Biddle and Mutrie, 1991). A further Cochrane Review has now focused on young people (Larun *et al.*, 2006). The review also included anxiety. The review found 16 studies and, although some promising results for exercise were noted for depression, the reviewers concluded that the effect of exercise on anxiety and depression for young people was not known at this time because of the lack of studies (Larun *et al.*, 2006). A recent prospective population study also found no evidence of a protective effect from physical activity on the onset of depression in adolescence (Stavrakakis *et al.*, 2013).

In a review of four systematic reviews concerning physical activity and depression in young people, Biddle and Asare (2011) concluded that physical activity had some potentially beneficial effects, but the evidence base was limited. Specifically, they highlighted low-quality intervention designs, with many reviews including cross-sectional studies that may distort associations or that failed to rule out reverse causality.

There is clearly more work to be done and there are two further registered systematic reviews in the Cochrane database in relation to physical activity and depression. The first is related to older adults and the second relates to the use of dance therapy as a mode of exercise for people with depression. We look forward to these results in this ever-expanding area of research.

Physical activity and depression: is there a causal connection?

Reflecting on the evidence for the third edition of this book takes us back to the sage words of A.B. Hill who first guided the public health community about how to make causal inferences in areas where the evidence was often incomplete. One seminal example concerns whether or not smoking caused lung cancer (Hill, 1965). Hill evolved eight principles or 'tests' which could be fulfilled at different levels. The eight criteria, framed here for testing whether or not it could be concluded that exercise causes a reduction in clinical depression, are as follows:

1. *Strength of association.* This refers to the strength of the association between the 'treatment' of exercise and the reduction in depression scores. This is shown by the effect sizes from meta-analyses. The highest is 1.1 from Lawlor and Hopker (2001) and the lowest is the adjusted ES from the four highest quality studies of 0.31 from the Rimer *et al.* (2012) Cochrane Review. Epidemiological studies suggest a relative risk of around 1.7 for the inactive reporting depression at a later date. This evidence is not quite as strong as that for exercise and coronary heart disease, where a range of relative risk between 1.5 and 2.5 for the inactive has been reported (Pate *et al.*, 1995). Nevertheless, the strength of association between exercise and depression is clear to see and is moderate to large in magnitude.

2. *Consistency of evidence.* This is the consistency of evidence concerning exercise as a treatment for depression from different places, with different populations and different approaches to exercise. Men and women have been studied, adults of middle and older age groups have been included, the data span three decades, and the circumstances include community, hospitals and primary care settings. So it does seem that the findings are consistent.

3. *The specificity of effect.* Specificity refers to whether or not other associations exist between depression and other conditions. Hill argues that if specificity can be claimed (i.e. limiting the conditions to the disease, such as smoking and lung cancer), this strengthens the argument for causation. In exercise studies specificity does not exist. Depression is not the only disease linked to inactivity, nor is inactivity the only environmental condition associated with depression. Furthermore, depression itself has multiple causes (Kaplan *et al.*, 1987). However, Hill also argued that if specificity is not present other criteria may supply extra evidence.

4. *Temporal sequence.* In order to conclude that there is a causal link between inactivity and depression we must demonstrate that inactivity precedes the onset of depression. Early cross-sectional studies could not provide an answer to this question because it was equally likely that depression preceded physical inactivity. However, there are now at least seven prospective populations studies showing that the inactive are more likely to develop depression (see Table 3.4) while three such studies failed to show this protective effect (see Table 3.5). Thus the weight of the evidence supports the notion of the temporal sequence being appropriate, thus strengthening the argument for causation (see earlier section on prevention). However, all of the trials in systematic reviews will have fulfilled this criterion because to begin with people are insufficiently active and then they become active.

5. *Dose response.* Hill's fifth criterion is evidence for a dose–response curve or biological gradient. Several of the prospective epidemiological studies have shown a dose–response gradient, with the least active at baseline being most at risk of developing depression at follow-up, while the most active had the lowest risk. In terms of experimental studies,

although both aerobic and non-aerobic exercise have produced an antidepressant effect, almost all the aerobic exercise has been based on moderate intensity (60 to 75%) levels with a typical prescription of three times per week for 20 to 60 minutes. Dunn *et al.*'s (2005) experimental study has provided evidence that, at least for aerobic exercise, the public health dose (equivalent to 30 minutes on most days of the week) produced an antidepressant effect, whereas a smaller dose did not. Thus, while there are a variety of 'doses' that have not yet been tested, there is evidence for a dose–response relationship which again adds to the evidence for a causal connection. However, we should be cautious because even more exercise may not continue to be beneficial.

6. *Plausibility.* The sixth criterion is biological plausibility. Here we are looking for the explanation of the observed association. There is agreement that the underlying mechanisms of the effects of exercise on mental illness are still being tested and debated (Ekkekakis, 2013). Several possible mechanisms, including biochemical changes, such as increased levels of endorphins, and psychological changes, such as an increased sense of mastery, have been proposed (La Forge, 1995; Petruzzello *et al.*, 1991). Much more work is needed in this area and technology may just be at the point of enabling human studies in which brain activities can be measured while people are moving. Many people know about the 'endorphin' theory but in an excellent review of this potential explanation the evidence remains unconvincing (Dishman and O'Connor, 2009). The studies showing an antidepressant effect for non-aerobic exercise suggest that improvement in aerobic fitness is not a key issue. However, objective measures of all possible fitness parameters (aerobic, strength, flexibility and body composition) should be included in studies to provide evidence that the exercise programme has had the desired fitness effect and to shed light on potential mechanisms.

    The fact that we do not know which mechanism operates should not prevent us from saying they remain 'plausible'. Dishman and O'Connor (2009) concluded that our lack of knowledge about the biological plausibility of the association between exercise and mental health is a major shortcoming. This may contribute to the lack of acceptance of the role of exercise by psychiatrists (Hale, 1997). However, Hill (1965) reminds us that we should not demand too much of this criterion because 'what is biologically plausible depends upon the biological knowledge of the day' (p. 298). Determining the mechanisms for the psychological effects of exercise in general and for depression in particular is perhaps the greatest challenge for exercise scientists trying to illuminate the relationship between exercise and mental health. It is clear that the answer to this complex question will not be found in exercise laboratories alone. We must collaborate with colleagues in neuroscience and psychological medicine to expand our knowledge.

7. *Coherence.* Coherence means that the possible mechanisms should not conflict with what is understood to be the natural history and biology of mental illness. While, as with many other aspects of these criteria, the evidence is far from complete, two examples might show coherence. More women than men report depression and women report less activity than men. In addition, the prevalence of depression increases with age and so does the prevalence of inactivity. The development of animal models to study inactivity and depression, and the use of exercise to combat depression, will provide further evidence for coherence. We also see evidence for this criterion in the suggestion that exercise mimics the action of antidepressant drugs such as serotonin reuptake inhibiting drugs (SSRIs).

8. *Experimental evidence.* Perhaps the best evidence comes under Hill's criterion of experimental evidence. This has already been discussed in the conclusions from the systematic

reviews. The experimental evidence supports a causal link between exercise programmes and depression reduction.

Thus, with this short overview, we suggest that the causal connection between exercise and reduced symptoms of clinical depression is strongly defended by the application of Hill's tests of causal inference. This again suggests to us that practitioners need not be cautious about suggesting exercise as a treatment for depression.

One of the most important lessons from the end of the seminal 1965 paper by Hill is a comment which we feel applies to many aspects of physical activity and health, and particularly to the issue of whether or not we can prove a causal link between exercise and reduction in depression:

> All scientific work is incomplete – whether it be observational or experimental. All scientific work is liable to be upset or modified by advancing knowledge. That does not confer upon us a freedom to ignore the knowledge we already have, or postpone the action that it appears to demand at a given time.
>
> (Hill, 1965, p. 12)

If we wait until the evidence is even more convincing and the designs of studies much improved we will have denied many people the varied benefits of physical activity. Even for those for whom increased activity may not alleviate depressive symptoms there are many and varied additional benefits that could be accrued and therefore we do not believe that practitioners should hesitate about promoting physical activity for good mental health. A further guiding principle is that interventions should do no harm. No negative effects have been noted in trials in which exercise has been used as a potential treatment, very few injuries have been reported and no trial has ever been stopped because people became more depressed when being encouraged to exercise.

The potential benefit of advocating the use of exercise as part of treatment for depression far outweighs the potential risk that no effect will occur. There are very few possible negative side effects (e.g. injury, exercise dependence). In addition, there are potential physical health benefits such as an increase in fitness, weight reduction and decreased cardiometabolic risk. Therefore, physical activity should be advocated as part of the treatment for clinically defined depression.

Other reviewers are less positive about this causal connection. For example, Landers and Arent (2001) said that 'It is premature ... to state with certainty that exercise causes reductions in depression', and O'Neal *et al.* (2000) stated that 'there is insufficient evidence to fully describe the relationship between exercise and depression'. In 2001, Dunn *et al.* said, 'At this point the evidence is suggestive but not convincing'. We have always argued that the evidence as it stands could be viewed either as a glass half empty or a glass half full. We favour the half-full view and believe that there really is a causal connection to be made.

While we would not want to overstate the evidence, we do wonder what the risk of looking at the evidence in a glass half-full and optimistic way really is. Some people might say that the evidence is not causal and that there are only associations or even a placebo effect. Such a response is difficult for researchers to refute without further evidence but should not stop people advocating the use of exercise for depression. Others might take the view that this will not work for everyone. Of course this is true and it is also true of many treatments in medicine. But exercise has an advantage here because it really is a 'win-win' scenario. Providing that people do increase their physical activity levels there are numerous health benefits that can be accrued even if it does not help with depression. There are very few treatments that can boast this kind of promise. Moreover, many with mental health problems display unhealthy profiles, such as obesity and low fitness.

There are those who are sceptical because we do not know exactly why exercise might have this positive effect on depression. Just because we do not know how a treatment works should not really stop us using it. For example, one treatment for depression that is still used for extreme cases in the UK is Electro Convulsive Therapy (ECT). This is still advocated even though it is not known how it works. Furthermore, there have been no negative effects reported from the use of exercise for depression which cannot be said for most of the antidepressant medications, which usually clearly state the risk of negative side effects.

The fact that the knowledge base is incomplete and that the evidence for a causal connection between inactivity and depression is not universally accepted should not prevent mental health practitioners of all kinds from advocating that their patients and clients should become more physically active. At best this may help them feel less depressed and at worst this could have a positive health impact on other aspects of their lives – what is there to lose? For example, it has been shown that those who experience bipolar disorder have increased risk of mortality from cardiovascular causes and pulmonary embolism, and increased risk of morbidity from obesity and Type 2 diabetes, in comparison to the general population (Morriss and Mohammed, 2005). In addition, such patients often have low exercise levels, so even if by exercising they do not improve the bipolar disorder (it is recognised that there may well be genetic factors that make it unlikely that exercise could be a stand-alone treatment for this disorder), they may decrease their overall health risks – exercise is a win-win scenario if used correctly.

Published guidelines

Several policy guidelines groups in the UK approached the topic of exercise and depression in the spirit of Hill's quoted advice. Such groups have also reviewed the evidence about the effectiveness of physical activity in the treatment of depression and they have reached more positive conclusions than the Lawlor and Hopker (2001) review. The National Institute for Health and Clinical Excellence reviewed the evidence in 2009 and recommended structured, supervised exercise programmes three times a week (of 45 minutes to one hour) over 10 to 14 weeks as an intervention for mild to moderate depression (NICE, 2009). A more recent guideline published by the Scottish Intercollegiate Guidelines Network (SIGN) in 2010 on the topic of non-pharmaceutical management of depression in adults also recommended that structured exercise could be considered as a treatment option for patients with depression. The evidence on which this recommendation was made was graded 'B' within the SIGN system (Scottish Intercollegiate Guidelines Network (SIGN), 2010). SIGN guidance uses an A B C D grading system. A set of evidence given a Grade A is awarded to a body of evidence with almost all studies or reviews or meta-analysis being judged to be well conducted with very little risk of bias. Grade B is given to evidence judged to be from high-quality systematic reviews of case control or cohort studies or high-quality studies with a very low risk of confounding/bias and a high probability that the relationship is causal. Thus SIGN is confident about the evidence, although we may want the evidence to be of even higher quality and achieve Grade A in future.

A further important policy document that has endorsed the use of exercise for the treatment and prevention of depression is the consensus document of the Chief Medical

Officers of England, Scotland, Wales and Northern Ireland (Department of Health, 2011) which underpinned national physical activity guidelines for the UK.

Increasing acknowledgement from mental health professionals of the role of physical activity and exercise

Over the past 20 or so years the literature on physical activity, exercise and depression has been growing. The evidence, however, has taken some time to filter down to professionals and organisations who might be involved with the treatment of depression. For example, in 1997 in the UK, an overview of depression and its treatment did not mention the value of exercise at all (Hale, 1997).

On a more positive note, there is some evidence that any reluctance to consider the 'body' in the treatment of mental health may be shifting. In the UK, the National Health Service has produced a website to enable users to understand a variety of conditions and to know what treatment choices they might have, including self-help strategies (see http://www.nhs.uk/Pages/HomePage.aspx). In describing treatment for mild depression the website suggests that 'there is evidence that exercise may help depression and it is one of the main treatments if you have mild depression. Your GP may refer you to a qualified fitness trainer for an exercise scheme, or you can find out more about starting exercise here.' (See http://www.nhs.uk/Conditions/Depression/Pages/Treatment.aspx.) In addition, recent leaflets about depression from the Royal College of Psychiatrists in the UK suggest that exercise is a good self-help strategy for depression (see Table 3.7 and http://www.rcpsych.ac.uk/expertadvice/treatmentswellbeing/physicalactivity.aspx). The Scottish Association for Mental Health (SAMH) has recently produced a video and website proposing five ways to better mental health (http://www.samh.org.uk/). These are evidence based and are:

- staying connected
- learning
- giving
- taking notice
- keeping active.

The emphasis on the importance of physical activity has been endorsed by Sir Chris Hoy, the Olympic cyclist, who has become an ambassador for SAMH.

Another aspect of the treatment of depression which suggests that it is worthwhile to pursue exercise is that of patient choice. In the UK, drugs continue to be the most frequently

Table 3.7   Advice from the Royal College of Psychiatrists about how to use exercise to help depression (see http://www.rcpsych.ac.uk/expertadvice/treatmentswellbeing/physicalactivity.aspx)

Physical activity should be:
- **Enjoyable** – if you don't know what you might enjoy, try a few different things.
- Help you to feel more **competent,** or **capable**. Gardening or DIY projects can do this, as well getting you more active.
- Give you a **sense of control** over your life – that you have choices you can make (so it isn't helpful if you start to feel that you *have* to exercise). The sense that you are looking after yourself can also feel good.
- Help you to **escape** for a while from the pressures of life.
- Be **shared.** The **companionship** involved can be just as important as the physical activity.

used treatment for depression, although psychotherapy and ECT are also used (Hale, 1997). Patients often report that they do not want drugs (Scott, 1996). Consequently, exercise is a reasonable option with few negative side effects and could be cost-effective in comparison to other non-drug options such as psychotherapy. Studies on the cost-effectiveness and cost-benefit of exercise versus drugs or other therapies must be undertaken so that the potential economic advantages of exercise can be measured. Perhaps the economic arguments will be the most powerful in persuading mental health professionals to include exercise as a treatment option.

Chapter summary

- The weight of evidence shows that prospective studies suggest a protective effect from physical activity on the development of depression, but not all studies show this.
- Systematic reviews with meta-analytic findings show a large to moderate effect size from studies that have used exercise as a treatment for depression.
- The weight of the evidence suggests that there is a causal connection between physical activity/exercise and reduction of depression.

References

American Psychiatric Association. (2013). *Diagnostic and Statistical Manual of Mental Disorders (DSM-5)* (5th edn).
Anspaugh, D.J., Hunter, S. and Dignan, M. (1996). Risk factors for cardiovascular disease among exercising versus nonexercising women. *American Journal of Health Promotion, 10*(3), 171–174.
Azevedo Da Silva, M., Singh-Manoux, A., Brunner, E.J., Kaffashian, S., Shipley, M.J., Kivimäki, M. and Nabi, H. (2012). Bidirectional association between physical activity and symptoms of anxiety and depression: The Whitehall II study. *European Journal of Epidemiology, 27*(7), 537–546.
Babyak, M., Blumenthal, J.A., Herman, S., Khatri, P., Doraiswamy, M. and Moore, K. (2000). Exercise treatment for major depression: Maintenance of therapeutic benefit at 10 months. *Psychosomatic Medicine, 62,* 633–638.
Beck, A.T., Ward, C.H., Mendelsohn, M., Mock, J. and Erbaugh, H. (1961). An inventory for measuring depression. *Archives of General Psychiatry, 4,* 561–571.
Beck, A.T., Steer, R.A., Ball, R. and Ranieri, W. (1996). Comparison of Beck Depression Inventories -IA and -II in psychiatric outpatients. *Journal of Personal Assessment, 67*(3), 588–597. doi: 10.1207/s15327752jpa6703_13.
Bernaards, C.M., Jans, M.P., van den Heuvel, S.G., Hendriksen, I.J., Houtman, I.L. and Bongers, P.M. (2006). Can strenuous leisure time physical activity prevent psychological complaints in a working population? *Occupational Environmental Medicine, 63*(1), 10–16.
Biddle, S.J.H. and Asare, M. (2011). Physical activity and mental health in children and adolescents: A review of reviews. *British Journal of Sports Medicine, 45,* 886–895. doi: 10.1136/bjsports-2011-090185.
Biddle, S.J.H. and Mutrie, N. (1991). *Psychology of Physical Activity and Exercise: A health-related perspective.* London: Springer-Verlag.
——. (2001). *Psychology of Physical Activity: Determinants, well-being, and interventions.* London: Routledge.
——. (2008). *Psychology of Physical Activity: Determinants, well-being, and interventions (2nd edn).* London: Routledge.
Blumenthal, J.A., Babyak, M.A., Moore, K.A., Craighead, W.E., Herman, S., Khatri, P. and Krishnan, K.R. (1999). Effects of exercise training on older patients with major depression. *Archives of International Medicine, 159*(19), 2349–2356.
Camacho, T.C., Roberts, R.E., Lazarus, N.B., Kaplan, G.A. and Cohen, R.D. (1991). Physical activity

and depression: Evidence from the Alameda County Study. *American Journal of Epidemiology, 134*(2), 220–231.

Chalder, M., Wiles, N.J., Campbell, J., Hollinghurst, S.P., Haase, A.M., Taylor, A.H. and Lewis, G. (2012). Facilitated physical activity as a treatment for depressed adults: Randomised controlled trial. *British Medical Journal, 344*, e2758. doi: 10.1136/bmj.e2758.

Cooney, G.M., Dwan, K., Greig, C.A., Lawlor, D.A., Rimer, J., Waugh, F.R. and Mead, G.E. (2013). Exercise for depression. *Cochrane Database Systematic Review, 9*, CD004366. doi: 10.1002/14651858. CD004366.pub6.

Cooper-Patrick, L., Ford, D.E., Mead, L.A., Chang, P.P. and Klag, M.J. (1997). Exercise and depression in midlife: A prospective study. *American Journal of Public Health, 87*(4), 670–673.

Daley, A.J., Crank, H., Saxton, J.M., Mutrie, N., Coleman, R. and Roalfe, A. (2007). Randomized trial of exercise therapy in women treated for breast cancer. *Journal of Clinical Oncology, 25*(13), 1713–1721.

Department of Health. (2011). *Start Active, Stay Active: A report on physical activity for health from the four home countries' Chief Medical Officers*. London: Author.

Dishman, R. and O'Connor, P.J. (2009). Lessons in exercise neurobiology: The case of endorphins. *Mental Health and Physical Activity, 2*(1), 4–9.

Dunn, A.L., Trivedi, M.H. and O'Neal, H.A. (2001). Physical activity dose–response effects on outcomes of depression and anxiety. *Medicine and Science in Sports and Exercise, 33*(6, Suppl.), S587–S597.

Dunn, A., Trivedi, M.H., Kampert, J., Clark, C.G. and Chambliss, H.O. (2005). Exercise treatment for depression: Efficacy and dose-response. *American Journal of Preventive Medicine, 28*(1), 1–8.

Ekkekakis, P. (ed.). (2013). *Routledge Handbook of Physical Activity and Mental Health*. London: Routledge.

Farmer, M.E., Locke, B.Z., Moscicki, E.K., Dannenberg, A.L., Larson, D.B. and Radloff, L.S. (1988). Physical activity and depressive symptoms: The NHANES I Epidemiologic Follow-up Study. *American Journal of Epidemiology, 128*(6), 1340–1351.

Gallegos-Carrillo, K., Flores, Y.N., Denova-Gutierrez, E., Mendez-Hernandez, P., Dosamantes-Carrasco, L.D., Henao-Moran, S. and Salmeron, J. (2013). Physical activity and reduced risk of depression: Results of a longitudinal study of Mexican adults. *Health Psychology, 32*(6), 609–615. doi: 10.1037/a0029276.

Global Advocacy Council for Physical Activity International Society for Physical Activity and Health. (2010). The Toronto Charter for Physical Activity: A Global Call to Action.

Hale, A.S. (1997). ABC of mental disorders: Depression. *British Medical Journal, 315*, 43–46.

Hasler, G., Pine, D.S., Kleinbaum, D.G., Gamma, A., Luckenbaugh, D., Ajdacic, V. and Angst, J. (2005). Depressive symptoms during childhood and adult obesity: The Zurich Cohort Study. *Molecular Psychiatry, 10*(9), 842–850.

Hill, A.B. (1965). The environment and disease: Association or causation? *Proceedings of the Royal Society of Medicine, 58*, 295–300.

Kaplan, G.A., Roberts, R.E., Camacho, T.C. and Coyne, J.C. (1987). Psychosocial predictors of depression. *American Journal of Epidemiology, 125*, 206–220.

Kritz-Silverstein, D., Barrett-Connor, E. and Corbeau, C. (2001). Cross-sectional and prospective study of exercise and depressed mood in the elderly: The Rancho Bernardo study. *American Journal of Epidemiology, 153*(6), 596–603.

Krogh, J., Videbech, P., Thomsen, C., Gluud, C. and Nordentoft, M. (2012). DEMO-II trial. Aerobic exercise versus stretching exercise in patients with major depression – a randomised clinical trial. *PLoS One, 7*(10), e48316. doi: 10.1371/journal.pone.0048316.

La Forge, R. (1995). Exercise-associated mood alterations: A review of interactive neurobiological mechanisms. *Medicine, Exercise, Nutrition and Health, 4*, 17–32.

Landers, D.M. and Arent, S.M. (2001). Physical activity and mental health. In R.N. Singer, H.A. Hausenblas and C. M. Janelle (eds), *Handbook of Sport Psychology* (2nd edn) (pp. 740–765). New York: John Wiley.

Larun, L., Nordheim, L.V., Ekeland, E., Hagen, K.B. and Heian, F. (2006). Exercise in prevention and treatment of anxiety and depression among children and young people. *Cochrane Database of Systematic Reviews, 3*. doi: 10.1002/14651858.CD004691.pub2.

Lawlor, D.A. and Hopker, S.W. (2001). The effectiveness of exercise as an intervention in the management of depression: Systematic review and meta-regression analysis of randomised controlled trials. *British Medical Journal, 322*(7289), 763–767.

Mammen, G. and Faulkner, G. (2013). Physical activity and the prevention of depression: A systematic review of prospective studies. *American Journal of Preventative Medicine, 45*(5), 649–657. doi: 10.1016/j.amepre.2013.08.001.

Mathers, C.D. and Loncar, D. (2006). Projections of global mortality and burden of disease from 2002 to 2030. *PLoS Medicine, 3*(11), e442. doi: 10.1371/journal.pmed.0030442.

Morriss, R. and Mohammed, F.A. (2005). Metabolism, lifestyle and bipolar affective disorder. *Journal of Psychopharmacology, 19*(6, Suppl.), 94–101.

Moussavi, S., Chatterji, S., Verdes, E., Tandon, A., Patel, V., and Ustun, B. (2007). Depression, chronic diseases, and decrements in health: results from the World Health Surveys. *Lancet, 370*(9590), 851-858. doi: 10.1016/S0140-6736(07)61415-9.

Murray, C.J. and Lopez, A.D. (1997). Alternative projections of mortality and disability by cause 1990–2020: Global Burden of Disease study. *The Lancet, 349*(9064), 1498–1504. doi: 10.1016/S0140-6736(96)07492-2.

National Institute for Health and Clinical Excellence. (2009). Depression: The treatment and management of depression in adults (updated edn). London: British Psychological Society and Royal College of Psychiatrists.

OECD. (2012). Health at a Glance: Europe 2012.

Office of National Statistics. (2001). Social Trends (Vol. 31). London: The Stationary Office.

O'Neal, H.A., Dunn, A.L. and Martinsen, E.W. (2000). Depression and exercise. *International Journal of Sport Psychology, 31*, 110–135.

Paffenbarger, R.S., Jr., Lee, I.M. and Leung, R. (1994). Physical activity and personal characteristics associated with depression and suicide in American college men. *Acta Psychiatr Scandinavian Supplement, 377*, 16–22.

Pate, R.R., Pratt, M., Blair, S.N., Haskel, W.L., Macera, C.A., Bouchard, C., Buchner, D., Ettinger, W., Heath, G., King, A.C., Kriska, A., Leon, A., Marcus, B.H., Morris, J., Paffenbarger, R.S., Patrick, K., Pollock, M.L., Rippe, J.M., Sallis, J.F. and Wilmore, J. H. (1995). Physical activity and public health: A recommendation from the Centers for Disease Control and Prevention and the American College of Sports Medicine. *Journal of the American Medical Association, 273*, 402–407.

Petruzzello, S.J., Landers, D.M., Hatfield, B.D., Kubitz, K.A. and Salazar, W. (1991). A meta-analysis on the anxiety-reducing effects of acute and chronic exercise: Outcomes and mechanisms. *Sports Medicine, 11*, 143–182.

Radloff, L.S. (1977). The CES-D scale: A self-report depression scale for research in the general population. *Applied Psychological Measurement, 1*, 385–401.

Rimer, J., Dwan, K., Lawlor, D.A., Greig, C.A., McMurdo, M., Morley, W. and Mead, G.E. (2012). Exercise for depression. *Cochrane Database Systematic Review, 7*, CD004366. doi: 10.1002/14651858. CD004366.pub5.

Robertson, R., Robertson, A., Jepson, R. and Maxwell, M. (2012). Walking for depression or depressive symptoms: A systematic review and meta-analysis. *Mental Health and Physical Activity, 5*, 66–75.

Scott, J. (1996). Cognitive therapy of affective disorders: A review. *Journal of Affective Disorders, 37*, 1–11.

Scottish Intercollegiate Guidelines Network (SIGN). (2010). *Non-pharmaceutical Management of Depression in Adults*. Edinburgh: Scottish Intercollegiate Guidelines Network.

Spitzer, R.L., Endicott, J. and Robins, E. (1978). Research diagnostic criteria. *Archives of General Psychiatry, 35*, 773–782.

Stavrakakis, N., Roest, A.M., Verhulst, F., Ormel, J., de Jonge, P. and Oldehinkel, A.J. (2013). Physical activity and onset of depression in adolescents: A prospective study in the general population cohort TRAILS. *Journal of Psychiatry Res*. doi: 10.1016/j.jpsychires.2013.06.005.

Strawbridge, W.J., Deleger, S., Roberts, R.E. and Kaplan, G.A. (2002). Physical activity reduces the risk of subsequent depression for older adults. *American Journal of Epidemiology, 156*(4), 328–334.

Trigo, M., Silva, D. and Rocha, E. (2005). Psychosocial risk factors in coronary heart disease: Beyond type A behavior. *Revista Portuguesa de Cardiologia, 24*(2), 261–281.

van Gool, C.H., Kempen, G.I., Penninx, B.W., Deeg, D.J., Beekman, A.T. and van Eijk, J.T. (2003). Relationship between changes in depressive symptoms and unhealthy lifestyles in late middle aged and older persons: Results from the Longitudinal Aging Study Amsterdam. *Age and Ageing, 32*(1), 81–87.

Waraich, P., Goldner, E.M., Somers, J.M. and Hsu, L. (2004). Prevalence and incidence studies of mood disorders: A systematic review of the literature. *Canadian Journal of Psychiatry, 49*(2), 124–138.

Weyerer, S. (1992). Physical inactivity and depression in the community. Evidence from the Upper Bavarian Field Study. *International Journal of Sports Medicine, 13*(6), 492–496.

World Health Organization. (2010). *International Statistical Classification of Diseases and Related Health Problems* (10th edn).

4 Physical activity and other mental health challenges

Schizophrenia, anxiety and dependencies

In the UK, the Royal College of Psychiatrists sets the standards for the education and training of psychiatrists with the overall aim of improving the lives of people with mental illness. Over recent years they have enhanced what they say about the role of physical activity in mental health. The current leaflet and website section that explores the role of physical activity suggests:

> If you keep active, you are:
> - less likely to be depressed, anxious or tense
> - more likely to feel good about yourself
> - more likely to concentrate and focus better
> - more likely to sleep better
> - more likely to cope with cravings and withdrawal symptoms if you try to give up a habit such as smoking or alcohol
> - more likely to be able to keep mobile and independent as you get older
> - possibly less likely to have problems with memory and dementia.
> (http://www.rcpsych.ac.uk, accessed 16 May 2014)

We have covered depression in Chapter 3 and most of the other topics have also been covered in other sections of this book. In this chapter we will take an in-depth look at how physical activity relates to schizophrenia and to anxiety, and to dependencies such as alcohol and tobacco.

Chapter objectives

The purpose of this chapter is to focus on how physical activity relates to the common mental health issue of anxiety, the very serious mental illness of schizophrenia, and the role of physical activity in helping people who are dependent on drugs, alcohol and tobacco. Specifically, in this chapter we aim to:

- describe the potential role of physical activity in the treatment of schizophrenia;
- define anxiety for clinical and non-clinical populations;
- summarise the evidence linking exercise with non-clinical states of anxiety;
- summarise the evidence about exercise and clinical anxiety disorders;
- explore the role of physical activity in helping those with dependency on alcohol, drugs or tobacco.

Schizophrenia

Schizophrenia is a psychotic illness affecting a small proportion of the population, but it is the most common serious mental illness and, as such, places a disproportionately heavy burden on resources in psychiatric care (Faulkner, 2005). We have included it in this chapter because of it is a well-known mental illness and because of the growing literature of the benefit of physical activity for this proportion of the population. Schizophrenia is characterised by thought disturbance such as delusions, speech disturbance, difficulties in interpersonal functioning, inappropriate behaviours and emotional responses, and is most commonly treated with antipsychotic medication. A brief description of the DSM-IV criteria for schizophrenia is as follows:

- A disturbance that lasts for at least six months and includes at least one month of active-phase symptoms (e.g. delusions, hallucinations, disorganised speech, grossly disorganised or catatonic behaviour, negative symptoms).
- There must be significant impairment in one or more major areas of functioning (e.g. work, interpersonal relationships) for most of the time since the onset of the disturbance, and the functioning must be significantly lower than that prior to the onset of the disorder.

Treatment for schizophrenia typically involves drugs that have an antipsychotic effect, although there is much debate about the effectiveness of these drugs. There is also concern about compliance. Some patients may have access to psycho-social interventions in addition to the drug therapy, while others may be hospitalised (Faulkner, 2005).

There is a potential role for exercise in the treatment of schizophrenia and there is a growing literature on this topic. The role for activity may involve improvements in physical and mental health functioning, but it is clear that physical activity is very unlikely to be a stand-alone treatment for this disorder. Instead, physical activity may have a very important adjunctive role in the treatment of schizophrenia.

Early studies were typically descriptive but provided the suggestion that physical activity might be an important consideration. Chamove (1986) noted that physical activity and fitness levels are known to be low in schizophrenic patients, especially those in psychiatric hospitals. We now know that such low activity levels will make these patients at risk for cardiovascular and metabolic diseases, depression and obesity, and so, for prevention of risk, increasing physical activity levels will be very important. Early studies of the effect of increasing activity for such patients had positive outcomes but these studies tended to be pre-experimental. Some of the positive effects for increased activity noted in a study of 40 schizophrenic patients were as follows:

- less psychotic features
- less movement disorder
- improved mood
- more social interest and competence (Chamove, 1986).

Patients seemed to understand these benefits themselves. For example, Falloon and Talbot (1981) reported that as many as 78 per cent of patients have used exercise as a way of reducing hallucinations. Pelham and Campagna (1991) reported three single-subject case studies which incorporated quantitative information from standard fitness tests, Beck

Depression Inventory and Mental Health Inventory scores with qualitative information from interviews. The results showed physiological and psychological benefits. Information was also gathered on long-term exercise adherence. The article concluded with a useful set of guide-lines on exercise programmes for schizophrenic patients.

The same researchers (Pelham *et al.*, 1993) also reported an experimental design which showed that psychiatric patients (diagnosed with schizophrenia or major affective disorder), who undertook a 12-week aerobic exercise programme, decreased depression scores and increased aerobic fitness. The control group undertaking non-aerobic exercise did not show these improvements. This does not support Martinsen's findings that both aerobic and non-aerobic exercise decreased depression scores for a group of hospitalised depressed patients (Martinsen, 1990a, 1990b). However, only five individuals were assigned to each group in the Pelham *et al.* study and the statistical conclusions may therefore not be valid. In addition, it may be that schizophrenic patients respond differently to exercise than other psychiatric patients or it may be that initially low fitness levels influenced the results. Furthermore, Pelham *et al.* seemed to focus on depression as the major dependent variable which is only one aspect of schizophrenia.

In reviewing the very limited evidence for the use of exercise in the treatment of psychoses such as schizophrenia, Plante (1993) concluded that 'exercise may assist these patients with mood and self-esteem factors much more than with thought disturbances associated with psychotic symptomatology' (p. 367). Similarly, Faulkner and Biddle (1999, p. 453) concluded from a review of eight pre-experimental, three quasi-experimental and one experimental study that:

> The existing research does not allow firm conclusions … as to the psychological benefits of exercise for individuals with schizophrenia. It does, however, support the potential efficacy of exercise in alleviating negative symptoms of schizophrenia and as a coping strategy for the positive symptoms.

Guy Faulkner and collaborators have made some very important contributions to the literature on this topic. For example, Faulkner and Sparkes (1999) have reported a quali-tative study of exercise as therapy for schizophrenia. Three patients who began a 10-week exercise programme implemented in their hostel setting were studied through an ethno-graphic approach. Two of the three patients perceived the exercise programme to be very beneficial, while the third patient ceased participation after seven weeks. One main theme which emerged from the analysis was the role of exercise in encouraging patients out of their 'internal world' and into the 'social world', such as a swimming pool or a walking route. Another theme was that exercise helped the secondary symptoms of depression and low self-esteem, helped control auditory hallucinations, and promoted better sleep patterns and general behaviour. The authors recommended that care plans for schizophrenic patients should include exercise, but commented on how difficult that is to achieve. In the hostel where the exercise programme was carried out the staff were very enthusiastic about the way in which exercise had helped patients and noted deterioration when the programme stopped. Despite this there were no plans to ensure that the exercise programme would become a routine element of treatment.

The lack of standard randomised controlled trial data on the physical and mental benefits of exercise for schizophrenic patients may be one reason for the reluctance to spend money on exercise as part of treatment packages. However, in this area it will be very difficult to find sufficient participants to conduct such a study and the environment of a hostel or hospital setting is not conducive to random assignment to groups without contamination or resentment. Thus, a qualitative approach is appropriate and the evidence from such studies indicates that there are many potential benefits for exercise programmes to be put in place.

An Australian study has provided further qualitative data on this topic (Fogarty and Happell, 2005). Six residents of a Community Care Unit in Melbourne took part in an exercise programme for three months. A focus group interview was conducted with the participants and various staff involved. Four themes emerged:

- participants had enjoyed the graduated and individualised programme;
- the benefit of increased physical fitness;
- the benefit of the group approach;
- the intention of participants to continue the programme.

This was also the case in Faulkner's study reported above but he reported that the programme had not been sustained. The evidence is beginning to build and it is hoped that policy for treatment may include the opportunity for schizophrenic patients to exercise. However, longer term evaluation of whether or not such programmes can be sustained, and therefore be of benefit to patients, beyond the realms of research projects, is now called for.

Researchers from Belgium have begun a series of studies looking at how interventions that focus on the body (or physical therapy) may have benefit for schizophrenic patients. A systematic review of the benefits of physical therapy for patients with schizophrenia has been reported (Vancampfort *et al.*, 2012). These authors found 10 studies that met their inclusion criteria. Some of the studies focused on exercise programmes, such as aerobic or strength programmes, while others focused on processes, such as yoga or relaxation that might reduce muscle tension. They concluded that the aerobic and strength exercises and yoga reduced psychiatric symptoms, state anxiety and psychological distress, and improved health-related quality of life. There was also a suggestion that aerobic exercise improved short-term memory. They also noted that progressive muscle relaxation reduced state anxiety and psychological distress. This led the same grouping of researchers to conduct a separate systematic review of the effects of progressive muscular relaxation with schizophrenic patients (Vancampfort *et al.*, 2013) and found only three trials. This is clearly a new but encouraging area of research because the authors concluded that progressive muscular relaxation might be a useful adjunctive treatment that could help reduce state anxiety and psychological distress and improve subjective well-being for patients with schizophrenia.

In 2013, a group of researchers from the Netherlands conducted one of the largest trials to date on the topic of exercise for schizophrenic patients. The researchers randomised 63 patients with schizophrenia to a structured exercise experience for two hours each week (n = 31) or to weekly occupational therapy (n = 32) for six months (Scheewe *et al.*, 2013). The results were analysed on an intention-to-treat basis and showed that the exercise therapy had a significant effect on cardiovascular fitness compared with occupational therapy. However, only 39 participants from a possible 63 completed the protocols and, when per-protocol analysis was conducted, more positive results emerged showing that exercise therapy reduced symptoms of schizophrenia, depression, need of care and increased cardiovascular fitness compared with occupational therapy. These differences between intention-to-treat and per-protocol analysis demonstrates the challenge of conducting randomised controlled trials which demand adherence to follow-up testing with patient groups for whom such procedures are difficult to negotiate. There is also concern that functional capacity is reduced in schizophrenic patients perhaps to do with inactive lifestyles and medication that may slow metabolism. This concern creates a further strong rationale for the role of regular physical activity for schizophrenic patients.

Future studies in this area must also evaluate exercise programmes in a variety of ways, including physical and mental health benefits, cost-effectiveness, and patient and staff perception of benefit. In addition, they need to include the issue of how to negotiate with administrators, psychiatrists and those in charge of care, in hospitals, hostels or in the community, about the inclusion of exercise in the management and treatment of schizophrenic patients. A recent guide to how to design and adapt physical activity programmes for psychiatric patients and provide them as part of normal treatment is now available (Richardson *et al.*, 2005).

In a recent review of the available evidence, Faulkner and colleagues (2013) provide a rationale for the need for physical activity for schizophrenic patients and review the various programmes that have been tried. They call for further research that focuses more on helping this patient group adhere to the programmes using what is known from behavioural science. They also note the lack of exploration of potential mechanisms of the beneficial effects of activity in this patient group and point out the need for distinction of the effects of physical activity on the positive symptoms of schizophrenia (such as delusions and thought disorders) and the negative symptoms (such as low mood, apathy and social withdrawal) in future studies. They conclude that good physical health should be a goal for this patient group. As studies progress in this area we may also see discussion about the most appropriate mode and dosage of physical activity which will parallel discussions in the much more developed field of physical activity and depression (see Chapter 3).

> Key point: Schizophrenic patients report benefit from physical activity, and further research on this patient group should explore what kind of physical activity and dose is best.

The Anxiety Continuum

There is a continuum in defining anxiety that ranges from feelings which are short-lived and do not interfere greatly with our lives to long-lasting symptoms that suggest a clinical diagnosis of a mental illness. We have therefore planned this chapter to cover the literature that suggests physical activity and exercise may have a role to play in prevention and treatment at both ends of this continuum. We will offer technical definitions of anxiety at an appropriate point but here we want to ensure that readers understand the spectrum we are considering. At one end of the spectrum, where feelings of anxiety or worry, or fretfulness or tension, are short-lived, we consider that physical activity may be able to minimise the duration of these events and encourage more positive moods. We consider this to be the promotion of good mental health. At this end of the spectrum people do not generally seek or need help for the alleviation of such feelings and so physical activity may be seen as a self-help strategy. At the other end of the spectrum, where feelings of anxiety last for a long time and interfere with normal functioning at work or at home, professional help is often sought. Here we are dealing with mental illness and we consider that physical activity may play a role in both prevention and treatment.

Physical activity and non-clinical anxiety

Most people experience feelings of worry from time to time and may say that they feel anxious, tense or worried. Such feelings are normal reactions to circumstances life presents us with, such as preparing for exams or realising that there is not as much in our bank account as we thought. However, if such feelings persist over time and begin to interfere with work or personal and family relationships, then these feelings may be classified as generalised anxiety disorder (GAD). This would require a medical (clinical) diagnosis. Related anxiety topics are panic attacks, phobias (persistent, excessive or irrational fear of things such as flying, spiders, or being out in open spaces or with other people), or post-traumatic stress disorder. So there is no one thing that can be clearly labelled as 'clinical anxiety'. GAD is common, with about one in 25 adults experiencing this anxiety disorder during their lifetime. It is more common in women than in men (see NHS choices at http://www.nhs.uk/conditions/anxiety/pages/introduction.aspx). In the following section of this chapter the relationship between physical activity and anxiety at a non-clinical level will be reviewed first. Then later in the chapter we will focus on the clinical end of the spectrum.

The study of the proposed anxiety-reducing effects – sometimes called anxiolytic effects – of physical activity has a long history in sport and exercise psychology, and has remained an area of considerable interest to researchers. Anxiety is defined in terms of both state (transitory) and trait (enduring) characteristics, and sometimes with reference to both cognitive (worry) and somatic (bodily tension) elements such as increased muscle tension or increased heart rate. In addition, exercise researchers have been interested in the psycho-physiological stress reactions of participants differing in fitness levels, and in the interaction of physical activity and stress on immune function (Edwards and Mills, 2013; Ekkekakis, 2013).

Most studies on exercise and anxiety have assessed state anxiety using either the state scale of the State-Trait Anxiety Inventory (STAI) (Spielberger *et al.*, 1970), POMS tension subscale (McNair *et al.*, 1971), or the MAACL anxiety subscale (Zuckerman and Lubin, 1965). When trait anxiety has been assessed, studies have used almost exclusively the trait scale of the STAI. Early studies showed that acute bouts of exercise were followed by anxiety reduction using these scales (Morgan, 1979), but such conclusions may be flawed because state anxiety may have been raised due to the lab situations or simply due to the relief of finishing a bout of exercise that may not have been very pleasant.

Using an entirely different paradigm for measuring mood, known as the circumplex model (see Chapter 2 for further details), Ekkekakis and colleagues have described and summarised the literature which suggests that anxiety-reducing effects are more likely at moderate intensities and self-selected intensity of activity (Ekkekakis *et al.*, 2011).

Meta-analytic findings

The results from four early meta-analyses (Long and van Stavel, 1995; McDonald and Hodgdon, 1991; Petruzzello *et al.*, 1991; Schlicht, 1994) all showed effects of exercise on anxiety. Schlicht (1994) located 22 sub-sample findings between 1980 and 1990, and found a small and non-significant effect size of -0.15, thus concluding that exercise had a minor effect on anxiety. However, Petruzzello (1995) criticised this paper strongly by pointing out that Schlicht had underrepresented the field by not locating all of the studies (Schlicht, 1995). Although Schlicht (1994) analysed 22 sub-samples from 20 studies, Petruzzello *et al.*'s (1991) meta-analysis used 50 for Schlicht's time period, and 104 overall. Consequently, Schlicht was unable to conduct moderator analyses and his meta-analysis lacked statistical power (see Schlicht, 1995).

Petruzzello *et al.* (1991) conducted one of the most comprehensive meta-analyses of the field. We review their findings alongside the more focused meta-analyses of McDonald and Hodgdon (1991) and Long and van Stavel (1995). Petruzzello *et al.* (1991) analysed data from 124 studies that examined the effect of exercise on anxiety. They included studies published between 1960 and 1989 that investigated state anxiety, trait anxiety and psychophysiological indicators of anxiety. Published and unpublished studies were included, as well as studies varying in methodological design. By coding such variables, the effect for methodological adequacy could be tested.

McDonald and Hodgdon (1991) restricted their meta-analysis to studies investigating the effects of aerobic fitness training on psychological outcomes in adults, one of which was anxiety. This yielded 36 effect sizes from 22 studies. They did not consider unpublished studies, abstracts and dissertations, and included only studies using standardised anxiety measures, as well as fitness measures, and pre- and post-test measures.

Long and van Stavel (1995) restricted their meta-analysis to adults involved in quasi-experimental or experimental training studies using standardised anxiety measures. Clinical studies (psychiatric and Type A) were omitted, leaving 40 studies and 76 effect sizes.

A more recent meta-analysis improved upon earlier versions by employing the current standards of the systematic review process and found 49 studies that met the inclusion criterion of being a randomised controlled trial (Wipfli *et al.*, 2008). In earlier meta-analyses fewer than half of the included studies would have met this criterion. Wipfli *et al.* report an effect size of -0.48 (95% confidence intervals -0.63, -0.33) for exercise versus no treatment and a much smaller effect size for exercise versus other treatments for anxiety (-0.19). A further step taken here was to investigate the dose of exercise. Here the meta-analytic findings show a u-shaped curve with the largest reductions in anxiety occurring with 'doses' of exercise equating to an energy expenditure which would approximately equate to the public health dose of 30 minutes of activity on most days of the week. Less than this dose or more than this dose created poorer reductions in anxiety. However, this quadratic relationship was not statistically significant and more studies that provide information on the dose of activity will be needed to provide sufficient power for this kind of analysis.

The main findings from these meta-analyses are summarised in Table 4.1 and show that exercise has a significant small to moderate effect on anxiety with effects ranging from a reduction of 0.15 to 0.56. Petruzzello *et al.* (1991) found that for state anxiety studies using no-treatment control groups and motivational control groups both showed a significant ES, but this was larger for studies utilising a pre-post within-subjects design. McDonald and Hodgdon (1991) found that observational survey studies produced a lower ES than experimental studies. These findings suggest that the internal validity of the study may not necessarily influence effect sizes but anxiety change may occur when motivational factors are controlled. In addition, Petruzzello *et al.* found that exercise was as effective as other anxiety-reducing treatments. This finding may be particularly important given the low cost of exercise.

Aerobic exercise showed greater effects than non-aerobic exercise, but caution must be expressed concerning this result, since only 13 effect sizes were used to calculate the effects of non-aerobic exercise by Petruzzello *et al.* (1991). They found no differences between types of aerobic exercise, a finding supported by McDonald and Hodgdon (1991).

Interestingly, the length of the exercise session may be related to anxiety. Petruzzello *et al.* (1991) showed superior effects for exercise lasting 21 to 30 minutes in comparison to

Table 4.1   Summary results from five meta-analyses on exercise and anxiety

Study	Outcome variables	Activity/fitness measure	No. of effect sizes	Mean effect size
McDonald and Hodgdon (1991)	State anxiety	Aerobic fitness training	13	-0.28[1]
	Trait anxiety	Aerobic fitness training	20	-0.25[1]
Petruzzello et al. (1991)	State anxiety	Exercise	207	-0.24[1]
	Trait anxiety	Exercise	62	-0.34[1]
	Psycho-physiological indicators	Exercise	138	-0.56[1]
Schlicht (1994)	State and trait anxiety	Exercise	22	-0.15[2]
Long and van Stavel (1995)	Any measure of anxiety in within-group pre-post studies	Exercise training	26	-0.45[1]
	Any measure of anxiety in contrast group studies	Exercise training	50	-0.36[1]
Wipfli et al. (2008)	Any measure of anxiety in exercise versus no treatment	Exercise	49	-0.48[1]
	Any measure of anxiety in exercise versus other treatments	Exercise	28	-0.19

Notes:
1. Effect size significantly different from zero.
2. Estimation of population effect size using the Hunter and Schmidt correlation effect sizes (Hunter and Schmidt, 1990): effect size of 0.1 = small, 0.3 = moderate, 0.5 = large (Cohen, 1988).

sessions shorter than this. However, when the effect sizes in the 0- to 20-minute category that were calculated from comparisons with other anxiety-reducing treatments were eliminated, the ES increased from -.04 to -.22, and was not significantly different from the -.41 for exercise of 21 to 30 minutes' duration.

When reviewing physical activity and affect in Chapter 2, we suggested that higher intensity exercise might not produce such positive effects as more moderate exercise. However, for state anxiety, Petruzzello *et al.* (1991) found that effect sizes for the intensity of exercise were homogeneous. For psychophysiological indices of anxiety, though, the meta-analysis showed the highest effect size for 40 to 59 per cent of HR_{max} or VO_{2max} (ES = -1.06; n = 13) and this was significantly different from 70 to 79 per cent intensity (ES = -.41; n = 24). All four intensity categories, including 80 per cent and above, showed effect sizes significantly different from zero. These results suggest that moderate intensity exercise may be particularly beneficial for anxiety reduction, but other, higher intensities may also be beneficial. This pattern was also suggested in Wipfli *et al.*'s (2008) analysis.

Key point: Exercise has a small to moderate effect on reducing non-clinical levels of anxiety.

Population surveys

The extensive secondary data analysis of physical activity and mental health reported by Stephens (1988) included evidence on anxiety. Data on over 10,000 adults in Canada showed that reporting symptoms of anxiety was less likely in more active individuals. This held for men of all ages, and for women over 40 years, but not for younger women. Other population surveys have found similar associations between higher physical activity and low levels of anxiety-related disorders such as panic attacks, GAD and phobias in over 6,000 participants (Goodwin, 2003). In this study the associations remained after controlling for potentially confounding characteristics from the population, such as education level or illness, and did not vary by gender.

There are very few population surveys in which anxiety is categorised separately from mental health but at a non-clinical level. In the UK we have examined cross-sectional relationships between physical activity and mental health as measured by the HADS (Zigmond and Snaith, 1983) anxiety and depression scores in a sample of 1,742 participants from the third wave of the Twenty07 Study: Health in the Community (Mutrie *et al.*, 2003). Respondents reported their levels of physical activity at work, in the home and during leisure time, and the intensity of activity was also determined. Physical activity was related to depression scores but not to anxiety scores.

Experimental trials

In a review of exercise and anxiety, Leith (1994) identified 20 experimental studies. Of these, 14 (70%) showed reduced anxiety from exercise, with the rest showing no change. None showed increased anxiety from exercise. A series of experimental trials in the UK by Steptoe and his colleagues provides a useful framework for drawing conclusions concerning experimental work on exercise and anxiety.

Steptoe and Cox (1988) studied the psychological responses of 32 female medical students to both high (cycle ergometry exercise of 50rpm against 2kg/100W) and low (0.5kg/25W) exercise intensities. They showed a significant increase in anxiety from pre- to post-test for the high-intensity condition and a non-significant decrease for low-intensity exercise.

Steptoe's data here and in other studies are particularly striking, as they suggest that it is moderate rather than high-intensity exercise that produces anxiety reduction during exercise, although anxiety has also been shown to reduce in the post-exercise recovery period. This is consistent with the discussion in Chapter 2 concerning the dual-mode model proposed by Ekkekakis (2003).

These findings regarding intensity point towards a physiological explanation of why some levels of exercise (typically those below the ventilatory threshold) provide a more pleasurable experience, and therefore one also of possible reduced feelings of anxiety. As with many other areas where we have evidence that physical activity produces positive outcomes in terms of mood or mental health, the exact mechanisms remain unknown. However, they are likely to be associated with many different possible mechanisms all at the same time. For example, for one person anxiety may be reduced primarily because they have experienced a pleasurable bout of activity in green surroundings, but for another the primary reason may be that they have had 'time out' from other activities. For both of these people neurobiological and physiological changes that could explain reduced perceptions of anxiety will also be occurring. It remains a challenge for exercise science to fully explain the 'feel-better' response from activity that many people report. A good overview of the possible alternative explanations of why exercise can have an anxiety-reducing effect may be found in Chapter 6 of Buckworth *et al.*'s excellent book (2013).

Exercise and stress reactivity

The study of physiological reactivity to psychosocial stressors has generated medical interest with the increase in the evidence base which suggests that stress, such as that which we may experience in the workplace, is a risk factor for cardiovascular disease (Kivimäki *et al.*, 2012). Studies have focused on acute responses where a single bout of physical activity is undertaken by participants to determine if this 'buffers' or attenuates responses (very often cardiovascular responses such as blood pressure) to laboratory-based stressors. Such studies consistently show that a bout of physical activity does have a buffering effect on stress responses (Hamer *et al.*, 2006). A national review and research consensus process in England on physical activity and psychological well-being (Biddle *et al.*, 2000) also considered reactivity to stress. After considering the evidence, Taylor (2000) concluded that 'single sessions of moderate exercise can reduce short-term physiological reactivity to and enhance recovery from brief psychosocial stressors'.

Another typical experimental design is for participants to be assigned to 'low' and 'high' aerobic fitness groups on the basis of laboratory tests of aerobic fitness and then to be assessed on their physiological reactivity (e.g. blood pressure) to a stressor such as cold water immersion. Crews and Landers (1987) conducted a meta-analysis of 34 such studies and reported a mean ES of -0.48, showing a moderate effect for fitness on stress reactivity, with fitter individuals showing less reactivity. Stronger effects were shown after acute exercise rather than chronic involvement in exercise. The majority of studies used blood pressure and heart rate as dependent measures, but these may be confounded with the independent variable of fitness measurement. However, more recent meta-analytic findings of 73 studies showed greater reactivity with increasing fitness but better recovery (Jackson and Dishman, 2006). These authors call for more ecologically valid ('real-life') studies rather than just laboratory-based studies, and for training studies in which effects of improving fitness levels may be studied. However, Hamer and Steptoe (2013) noted that such studies have been inconclusive thus far. It is therefore difficult to make a clear conclusion on whether or not fitness per se has a stress-buffering effect.

If physical activity, or exercise, or fitness, do affect stress reactivity or recovery from stress, then further knowledge is needed on the underlying mechanisms of such effects. Hamer and Steptoe (2013) have provided an excellent overview of potential mechanisms and conclude that exercise may indeed have an effect on biological responses to stress, and point to the potential role of inflammatory markers as a mediating mechanism.

Clinical anxiety disorders

There is evidence for the anxiety-reducing effects of physical activity from several meta-analytic reviews which we discussed earlier in this chapter. However, almost none of the studies included in these reviews involved clinically diagnosed anxiety disorders. Taylor (2000) noted that for studies of acute exercise, the majority of study participants were college students, and that for chronic exercise only three studies (out of 27 reviewed) focused on groups with an anxiety disorder. Presenting symptoms for a person with a clinical level of anxiety might include fear, worry and inappropriate thoughts or actions that prevent them from functioning properly in work or family life. Diagnosis may include phobias (such as agoraphobia or social phobia), panic attacks, obsessive-compulsive disorder, stress disorders (such as post-traumatic stress) and generalised anxiety. The ICD-10 (1993) section on neurotic, stress-related and somatoform disorders (codes F40–F48) covers phobias, anxiety disorders, obsessive-compulsive disorders, reactions to severe stress, dissociative disorders (i.e. lack of integration of past and present), and somatoform dysfunctions, such as unexplained pain.

Anxiety itself is therefore an inadequate heading but one that is commonly used in the literature. DSM-5 provides criteria for the following types of anxiety (American Psychiatric Association, 2013): Separation Anxiety Disorder; Selective Mutism; Specific Phobia; Social Anxiety Disorder (Social Phobia); Panic Disorder; Panic Attack; Agoraphobia; Generalised Anxiety Disorder; Substance/Medication-Induced Anxiety Disorder; Anxiety Disorder Due to Another Medical Condition.

An example of the diagnostic criteria used for Generalised Anxiety Disorder is as follows:

A   Excessive anxiety and worry, for more days than not, that are out of proportion to the likelihood or impact of feared events.
B   The worry is pervasive and difficult to control.
C   The worry is associated with symptoms of motor tension (e.g. trembling, muscle tension), autonomic hypersensitivity (e.g. dry mouth, palpitations), or hyper-arousal (e.g. exaggerated startle response, insomnia).
D   The anxiety, worry or physical symptoms cause clinically significant distress or impairment in social, occupational or other important areas of functioning.
E   The condition has lasted for at least six months.

Treatments for these disorders might include cognitive-behavioural and counselling approaches or medication. However, many people may not be receiving any treatment for these conditions, since 'talk' therapy is not always widely available or accessible, and many people may not want drugs which have some noted side effects.

Asmundson and colleagues (2013) conducted a narrative review and commentary on the potential effects of exercise for anxiety and its disorders. They concluded that:

> the majority of studies are characterized by small samples, lack of adequate controls, lack of systematic attention to possible dose–response relationships, limited consideration of maintenance of gains following treatment, and primary focus on aerobic activity. These issues are to be expected in an emerging area of inquiry and provide opportunity for future investigation.
>
> (Asmundson *et al.*, 2013, p. 365)

To our knowledge only one meta-analysis has been conducted in which the participants of the trials had a diagnosed anxiety disorder. Jayakody and colleagues (2014) located eight randomised controlled trials in which exercise was compared with other treatments for anxiety disorders. They found that for panic disorders exercise did reduce anxiety but antidepressive medication was more effective. They also found an added benefit of exercise for social phobia which was being treated with cognitive behavioural therapy. With so few trials available for this meta-analysis, the authors were unable to make conclusions about the optimal mode or intensity of exercise.

Populations surveys

Very few population surveys actually measure anxiety disorders. A large cross-sectional analysis of 8,098 US adults, conducted as part of the National Comorbidity Survey, measured a range of anxiety disorders and the relationship with physical activity (Goodwin, 2003). The results showed a significant association between regular physical activity and lower prevalence of current major depression (odds ratio, OR = 0.75 (0.6, 0.94)), panic attacks (OR = 0.73 (0.56, 0.96)), social phobia (OR = 0.65 (0.53, 0.8)), specific phobia (OR = 0.78 (0.63, 0.97)), and agoraphobia (OR = 0.64 (0.43, 0.94)), after adjusting for differences in socio-demographic characteristics, self-reported physical disorders, and co-morbid mental disorders. This study also showed evidence of a dose–response effect, with those reporting the highest physical activity also reporting the lowest prevalence of mental disorders.

Both anxiety and depression were measured in a Scandinavian study of 20,207 men using the HADS scale (Thorsen *et al.*, 2005). The prevalence of HADS-defined depression and anxiety was lower among those who were physically active than in those who were physically inactive. However, when multivariate analysis was used to confirm these associations, with adjustments for various confounding variables, only the link with depression remained significant (adjusted odds ratio = 0.58; 95% CI (0.51, 0.65)).

Such cross-sectional studies could be interpreted in two ways: first, that physical activity is protective; or second, that those with anxiety and depression disorders are not inclined to be active. As we discussed in the chapter on depression (see Chapter 3), this limitation of cross-sectional surveys must be considered because lethargy or fear of going out of the house may indeed be symptoms of depression and anxiety that would inhibit movement and activity. When reviewing the literature on the preventative effect of physical exercise on depression (Chapter 3), we limited the studies to those that had at least two time points so that the issue of whether activity precedes reduced depression or depression precedes reduced activity could be studied. However, until recently such prospective studies have not been available with a focus on anxiety. Azevedo Da Silva and colleagues (2012) have provided a prospective examination of physical activity and anxiety, and depression symptoms with data from the Whitehall II study. These authors used variables to provide a binary categorisation of those who achieve currently recommended levels of physical activity and those who do not for over 9,000 participants (Azevedo Da Silva *et al.*, 2012). This resulted in 13.4 per cent of participants being classified as meeting the physical activity recommendations. They were also able to determine that 20 per cent experienced anxiety or depression, or both, by using established thresholds for responses from the General Health Questionnaire. These descriptors came from baseline data but there were two further time points at which all data were collected. At baseline it was found that participants who were active at recommended levels were less likely to have anxiety symptoms (OR = 0.71, 95% CI, 0.54–0.91), depressive symptoms (OR = 0.63, 95% CI, 0.48–0.81) and both (OR = 0.72, 95% CI, 0.54–0.97). These results are similar to those reported above from earlier studies.

Azevedo Da Silva and colleagues (2012), however, have three important results about the protective effect of physical activity because of the longitudinal nature of the data:

1.   They found that physical activity at baseline was not predictive of anxiety or depression scores at follow-up.

2.   But they were also able to show that if participants had regularly been active over all three time periods there was a protective effect for depression (OR = 0.72, 95% CI, 0.52–0.99 in comparison to those who were not regularly active) but not for anxiety.
3.   They also conducted the converse analyses and showed that if participants had experienced anxiety or depressive symptoms over the three time periods they were less likely to meet the recommended levels of activity. The authors concluded that there is a bi-directional relationship between anxiety and depression and physical activity, with activity having a protective effect (for depression) and existing anxiety or depression having a negative effect on physical activity levels.

Clear conclusions about the role of physical activity in protecting against anxiety therefore remain elusive. As seen in Chapter 3, clearer conclusions may be drawn about the protective role of physical activity on depression because there are many more prospective studies on this topic.

> Key point: Clear conclusions about the protective role of physical activity on anxiety are difficult to draw and more longitudinal population studies are required.

Intervention studies

A recent review of experimental studies on various patient groups with mental disorders, including anxiety and eating and substance abuse disorders, concluded that after more than a decade of research in this area there are very few controlled studies in most of the categories of mental disorder (Zschucke *et al.*, 2013). An early study by Orwin (1981) focused on eight patients diagnosed as agoraphobic who were treated with a running programme. Patients were asked to run to situations that they found fearful, such as supermarkets. Such places normally create feelings of anxiety for those with agoraphobia, but these patients were taught to attribute increased respiration and heart rate to the running and not to their phobic response. Orwin (1981) reported that all eight patients recovered from such repeated exposure after running and had similar success with situational phobias. Here the running seemed to be operating as a method of desensitising patients to the onset of anxiety symptoms by attributing bodily changes to the demands of the exercise. However, no other studies in which phobic patients have been treated in this way have been reported. Of course, Orwin's studies were pre-experimental with no control group, thus providing little evidence that exercise could be used as a treatment for phobias.

A series of Norwegian studies have tried to unravel some of the issues in the use of exercise for treating anxiety disorders. Martinsen and colleagues (1989c) included patients with agoraphobia in an exploratory study of the value of exercise for 92 non-psychotic patients who had various different psychiatric diagnoses. Exercise involved an eight-week programme which was an adjunct to other treatment. There was no control group. Results showed short-term gains for those diagnosed with agoraphobia with panic disorder but these were not maintained at the one-year follow-up. At the end of the programme, fitness improvement and symptom reductions were significant. However, without a control group it is not clear if the symptom reductions were part of the normal course of recovery or accelerated by the exercise.

Martinsen and colleagues (1989a) undertook a further study of exercise in the treatment of anxiety disorders. The anxiety disorder was diagnosed by clinical interview (using DSM-III criteria), and patients (n = 79) in a Norwegian psychiatric hospital were participants. The patients were randomly assigned to aerobic exercise (jogging or walking) or non-aerobic exercise (strength and flexibility training). Both training programmes lasted about 60 minutes for three times each week for eight weeks. Both groups decreased anxiety as rated by therapists blind to treatment conditions, but only the aerobic exercise group increased maximum oxygen consumption. These results are identical to those reported for the depressed patients by the same authors (Martinsen *et al.*, 1989b). The results suggest a beneficial effect of both aerobic and non-aerobic exercise on anxiety disorder. The fact that aerobic fitness improvement was not required to produce the beneficial effects suggests that the explanatory mechanisms are more likely to be psychological than physiological. However, one major drawback of this design is the lack of a control group. The exercise was alongside other treatment but did involve work with specialist instructors. The psychological effect of gaining extra attention and support from these instructors was therefore not controlled.

Another Norwegian study examined the effects of different intensities of aerobic exercise on anxiety disorders (Sexton *et al.*, 1989). Participants were 52 in-patients in a three- to four-week programme in a psychiatric hospital and were diagnosed by DSM-III criteria as having non-psychotic anxiety disorders. Patients were randomly assigned to moderate (walking) or vigorous activity (jogging) and had supervised exercise (30 minutes four to five times each week) for the duration of their programme. They were expected to continue the activity unsupervised for a total of eight weeks and were also followed up at six months. Both intensities of exercise showed reductions in anxiety symptoms at eight weeks and six months. Fitness gains were greater for the jogging group at eight weeks but the difference between groups had disappeared by six months. Aerobic gain did not correlate with reduction in anxiety. More joggers than walkers dropped out of the programme. This led the authors to recommend moderate rather than vigorous activity for other therapy programmes. Despite several good design features this study did not have a non-exercising control group to show that the exercise had an effect over and above the normal treatment effect of the psychiatric programme.

A more recent study employed good design features to study the effects of exercise training on patients diagnosed with Generalised Anxiety Disorder (GAD) (Herring *et al.*, 2012). In this study, 30 women diagnosed with GAD were randomly assigned to receive six weeks of resistance training or aerobic training, or a waiting list control group. One of the main outcome measures was worry symptoms, and it was found that both of the exercise training modes (combined in the analysis) reduced worry symptoms in comparison to the waiting list group. Despite the low numbers in each group and lack of follow-up of this short intervention, this study does show some promise for both resistance training and aerobic exercise to be used as a treatment for GAD. Studies with more participants and longer follow-up are needed in this area.

From these studies we can conclude that both aerobic and non-aerobic exercise can help reduce clinical anxiety symptoms. Moderate intensity exercise seems best for adherence and higher levels of intensity do not necessarily improve the outcome. However, since only one of the studies included a non-exercising control group it is difficult to conclude that there is a causal link.

Early on in the development of this area of research there was a suggestion that exercise might be contra-indicated for those suffering from anxiety neurosis. Pitts and McLure (1967) proposed that exercise could lead to the onset of anxiety symptoms in such patients, due to increases in lactate levels in the bloodstream. This hypothesis was refuted by Morgan (1979), but the evidence for the refutation came from studies on non-clinical participants. For some reason, perhaps an ethical one, the Pitts-McLure hypothesis has not been properly tested in a well-designed study involving patients with clinical anxiety. However, O'Connor *et al.* (2000) conducted a review of all studies where participants were diagnosed with a panic disorder and noted that only five panic attacks had occurred in 444 exercise bouts performed by 420 panic disorder patients. They concluded that the weight of the published evidence shows that acute physical activity does not provoke panic attacks in panic disorder patients and thus refuted the Pitts-McLure hypothesis.

Many patients with chronic medical conditions may suffer from anxiety which is unrecognised because attention is being paid to the primary medical condition. Herring and colleagues conducted a systematic review of studies that used exercise training as a treatment for anxiety symptoms in patients with chronic medical conditions (Herring *et al.*, 2010). They found that the average effect size for exercise training for reducing symptoms of anxiety was -0.29. While this is modest at best, this is a promising new line of research that could help many patient groups cope with chronic medical conditions.

> Key point: There is a promising literature on the use of exercise in the treatment of anxiety disorder but much more research is needed in this area.

Could physical activity help with dependencies?

The topic of dependence on alcohol and drugs falls into all of the commonly used classifications of mental illness. Using ICD-10 (World Health Organization, 1993), a diagnosis of dependence is made through noting various dependence syndromes. These features are noted in Table 4.2. If three or more of these features are present, a diagnosis of dependence is made.

Even if a clinical diagnosis is not made, amounts of alcohol and drug use below this level are still a concern to health, to health care costs and to social order. There is particular concern about the increasing incidence of both alcohol and drug use among young people, since a variety of health problems may follow but also because of the possible social disorder that may result (Sutherland and Shepherd, 2001). We will also discuss dependence on tobacco in this section. While it is not normally considered as a clinical condition, tobacco use is

Table 4.2   ICD-10 classification of dependence syndrome (World Health Organization, 1993)

Classification	Dependence syndrome
Compulsion	Desire/compulsion to take the substance
Impaired control	Difficulty in controlling behaviour in regard to onset, termination and level of substance taking
Withdrawal	Physiological withdrawal states occur when substance withdrawn
Relief use	Substance used to avoid or relieve withdrawal symptoms
Tolerance	Increased amount of substance required to achieve effect similar to lower dose
Salience	Increased amounts of time spent in obtaining or taking substance or recovering from its effects Persistence despite awareness of harmful response

universally seen as a major health risk with high prevalence. Several researchers have now looked at how exercise might help people quit smoking and therefore improve health.

Alcohol dependence

Alcohol dependence is a common problem and one that is growing in prevalence. In 1992, a national survey showed that 24 per cent of men and 7 per cent of women were drinking at levels above the recommendations for safe limits (HMSO, 1992). A decade later these figures had risen to 44 per cent of men and 30 per cent of women exceeding recommended levels (Office for National Statistics, 2004), indicating a large percentage of the population who are at risk of becoming dependent and whose health may suffer as a result of high levels of alcohol consumption.

The topic of appropriate treatment for alcohol abuse has received much discussion with no one method showing distinct advantages (Heather *et al.*, 1985). Rehabilitation from an addictive behaviour involves establishing self-control strategies and finding coping strategies for the emotions involved with withdrawal and continued abstinence (Marlatt and Gordon, 1985). Three stages of treatment have been recognised as follows:

- stage 1: detoxification, emergency treatment and screening;
- stage 2: rehabilitation, including primary and extended care;
- stage 3: relapse prevention and care required for maintenance (Institute of Medicine, 1990).

In considering why physical activity might be included as part of any stage of treatment, as with other topics in this chapter, both physical and mental health reasons are viable. Self-esteem is often very low as the problem drinker faces the need for treatment and realises the physical and mental damage that alcohol may have caused (Beck *et al.*, 1976). It is intriguing to note that one of the earliest documented pieces of research in exercise psychology was in the area of alcohol rehabilitation, although several decades passed before the research was replicated (Cowles, 1898). Cowles' conclusion provides a challenge to current researchers to provide experimental evidence of the declared benefits of exercise:

> The benefits accruing to the patients from the well-directed use of exercise and baths is indicated by the following observed symptoms: increase in weight, greater firmness of muscles, better colour of skin, larger lung capacity, more regular and stronger action of the heart, clearer action of the mind, brighter and more expressive eye, improved carriage, quicker responses of nerves, and through them of muscle and limb to stimuli. All this has become so evident to them that only a very few are unwilling to attend the classes and many speak freely of the great benefits derived.
>
> (Cowles, 1898, p. 108)

Problem drinkers often have low levels of cardiorespiratory fitness and muscle strength, and appropriate programmes of exercise have been shown to be effective in improving these physical parameters (Donaghy *et al.*, 1991; Tsukue and Shohoji, 1981). Since regular exercise has been associated with improved mental health, decreased levels of depression and anxiety and increased self-esteem, and these are commonly reported problems in alcohol rehabilitation, the use of exercise as part of the treatment for alcohol rehabilitation has been piloted in several locations (Donaghy *et al.*, 1991; Frankel and Murphy, 1974; Gary and Guthrie,

1972; Murphy *et al.*, 1986; Palmer *et al.*, 1988; Sinyor *et al.*, 1982). In these studies, the exercise programmes may be considered to be lifestyle interventions providing the problem drinker with the skills to undertake a positive health promoting behaviour (exercise), simultaneously providing self-control strategies, coping strategies and an alternative to drinking (Marlatt and Gordon, 1985; Murphy *et al.*, 1986).

Donaghy and Mutrie (1997) reported a randomised controlled trial in which 117 problem drinkers were assigned to either a three-week supervised exercise programme (followed by a 12-week home-based programme) or a placebo group. The latter received a stretching programme for three weeks and advice to continue exercising for the next 12 weeks. The exercise group improved scores on physical self-worth and perceptions of strength and physical condition at one and two months after entry to the programme. The between-groups difference in physical self-perceptions was not evident at five months, but this may be due to drop-off in exercise adherence (Donaghy and Mutrie, 1997). Evidence exists, therefore, that a structured exercise programme added to a three-week treatment programme can help problem drinkers improve their perception of physical self-worth.

Adherence to exercise was a problem, with 26 per cent having left the treatment programme (not just the exercise) at the end of three weeks and by the second month follow-up a further 30 per cent had dropped out. Activity levels were sustained for the exercise groups for 8 to 12 weeks following the three-week programme but had dropped to the level of the control group by five months.

Donaghy and Ussher (2005) summarised the available evidence on this topic and concluded that the support for the physical benefits of an exercise programme as part of alcohol rehabilitation, such as improved aerobic fitness and strength, is strong. However, the evidence for mental health benefits and for any effect on improving abstinence from alcohol is weaker (Donaghy and Ussher, 2005). Special challenges for this population include low starting levels of fitness and muscle weakness, relapse to drinking with consequent effects on exercise behaviour, social isolation and lack of support. There is clearly a need for help, such as telephone contact or regular meetings, to sustain activity levels initiated in treatment programmes for this patient group. There is also a need to integrate the exercise into other treatments such as discussion groups, self-help groups or forms of cognitive behavioural therapy. Reinforcing the value of exercise and encouraging adherence could be topics for group leaders and therapists in these other forms of treatment.

> Key point: Evidence suggests that problem drinkers can benefit from exercise programmes in terms of physical outcomes. However, evidence for mental health benefits or any advantage to reducing alcohol intake is weaker.

Drug dependence

Illegal drugs are used for recreational purposes worldwide. Substance misuse in which a dependence has become apparent is a growing problem and is one of the most prevalent psychiatric disorders in modern society. Opiates, tranquillisers and crack cocaine are the three most common drugs that create problems of dependence for users in the UK.

Treatment for drug dependence can take place in primary care or in specialist drug treatment services, and often involves prescribing substitute drugs such as methodone. The Department of Health (1999) suggested the following aims for the treatment of drug misuse:

- Assist the patient to remain healthy, until, with appropriate care and support, he or she can achieve a drug-free life.
- Reduce the use of illicit or non-prescribed drugs by the individual.
- Deal with problems related to drug misuse.
- Reduce the dangers associated with drug misuse, particularly the risk of HIV, hepatitis B and C, and other blood-borne infections from injecting paraphernalia.
- Reduce the duration of episodes of drug misuse.
- Reduce the chance of future relapse from drug misuse.
- Reduce the need for criminal activity to finance drug misuse.
- Reduce the risk of prescribed drugs being diverted on to the illegal drug market.

It is clear from these treatment aims that physical activity could not be a panacea but that it could have a possible role such as improving physical health, providing a diversion from drugs, providing an alternative social network and possibly helping prevent relapse. However, evidence for the use of exercise in drug rehabilitation programmes is very hard to find. One review found six studies published between 1991 and 2002 (Donaghy and Ussher, 2005). Five of the studies were from North America and one from China. Only two of these studies had control groups, showing the difficulty of finding adequate numbers in most treatment settings to mount a randomised trial. A more recent pilot study recruited only 16 participants from a potential pool of 35 for a 12-week individually tailored exercise programme (Brown *et al.*, 2010). In this pre-post design the 16 participants showed benefits in increased number of days they were abstinent and improved fitness. However, while the authors suggest that fully powered randomised trials are warranted, they also note challenges of recruitment and adherence to the programme. These issues call into question the idea that a randomised trial is the best way forward in this area.

A study conducted in Scotland attempted a multiple baseline design to overcome some of the challenges of a RCT. Participants were clients attending a special exercise programme organised by the Community Drug Team in Greenock (Smith, 2006). Qualitative data were also collected from clients and service providers. Twenty-one participants, who were all misusing more than one substance, attended some or all of a 10-week exercise programme. Baseline measures were taken on a minimum of three occasions to establish whether or not a stable condition was present and then clients began the exercise programme. The main changes over time were improvements in the distance walked in six minutes and self-perceived physical health benefits. However, adherence was so varied that it was difficult to conclude that the exercise programme was related to these outcomes. Thus, even a multiple baseline design proved difficult to enact in this setting. It was also noted that the clients had high levels of lifestyle activity because they walked to most places for transport.

One of the most interesting studies reviewed by Donaghy and Ussher (2005) involved a Chinese martial art form, and perhaps an activity such as Tai Chi would be appropriate to consider. The qualitative results in the Scottish study were interesting. Clients attending the group perceived a number of benefits such as something to look forward to, something that helped them feel fitter and something that improved mental health. The following quote from one user shows some of this effect:

> Well, it didnae [did not] cost any money to feel good an' stuff. So, em, feeling good, about feeling good without taking drugs, made you feel good anyway!

Staff members also felt that the programme was worthwhile, although it was acknowledged that there are many barriers to overcome for those in drug rehabilitation to attend regular exercise classes (Smith, 2006). This study has provided some new evidence for the role of exercise in a drug rehabilitation programme in the UK but it is clear that it is still very difficult to mount a service for clients and even more difficult to evaluate it. The qualitative approach remains the best research methodology in this setting.

From these various study designs there is promising evidence that including an exercise programme for those in drug rehabilitation has the potential to increase abstinence, reduce withdrawal symptoms, positively influence fitness levels and self-esteem, and reduce relapse. The problems faced in drug rehabilitation are similar to those in alcohol rehabilitation; high levels of anxiety and depression are often reported as well as low self-esteem (Banks and Waller, 1988), and thus it might be assumed that exercise could have the same potentially therapeutic effect. One unique problem for drug rehabilitation is the variety of drugs and their effects both during addiction and withdrawal. In addition, drug misuse often involves the use of many drugs by the same person (Arif and Westermeyer, 1988). It may be that this variety of responses makes the standard 'clinical' trial experiment untenable, because there is likely to be a large variation in the dependent variables but only small numbers of participants available because of the nature of the treatment programmes. In addition, these are often residential. Again, qualitative methodology may therefore be the best way to gather information.

Exercise programmes for those attempting to withdraw from drugs present a particular challenge in overcoming adverse withdrawal effects from drugs. Such patients are liable to forget appointments for exercise, and the withdrawal effects may prevent exercise completely on some days or they may have an inability to leave the house to go to an exercise facility. Keeping in regular contact with these patients is very helpful to them. Perhaps home-based exercise, such as through an exercise video or web page, could provide some support through difficult phases, but regular phone calls, prompts and visits may also be required.

> Key point: Exercise programmes for those attempting to withdraw from drugs are challenging to deliver but have many potential benefits. Standard research designs are also challenging with this patient group and researchers need creative designs to provide service providers with appropriate evidence for the suggested benefits.

Tobacco dependence

A more recent question regarding the role of exercise in drug dependence relates to whether or not physical activity can play a role in helping people who are trying to give up cigarette smoking. Of course tobacco use is not normally considered as a clinical problem, but nicotine dependence remains a major health risk. Governments around the world have taken strong policy stances, such as banning smoking in public places, as a means to reducing the percentage of the population who smoke. Many people do seek help to attempt to quit, and the NHS in the UK offers many services to help people who want to quit. Is it possible that physical activity could help people who want to quit?

Taylor and Ussher (2013) have provided a summary of the literature on the role of physical activity in coping with withdrawal from tobacco. Their thorough review of the growing literature covers the effects of regular physical activity on smoking cessation, acute effects of single bouts of exercise, the possible mechanisms of such effects and the design of interventions that involve physical activity and engage smokers. The strongest findings relate to single sessions of exercise at a low to moderate level of intensity, such as walking, helping people with withdrawal symptoms and nicotine cravings.

A meta-analysis of 15 studies that measured effects of a single bout of exercise on strength of desire to smoke showed a very large effect size in favour of exercise (Haasova *et al.*, 2013). Given the substantial evidence on the health benefits of quitting smoking and the known difficulty of overcoming dependence on tobacco, this new approach of using physical activity must be encouraged and further research carried out. Even if it does not help in a direct way, the positive health benefits of increasing activity must be considered as evidence enough that exercise should be an important adjunct to any attempts to quit smoking.

> Key point: Smoking is a high-risk health behaviour with high prevalence. Many approaches are needed to help those who want to quit and there is promising evidence that physical activity has a role to play in smoking cessation.

Chapter summary

- There has been a growing literature on the potential beneficial effects of activity for those with schizophrenia. At the very least we can be clear that physical activity is good for the physical health of these patients.
- Meta-analytic findings suggest that exercise is associated with a significant small to moderate reduction in non-clinical anxiety. This holds for acute and chronic exercise, state and trait anxiety, psychophysiological indices of anxiety, and groups differing by gender and age.
- Experimental studies support an anxiety-reducing effect for exercise and mainly for moderate rather than high-intensity exercise.
- The most recent evidence concerning stress and exercise suggests that exercise helps us recover faster from stressful events that have been created in laboratory conditions. The mechanisms for all such effects remain speculative at this point in time.
- Population studies do not provide convincing evidence that physical activity is associated with reduced risk of clinically defined anxiety and experimental studies do not provide much more evidence.
- There is no evidence that exercise might induce further anxiety or panic in participants who have anxiety disorders.
- Problem drinkers can benefit from exercise programmes in terms of physical outcomes, but the evidence for mental health benefits or any advantage to reducing alcohol intake is weaker.
- There are many potential benefits to include physical activity in programmes that are helping people withdraw from drug addiction. However, standard research designs are challenging with this patient group and so it has been difficult to provide evidence for these benefits.
- There is promising evidence that physical activity can help people who are attempting to quit smoking.

References

American Psychiatric Association. (2013). *Diagnostic and Statistical Manual of Mental Disorders (DSM-5)* (5th edn).

Arif, A. and Westermeyer, J. (1988). *Manual of Drug and Alcohol Abuse Guidelines for Teaching in Medical and Health Institutions.* New York: Plenum.

Asmundson, G.J., Fetzner, M.G., Deboer, L.B., Powers, M.B., Otto, M.W. and Smits, J.A. (2013). Let's get physical: A contemporary review of the anxiolytic effects of exercise for anxiety and its disorders. *Depress Anxiety, 30*(4), 362–373. doi: 10.1002/da.22043.

Azevedo Da Silva, M., Singh-Manoux, A., Brunner, E.J., Kaffashian, S., Shipley, M.J., Kivimäki, M. and Nabi, H. (2012). Bidirectional association between physical activity and symptoms of anxiety and depression: The Whitehall II study. *European Journal of Epidemiology, 27*, 537–546.

Banks, A. and Waller, T.A.N. (1988). *Drug Misuse: A practical handbook for GPs.* London: Blackwell Scientific Publications.

Beck, A.T., Weissman, M. and Kovacs, M. (1976). Alcoholism, hopelessness and suicidal behavior. *Journal of Studies on Alcohol, 37*, 66–67.

Biddle, S.J.H., Fox, K.R. and Boutcher, S.H. (eds). (2000). *Physical Activity and Psychological Well-being.* London: Routledge.

Brown, R.A., Abrantes, A.M., Read, J.P., Marcus, B.H., Jakicic, J., Strong, D.R. and Gordon, A.A. (2010). A pilot study of aerobic exercise as an adjunctive treatment for drug dependence. *Mental Health and Physical Activity, 3*(1), 27–34. doi: 10.1016/j.mhpa.2010.03.001.

Buckworth, J., Dishman, R., O'Connor, P.J. and Tomporowski, P.D. (2013). *Exercise Psychology* (2nd edn). Champaign, IL: Human Kinetics.

Chamove, A.S. (1986). Positive short-term effects of activity on behaviour in chronic schizophrenic patients. *British Journal of Clinical Psychology, 25*, 125–133.

Cohen, J. (1988). *Statistical Power Analysis for the Behavioral Sciences.* Hillsdale, NJ: Erlbaum.

Cowles, E. (1898). Gymnastics in the treatment of inebriety. *American Physical Education Review, 3*, 107–110.

Crews, D.J. and Landers, D.M. (1987). A meta-analytic review of aerobic fitness and reactivity to psychosocial stressors. *Medicine and Science in Sports and Exercise, 19*(5, Supplement), S114–S120.

Department of Health. (1999). *Drug Misuse and Dependence. Guidelines on clinical management.*

Donaghy, M. and Mutrie, N. (1997). Physical self-perception of problem drinkers on entry to an alcohol rehabilitation programme. *Physiotherapy, 83*(7), 358.

Donaghy, M.E. and Ussher, M.H. (2005). Exercise interventions in drug and alcohol rehabilitation. In G.E.J. Faulkner and A.H. Taylor (eds), *Exercise, Health and Mental Health: Emerging relationships* (pp. 48–69). London: Routledge.

Donaghy, M., Ralston, G. and Mutrie, N. (1991). Exercise as a therapeutic adjunct for problem drinkers (abstract). *Journal of Sports Sciences, 9*, 440.

Edwards, K.M. and Mills, P. (2013). Physical activity, stress and immune function. In P. Ekkekakis (ed.), *Routledge Handbook of Physical Activity and Mental Health* (pp. 342–355). Abingdon, Oxon: Routledge.

Ekkekakis, P. (2003). Pleasure and displeasure from the body: Perspectives from exercise. *Cognition and Emotion, 17*, 213–239.

——. (2013). *Routledge Handbook of Physical Activity and Mental Health.* Abingdon, Oxon: Routledge.

Ekkekakis, P., Parfitt, G. and Petruzzello, S.J. (2011). The pleasure and displeasure people feel when they exercise at different intensities: Decennial update and progress towards a tripartite rationale for exercise intensity prescription. *Sports Medicine, 41*(8), 641–671. doi: 10.2165/11590680-000000000-00000.

Falloon, I.R.H. and Talbot, R.E. (1981). Persistent auditory hallucinations: Coping mechanisms and implications for management. *Psychological Medicine, 11*, 329–339.

Faulkner, G.E.J. (2005). Exercise as an adjunct treatment for schizophrenia. In G.E.J. Faulkner and A.H. Taylor (eds), *Exercise, Health and Mental Health: Emerging relationships* (pp. 27–47). London: Routledge.

Faulkner, G.E.J. and Biddle, S.J.H. (1999). Exercise as an adjunct treatment for schizophrenia: A review of literature. *Journal of Mental Health, 8*, 441–457.

Faulkner, G.E.J. and Sparkes, A. (1999). Exercise as therapy for schizophrenia: An ethnographic study. *Journal of Sport and Exercise Psychology, 21*, 52–69.

Faulkner, G., Gorczynski, P. and Arbour-Nicitopoulos, K. (2013). Exercise as an adjunct treatment for schizophrenia. In P. Ekkekakis (ed.), *Routledge Handbook of Physical Activity and Mental Health* (pp. 541–555). Abingdon, Oxon: Routledge.

Fogarty, M. and Happell, B. (2005). Exploring the benefits of an exercise program for people with schizophrenia: A qualitative study. *Issues in Mental Health Nursing, 26*(3), 341–351.

Frankel, A. and Murphy, J. (1974). Physical fitness and personality in alcoholism: Canonical analysis of measures before and after treatment. *Quarterly Journal of Studies on Alcohol, 35*, 1271–1278.

Gary, V. and Guthrie, D. (1972). The effects of jogging on physical fitness and self-concept in hospitalized alcoholics. *Quarterly Journal of Studies on Alcoholism, 33*, 1073–1078.

Goodwin, R.D. (2003). Association between physical activity and mental disorders among adults in the United States. *Preventive Medicine, 36*(6), 698–703.

Haasova, M., Warren, F.C., Ussher, M., Janse Van Rensburg, K., Faulkner, G., Cropley, M. and Taylor, A.H. (2013). The acute effects of physical activity on cigarette cravings: Systematic review and meta-analysis with individual participant data. *Addiction, 108*(1), 26–37. doi: 10.1111/j.1360-0443.2012.04034.x.

Hamer, M. and Steptoe, A. (2013). Physical activity, stress reactivity, and stress-mediated pathophysiology. In P. Ekkekakis (ed.), *Routledge Handbook of Physical Activity and Mental Health* (pp. 303–315). Abingdon, Oxon: Routledge.

Hamer, M., Taylor, A. and Steptoe, A. (2006). The effect of acute aerobic exercise on stress related blood pressure responses: A systematic review and meta-analysis. *Biology and Psychology, 71*(2), 183–190. doi: 10.1016/j.biopsycho.2005.04.004.

Heather, N., Roberston, I. and Davies, P. (1985). *The Misuse of Alcohol: Crucial issues in dependence treatment and prevention.* London: Croom Helm.

Herring, M.P., O'Connor, P.J. and Dishman, R.K. (2010). The effect of exercise training on anxiety symptoms among patients: A systematic review. *Archives of International Medicine, 170*(4), 321–331. doi: 10.1001/archinternmed.2009.530.

Herring, M.P., Jacob, M.L., Suveg, C., Dishman, R.K. and O'Connor, P.J. (2012). Feasibility of exercise training for the short-term treatment of generalized anxiety disorder: A randomized controlled trial. *Psychotherapy and Psychosomatics, 81*(1), 21–28. doi: 10.1159/000327898.

HMSO. (1992). *Scotland's Health – A challenge to us all: A policy statement.* Edinburgh: HMSO.

Hunter, J. and Schmidt, F.L. (1990). *Methods of Meta-analysis: Correcting error and bias in research findings.* Newbury Park, CA: Sage.

Institute of Medicine. (1990). *Broadening the Base of Treatment for Alcoholism.* New York: Wiley.

Jackson, E.M. and Dishman, R.K. (2006). Cardiorespiratory fitness and laboratory stress: A metaregression analysis. *Psychophysiology, 43*(1), 57–72. doi: 10.1111/j.1469-8986.2006.00373.x.

Jayakody, K., Gunadasa, S. and Hosker, C. (2014). Exercise for anxiety disorders: Systematic review. *British Journal of Sports Medicine, 48*(3), 187–196. doi: 10.1136/bjsports-2012-091287.

Kivimäki, M., Nyberg, S.T., Batty, G.D., Fransson, E.I., Heikkila, K., Alfredsson, L. *et al.*, (2012). Job strain as a risk factor for coronary heart disease: A collaborative meta-analysis of individual participant data. *Lancet, 380*(9852), 1491–1497. doi: 10.1016/S0140-6736(12)60994-5.

Leith, L. (1994). *Foundations of Exercise and Mental Health.* Morgantown, WV: Fitness Information Technology.

Long, B.C. and van Stavel, R. (1995). Effects of exercise training on anxiety: A meta-analysis. *Journal of Applied Sport Psychology, 7*, 167–189.

Marlatt, G.A. and Gordon, G.R. (1985). *Relapse Prevention.* New York: Guilford Press.

Martinsen, E.W. (1990a). Benefits of exercise for the treatment of depression. *Sports Medicine, 9*(6), 380–389.

———. (1990b). Physical fitness, anxiety and depression. *British Journal of Hospital Medicine, 43*(194), 196–199.

Martinsen, E.W., Hoffart, A. and Solberg, O. (1989a). Aerobic and non-aerobic forms of exercise in the treatment of anxiety disorders. *Stress Medicine, 5*, 115–120.

Martinsen, E. W., Hoffart, A. and Solberg, O. (1989b). Comparing aerobic and non-aerobic forms of exercise in the treatment of clinical depression: A randomized trial. *Comprehensive Psychiatry, 30*, 324–331.

Martinsen, E.W., Sandvik, I. and Kolbjornsrud, O.B. (1989c). Aerobic exercise in the treatment of non psychotic mental disorders: An exploratory study. *Nordic Journal of Psychiatry, 43*, 411–415.

McDonald, D.G. and Hodgdon, J.A. (1991). *Psychological Effects of Aerobic Fitness Training: Research and theory*. New York: Springer-Verlag.

McNair, D.M., Lorr, M. and Droppleman, L.F. (1971). *Profile of Mood States Manual*. San Diego, CA: Educational and Industrial Testing Service.

Morgan, W.P. (1979). Anxiety reduction following acute physical activity. *Psychiatric Annals, 9*, 36–45.

Murphy, T.J., Pagano, R.R. and Marlatt, G.A. (1986). Lifestyle modification with heavy alcohol drinkers: Effects of aerobic exercise and mediation. *Addictive Behaviours, 11*, 175–186.

Mutrie, N., Hannah, M.K. and Berger, U. (2003). The relationship among different modes of physical activity and non-clinical depression. *Journal of Sports Sciences, 21*(4), 355.

O'Connor, P.J., Smith, J.C. and Morgan, W.P. (2000). Physical activity does not provoke panic attacks in patients with panic disorder: A review of the evidence. *Anxiety, Stress, and Coping, 13*, 333–353.

Office for National Statistics. (2004). Social Trends. *32*.

Orwin, A. (1981). The running treatment: A preliminary communication on a new use for an old therapy (physical activity) in the agorophobic syndrome. In M.H. Sacks and M. Sacks (eds), *Psychology of Running* (pp. 32–39). Champaign, IL: Human Kinetics.

Palmer, J., Vacc, N. and Epstein, J. (1988). Adult inpatient alcoholics: Physical exercise as a treatment intervention. *Journal of Studies on Alcohol, 49*(5), 418–421.

Pelham, T.W. and Campagna, P.D. (1991). Benefits of exercise in psychiatric rehabilitation of persons with schizophrenia. *Canadian Journal of Rehabilitation, 4*(3), 159–168.

Pelham, T.W., Campagna, P.D., Ritvo, P.G. and Birnie, W.A. (1993). The effects of exercise therapy on clients in a psychiatric rehabilitation programme. *Psychosocial Rehabilitation Journal, 16*(4), 75–84.

Petruzzello, S.J. (1995). Does physical exercise reduce anxious emotions? A reply to W. Schlicht's meta-analysis. *Anxiety, Stress and Coping, 8*, 353–356.

Petruzzello, S.J., Landers, D.M., Hatfield, B.D., Kubitz, K.A. and Salazar, W. (1991). A meta-analysis on the anxiety-reducing effects of acute and chronic exercise: Outcomes and mechanisms. *Sports Medicine, 11*, 143–182.

Pitts, F.N. and McClure, J.N. (1967). Lactate metabolism in anxiety neurosis. *The New England Journal of Medicine, 277*, 1329–1336.

Plante, T.G. (1993). Aerobic exercise in prevention and treatment of psychopathology. In P. Seraganian (ed.), *Exercise Psychology. The influence of physical exercise on psychological processes* (pp. 358–379). New York: John Wiley.

Richardson, C.R., Faulkner, G., McDevitt, J., Skrinar, G.S., Hutchinson, D.S. and Piette, J.D. (2005). Integrating physical activity into mental health services for persons with serious mental illness. *Psychiatric Services, 56*(3), 324–331.

Scheewe, T.W., Backx, F.J., Takken, T., Jorg, F., van Strater, A.C., Kroes, A.G. and Cahn, W. (2013). Exercise therapy improves mental and physical health in schizophrenia: A randomised controlled trial. *Acta Psychiatrica Scandinavica, 127*(6), 464–473. doi: 10.1111/acps.12029.

Schlicht, W. (1994). Does physical exercise reduce anxious emotions? A meta-analysis. *Anxiety, Stress and Coping, 6*, 275–288.

———. (1995). Does physical exercise reduce anxious emotions? A retort to Steven J. Petruzzello. *Anxiety, Stress and Coping, 8*, 357–359.

Sexton, H., Maere, A. and Dahl, N.H. (1989). Exercise intensity and reduction in neurotic symptoms: A controlled follow-up study. *Acta Psychiatrica Scandinavica, 80*, 231–235.

Sinyor, D., Brown, T., Rostant, L. and Seraganian, P. (1982). The role of physical exercise in the treatment of alcoholism. *Journal of Studies on Alcohol, 43*, 380–386.

Smith, J.F. (2006). *Is Exercise Beneficial in the Rehabilitation of Drug Users?* M.Phil., University of Strathclyde, Glasgow.

Spielberger, C.D., Gorsuch, R.L. and Lushene, R. (1970). *State-trait Anxiety Inventory Manual*. Palo Alto, CA: Consulting Psychologists Press.

Stephens, T. (1988). Physical activity and mental health in the United States and Canada: Evidence from four population surveys. *Preventive Medicine, 17*, 35–47.

Steptoe, A. and Cox, S. (1988). Acute effects of aerobic exercise on mood. *Health Psychology, 7*, 329–340.

Sutherland, I. and Shepherd, J.P. (2001). The prevalence of alcohol, cigarette, and illicit drug use in a stratified sample of English adolescents. *Addiction, 96*, 637–640.

Taylor, A.H. (2000). Physical activity, anxiety, and stress. In S.J.H. Biddle, K.R. Fox and S.H. Boutcher (eds), *Physical Activity and Psychological Well-being* (pp. 10–45). London: Routledge.

Taylor, A.H. and Ussher, M.H. (2013). Physical activity as an aid in smoking cessation. In P. Ekkekakis (ed.), *Routledge Handbook of Physical Activity and Mental Health* (pp. 451–464). Abingdon, Oxon: Routledge.

Thorsen, L., Nystad, W., Stigum, H., Dahl, O., Klepp, O., Bremnes, R.M. and Fossa, S.D. (2005). The association between self-reported physical activity and prevalence of depression and anxiety disorder in long-term survivors of testicular cancer and men in a general population sample. *Supportive Care in Cancer, 13*(8), 637–646.

Tsukue, I. and Shohoji, T. (1981). Movement therapy for alcoholic patients. *Journal of Studies on Alcohol, 42*, 144–149.

Vancampfort, D., Probst, M., Skjaerven, L.V., Catalán-Matamoros, D., Lundvik-Gyllensten, A., Gomez-Conesa, A. and De Hert, M. (2012). Systematic review of the benefits of physical therapy within a multidisciplinary care approach for people with schizophrenia. *Physical Therapy, 92*, 11–23.

Vancampfort, D., Correll, C.U., Scheewe, T.W., Probst, M., De Herdt, A., Knapen, J. and De Hert, M. (2013). Progressive muscle relaxation in persons with schizophrenia: A systematic review of randomized controlled trials. *Clinical Rehabilitation, 27*(4), 291–298. doi: 10.1177/0269215512455531.

Wipfli, B.M., Rethorst, C.D. and Landers, D.M. (2008). The anxiolytic effects of exercise: A meta-analysis of randomized trials and dose–response analysis. *Journal of Sport Exercise Psychology, 30*(4), 392–410.

World Health Organization. (1993). *The ICD-10 Classification of Mental and Behavioral Disorders: Diagnostic criteria for research*. Geneva: WHO.

Zigmond, A.S. and Snaith, R.P. (1983). The hospital anxiety and depression scale. *Acta Psychiatrica Scandinavia, 67*, 361–370.

Zschucke, E., Gaudlitz, K. and Strohle, A. (2013). Exercise and physical activity in mental disorders: Clinical and experimental evidence. *Journal of Preventative Medical Public Health, 46 Suppl. 1*, S12–21. doi: 10.3961/jpmph.2013.46.S.S12.

Zuckerman, M. and Lubin, B. (1965). *Manual for the Multiple Affect Adjective Checklist*. San Diego, CA: Educational and Industrial Testing Service.

5 Physical activity and cognitive functioning
Can physical activity help the brain function better?

Anecdotal reports from many exercisers often suggest that after physical activity they are able to think 'better', more clearly, or simply feel that their alertness is improved. Similarly, it is often claimed that active children 'do better' at school. A grand claim! These suggest that physical activity can have a positive effect on some forms of cognitive functioning its importance is clear across the age span. For example, for young people the potential for cognitive and academic growth at this important life stage, including brain development, is clear to see and justify. Moreover, for older adults cognitive decline is possible and therefore physical activity may be a strategy to slow or prevent such a decline. Indeed, the huge personal, social and health care costs of cognitive impairment in later life – something only increasing as the population ages at an increasing rate – means that physical activity could be a particularly important health behaviour to promote. For these reasons, this chapter will address physical activity and cognitive functioning by reviewing the evidence with an emphasis on young people and older adults.

Specifically, in this chapter, we aim to:

- introduce and define the concept of cognitive functioning;
- review the evidence linking physical activity with cognitive functioning in young people, including measures of academic achievement;
- review the evidence linking physical activity with cognitive functioning in adults and older adults;
- review the evidence concerning the role of physical activity in reducing the risk of cognitive decline in older adults.

What is cognitive functioning?

The term cognitive functioning is concerned with our mental processes required for day-to-day and 'higher order' functioning, such as difficult problem-solving. Other functions may include attention, memory, use of language, learning of skills, inhibition and decision-making. Cognitive inhibition refers to the holding back or overriding of a psychological process, such as slowing down or reducing the chance of a behaviour or action occurring. This requires memory and ability to process possible consequences of actions.

Key point: Cognitive functioning refers to our mental processes required for both day-to-day tasks and more difficult 'higher order' functioning.

Cognitive functioning may also range from performing quite easy tasks, such as simple reaction time, to much more complex information processing requiring higher levels of cognitive functioning. These functions may affect daily performance, such as school, work or in performing tasks of daily living. As such, some studies have investigated whether physical activity affects such outcomes, with school or academic performance a common measure.

This area of study is complex. The exposure variable may be total physical activity, physical fitness, sports participation, physical education, or other discrete forms of physical activity. All of these activities can vary by intensity, duration and context. Some may also involve high cognitive requirements, such as in playing games. At the same time, studies may assess a plethora of outcome variables, ranging across well-validated laboratory and psycho-logical tests of cognitive function to performance and outcome measures such as classroom behaviour, test scores and school marks (grades) or overall academic achievement. Some studies have also investigated behavioural issues, such as behaviour in the school classroom. From a neuroscience perspective, the dorsolateral prefrontal cortex has been identified as a key area of the brain for information processing, including the integration of different aspects of cognition and behaviour.

Physical activity and cognitive functioning in young people

The study of physical activity and cognitive functioning in children and adolescents has been justified on the basis that people of this age are still developing, physically and mentally, and that physical activity may have important developmental benefits. Kirkendall (1986), for example, concluded that a modest positive relationship existed between motor perfor-mance and intellectual performance in children and that this relationship was strongest in the early stages of development. Research in perceptual-motor development has suggested that the early development of psychomotor function and neuromuscular control could assist academic learning in young children. Increases in cerebral blood flow have been documented after physical activity, and this could assist in cognitive functioning. Similarly, activity will increase blood flow in the prefrontal somatosensory and primary motor cortices of the brain (Williams, 1986). However, despite these plausible mechanisms, the studies of cognitive change in children exposed to physical activity interventions have been poorly controlled and open to clear methodological criticism. Best (2010, p. 333) also argues in favour of the plausible link between physical activity and cognitive functioning at these ages by saying:

> [The] protracted cognitive and neural development may be one clue to understanding why children's executive function (EF) is sensitive to the effects of aerobic exercise. Both EF and the underlying neural circuitry are still immature in late childhood and even adolescence, and therefore, certain experiences may facilitate their development or temporarily enhance their functioning. Aerobic exercise appears to be such an experience that would positively impact EF and the supporting neural circuitry.

Evidence from systematic reviews

Research concerning physical activity and wider aspects of cognitive functioning in children, or at least school performance, is not new, with studies going back to the 1950s (Howie and Pate, 2012). Moreover, there has been considerable growth since then with many systematic reviews, including meta-analyses, in the past decade or so (Biddle and Asare, 2011).

One of the first meta-analyses to address a topic in physical activity research was one investigating interventions for learning disabled children (Kavale and Mattson, 1983). A meta-analysis of 180 studies showed no positive effect on academic, cognitive or perceptual motor performance from perceptual-motor training on children whose average IQ was 88 at the age of 8. However, given that there were no effects on (perceptual) motor performance itself, it is difficult to conclude whether the null findings were due to lack of intervention fidelity or a genuine lack of influence on cognitive outcomes. Without a change in perceptual-motor performance, this cannot be answered.

Sibley and Etnier (2003) reported a meta-analysis on acute and chronic physical activity and cognition in children. All research designs were included, including experimental and cross-sectional studies. A small but significant overall effect size was found (ES = 0.32) across 44 studies. Stronger effect sizes were reported for unpublished rather than published studies, for some age groups over others (although there was no obvious linear age trend), and for some types of cognitive assessment. Outcomes measures of perceptual skills (ES = 0.49) and developmental level/academic readiness (ES = 0.39) appeared to have higher effects. The only assessment that did not differ from zero was for memory tests, and very low effects were noted for mathematical and verbal tests. There were no differences across types of activity (e.g. resistance/circuit training, PE programmes and aerobic exercise). The authors concluded that much more research was required to clarify these trends.

At the same time as the meta-analysis by Sibley and Etnier, a semi-systematic review was published by Tomporowski (2003) in which he looked at only acute exercise studies and their effect on cognitive and behavioural outcomes in young people, including those with clinical disorders, such as attention deficit hyperactivity disorder (ADHD). For those without clinical disorders, but through an analysis of only four studies, Tomporowski concluded that acute physical activity facilitates cognitive performance. Moreover, through an analysis of 16 papers on young people with clinical disorders, he also concluded that exercise interventions 'are associated with reductions in disruptive behaviours and improvements in desirable behaviours and cognitive function' (p. 354). This extends previous reviews by highlighting possible effects not only for cognition but also for certain behaviours. However, Tomporowski did say that his conclusions were 'tentative' due to rather few studies and the differences in outcomes measures used across studies.

Tomporowski et al. (2008) built on the meta-analysis by Sibley and Etnier (2003) by investigating effects for chronic physical activity participation on three outcomes: intelligence, cognition and academic achievement. In summarising studies using experimental and prospective designs, improvements in outcome variables were shown in all three studies for intelligence, in three of four studies for cognition, but only in one of five studies on academic achievement. Not all studies showing positive effects did so for all outcome variables. Similarly, three of four cross-sectional studies reported positive associations between physical fitness and academic achievement. Again, the authors of this review urged caution in drawing firm conclusions due to weak research designs and the possibility of teacher expectancy effects. Moreover, it was argued that the lack of consistency between studies may have been due to: (1) the use of some cognitive outcome tests that are not sensitive to changes in physical activity; (2) some physical activities may have better effects than others; (3) the wide range of population samples; and (4) the effects may be a function of developmental stage and age of the participants. Nevertheless, Tomporowski *et al.* concluded that 'systematic exercise programs may actually enhance the development of specific types of mental processing known to be important for meeting challenges encountered both in academics and throughout the lifespan' (p. 127).

The reviews summarised thus far tend to show some effects, but equally have many limitations. One of the problems may be that not only are many different outcomes assessed in these studies, but different domains of 'cognition' are addressed. For example, many of the reviews look at cognitive functioning test scores, while others report broader outcomes reflecting academic performance. The latter is likely to be influenced by myriad factors which may be difficult to control for in analyses. At the same time, it is exactly these kinds of outcomes that most interest educators and policy-makers. School physical education (PE), for example, has long been seen as a 'marginal' subject and given less priority than so-called 'core academic' subjects, particularly those involving numeracy and literacy. For these reasons, identifying the state of the evidence on just academic performance outcomes in relation to physical activity is important.

> Key point: Physical activity is associated with better cognitive functioning in young people, although there is much more that we need to learn.

Academic achievement outcomes

A number of reviews have now been published synthesising evidence on the relationship between physical activity and wider academic achievement outcomes and performance in children (Fedewa and Ahn, 2011; Keeley and Fox, 2009; Rasberry *et al.*, 2011; Singh *et al.*, 2012; Trudeau and Shephard, 2008). Trudeau and Shephard (2008) concluded from seven quasi-experimental studies that additional time spent in physical activity at school did not harm academic achievement, even with less time allocated to academic learning in the classroom. This conclusion was supported by a review of similar studies by Keeley and Fox (2009).

More recently, Fedewa and Ahn (2011) updated the meta-analysis by Sibley and Etnier (2003) by analysing 59 studies that addressed cognitive outcomes, most of which were academic achievement measures. The overall ES was 0.28, which is small and significant and similar to that reported by Sibley and Etnier. Larger effects were noted for outcome measures of maths achievement, IQ and reading scores. Larger effects were also noted for small group interventions, aerobic fitness programmes, and when participation was three days per week. The authors concluded that more needs to be known about potential moderators of effects, including effects for socio-economically disadvantaged youth.

In 2010, a large review was published by the US Centers for Disease Control and Prevention (Centers for Disease Control and Prevention, 2010). This was subsequently published as a peer-reviewed paper (Rasberry *et al.*, 2011). This was a far-reaching review addressing academic performance in all school-based physical activity contexts, and results were analysed by each context, including physical education, break-time (recess), classroom physical activity (e.g. activity breaks), extra-curricular physical activity (e.g. sport), and 'other school-related extra-curricular physical activity' (e.g. exercise programmes). The results are summarised in Table 5.1.

Table 5.1 shows that by using a simple head count, positive and null outcomes are fairly evenly matched. There are very few negative outcomes. However, there are many methodological issues that plague this area. First is the measurement of the key academic outcomes. Simple achievement tests may be fairly blunt instruments and a better case could be made for specific cognitive tests, especially those conducted under well-controlled lab conditions. Second, many studies use either cross-sectional designs or interventions with no blinding. The latter issue could be a serious limitation if teachers are asked to collect data and where they may be expecting positive outcomes. Third, academic achievement will be affected by many factors, and not just physical activity. These moderators or confounders are rarely studied.

One review which attempted to overcome some of these limitations was reported by Singh *et al.* (2012). They only reviewed prospective studies, with 10 being observational and four being interventions. They evaluated results using the 'best evidence synthesis' approach advocated by Slavin (1995). For a conclusion to be made that there is 'strong evidence', there must be consistent findings across at least two high-quality studies. Consistency was defined as at least 75 per cent of studies showing results in the same direction. The authors, by combining observational and intervention studies, found that there was 'strong evidence' for an association between physical activity and academic performance. However, this was based on the minimum criterion of two high-quality studies (one observational and one intervention) so may be a little optimistic. When findings are broken down, sport-related physical activity observational studies show inconsistent findings, while the three intervention studies are positive.

Verburgh *et al.* (2013) conducted a meta-analysis concerning both acute and chronic exercise but focusing only on executive functioning outcomes. They also differentiated between pre-adolescent children, adolescents and younger adults. We discuss the adult data later in the chapter. Where possible, they tried to distinguish effects for different types of executive functioning (see Table 5.3 in a later section on adults for definitions).

Acute bouts of exercise showed positive effects for children aged 6 to 12 years (ES = 0.57) and adolescents aged 13 to 17 years (ES = 0.52). However, these are all for the executive function domain of inhibition (see Table 5.3) and involved only two studies for children and three for adolescents. The only effect size for chronic exercise studies was for children (not adolescents) focusing on the executive function task of 'planning' (see Table 5.3), and this showed a small non-significant effect (ES = 0.14).

Physical activity and cognitive functioning in young people: conclusions

The association between physical activity and cognitive functioning in young people is complex. People in this age range are developing rapidly and being influenced by many factors. Moreover, studies are employing a wide range of physical activities and cognitive outcome measures, some being simple field measures of academic performance. These factors lead any conclusions to be necessarily tentative. That said, the literature does hint at the possibility of beneficial cognitive outcomes from physical activity. At worse, we may conclude that extra physical activity in schools, whether it is 'educational' (e.g. physical education) or simply 'active' (e.g. after-school activity clubs or exercise sessions), will not harm academic development. More optimistically, we may conclude that such physical activity will yield small but significant positive effects. Summary findings are shown in Table 5.2.

Key point: Physical activity has been shown to be associated with positive academic outcomes for young people. However, research designs are weak and open to bias.

Table 5.1   Summary of findings from Rasberry *et al.* (2011) for academic achievement across different school physical activity contexts.

Physical activity context	Type of study	Outcome measures	Positive outcomes[1]	Null outcomes	Negative outcomes	Comments
Physical education	Intervention	Academic achievement	11	9	1	Significant limitations in research designs and measurement. Results suggest plausibility of links between PE and academic achievement, or, at worse, no academic detriment from reallocating some classroom time to physical education.
	Non-intervention	Academic achievement	14	13	0	
Break/recess[2]	Intervention	Cognitive skills and attitudes	4	6	0	None studied academic achievement. The role of social interaction and nature of physical activity undertaken in recess needs investigating.
Classroom physical activity	Intervention	Academic achievement	5	3	0	Design limitations (e.g. lack of blinding) likely to be important. Few studies employing activity breaks, but this could be beneficial for concentration and attention. Needs investigating alongside breaks to extended sedentary (sitting) time.
Extra-curricular physical activity	Intervention	Academic achievement	1	5	0	Mixed findings suggestive of the importance of investigating the nature of this type of physical activity. Competitive sport programmes will vary in nature and type of physical activity as well as social context.
	Non-intervention	Academic achievement	13	10	1	

Notes:
1. Outcomes are numbered by total performance outcomes rather than numbers of studies.
2. Break/recess time had very few outcomes to assess beyond those studying cognitive skills in interventions studies. Results for cognitive skills are not listed here for other physical activity contexts.

Table 5.2 Summary of key findings from systematic reviews investigating the relationship between physical activity and cognitive outcomes in young people

Author (date)	Number of studies	Types of physical activity	Cognitive outcome measures	Key conclusions	Comments
Kavale and Mattson (1983)	180	Perceptual motor training	Visual perception skills, reading achievement; academic achievement; cognitive aptitude	No effects (ES = 0.082).	Meta-analysis on learning disabled children only. No motor performance effects from interventions.
Sibley and Etnier (2003)	44	PE, resistance training, aerobic, perceptual-motor	Perceptual skills, IQ, academic achievement verbal, maths, memory, academic readiness	ES = 0.32. Suggestive of PA is related to improved cognitive performance and academic achievement.	Meta-analysis of acute, chronic and cross-sectional studies.
Tomporowski (2003)	21	Various physical activities	Academic performance; cognitive performance; behaviour	Tentative conclusion that PA can have short-term positive effects on children's behaviour and cognitive performance.	Semi-systematic review investigating children with and without clinical disorders.
Tomporowski *et al.* (2008)	16	'Chronic exercise'; 'habitual PA'	Intelligence, cognition, academic achievement	No association between PA and IQ. Physical fitness associated with better cognitive processing. Tentative support for link between chronic PA and academic achievement.	Semi-systematic review.
Trudeau and Shephard (2008)	17	PE, school PA, school sports	Academic performance	PA is cross-sectionally associated with concentration, memory and classroom behaviour. Interventions show that allocation of time to PA will not harm academic performance.	Systematic review.
Keeley and Fox (2009)	17	PA	Academic performance; cognitive performance	PA cross-sectional studies: weak relationship with academic achievement. Interventions show allocation of time to PA will not harm academic performance.	Systematic review.

Fedewa and Ahn (2011)	59	PA (but coded for analysis by different types)	Academic performance; cognitive performance	ES = 0.28 (95% CI = 0.20–0.37). PA has significant positive impact on children's cognitive outcomes and academic performance.	Meta-analysis.
Rasberry et al. (2011)	50	PE, break/recess, classroom PA, extra-curricular PA	Academic performance	Mixed findings with 50% showing a positive association and 48% no association.	Systematic review.
Singh et al. (2012)	14	PA; physical fitness	Academic performance	'Strong evidence' for an association between PA and academic performance; based on the minimum criterion of two high-quality studies (one observational and one intervention).	Systematic review of prospective studies only. Physical fitness may have different outcomes from PA and should be treated separately.
Verburgh et al. (2013)	10	Acute and chronic exercise	Executive functioning	Moderate effects for acute exercise but no effect for chronic exercise.	Very a few studies when analysed separately for children and adolescents.

Notes:
PA: physical activity.
PE: physical education.

Physical activity and cognitive functioning in young people: an illustrative study

Davis and colleagues (2011) conducted a well-controlled experiment testing the effects of two doses of exercise on inactive, overweight 8- to 10-year-old children. Three groups were randomised from a sample of 171 children:

- control group (n = 60): no exercise control;
- low-dose exercise experimental group (n = 55): daily 20 minutes of exercise for 13 weeks, with 20 minutes of sedentary pursuits;
- high-dose exercise experimental group (n = 56): daily two periods of 20 minutes of exercise for 13 weeks.

The outcome variables assessed reflected three types of cognitive assessments. First, a standardised test battery was used that yielded two types of scores: (1) executive function (planning score); (2) cognitive performance through measures of attention, 'simultaneous' tests (spatial and logical questions), and 'successive' tasks (analysis or recall of stimuli arranged in sequence and formation of sounds in order); and (3) academic performance tests of mathematics and reading.

The primary study hypothesis was that exercise would improve scores on executive function but not the other cognitive tests. The academic achievement scores were analysed without a specific hypothesis. In addition to these tests, a sub-sample of children (n = 20; n = 11 in experimental conditions) was also tested for changes in brain activation through the use of functional magnetic resonance imaging (fMRI). Post-test scores, adjusted for confounders including baseline, are shown in Figure 5.1. Those in the high exercise group scored significantly higher than those in the control group on executive function and maths, and a dose–response relationship was seen. Such effects were consistent with the data from the fMRI insofar as significant changes were noted in the exercising children in the bilateral

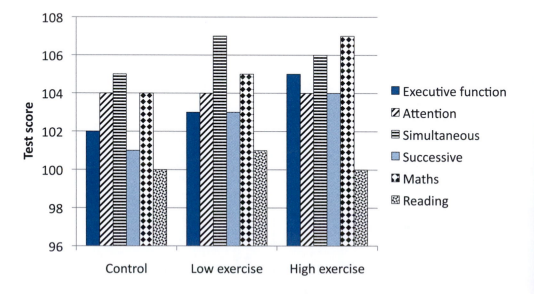

Figure 5.1   Adjusted post-test mean scores from exercise intervention

Source: Davis *et al.* (2011).

prefrontal cortex and bilateral posterior parietal cortex. For example, the prefrontal cortex is associated with planning complex cognition and decision-making. Moreover, the non-executive function measures did not show significant changes, and the scores for reading showed no change.

This is a strong study with good research design features. For example, testers were blind to group allocation and intention-to-treat analyses were used. Two levels of exercise load allowed for the testing of dose–response effects and a combination of standardised cognitive tests, academic achievement scores and objective neuro-imaging data were used. This study, therefore, provides the most convincing case to date of the effects of physical activity on cognitive functioning in children.

Physical activity and cognitive functioning in adults and older adults

The association between physical activity and cognitive functioning in adults has recently gathered momentum due to the rapidly ageing population in developed countries. This has led to a great deal of interest in cognitive decline that may accompany ageing, and whether physical activity has a role in slowing or even preventing such cognitive changes (Hogervorst *et al.*, 2012). However, not all studies have focused on the older adult range. For example, Etnier and colleagues (1997) conducted a wide-ranging meta-analysis of 134 studies and reported a mean overall ES of 0.25 – a relatively small, though significant, effect. This involved all ages, including young people. However, effect sizes differed considerably across the adult age range, with no clear age-dependent pattern (see Figure 5.2). This may be due to combining various physical activity types and contexts, including acute and chronic studies, with various measures of cognitive functioning. The number of effect sizes used in the calculation of these means is also highly variable. The effect was small for acute (ES = 0.16) and chronic (ES = 0.33) designs, but larger for cross-sectional (ES = 0.53) and mixed designs

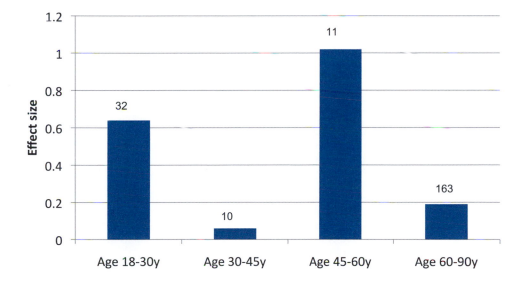

Figure 5.2   Mean effect sizes by age from meta-analysis on physical activity and cognitive functioning
Source: Etnier *et al.* (1997).

(ES = 0.54). More threats to the internal validity of both acute and chronic exercise studies yielded larger effect sizes.

As reported for young people, Verburgh *et al.* (2013) conducted a meta-analysis focusing only on executive functioning outcomes from physical activity. They differentiated between acute and chronic exercise and also between pre-adolescent children, adolescents and younger adults (aged 18 to 35 years). Where possible, they tried to distinguish effects for different types of executive functioning, including inhibition, working memory, set-shifting, cognitive flexibility, contextual memory and planning (see Table 5.3).

Results for young adults showed a moderate positive effect size for acute exercise on executive functioning (ES = 0.54). Different effects were seen for different types of executive functioning in this age group, with a small to moderate effect for inhibition from seven studies (ES = 0.42) but no effect for working memory from four studies (ES = 0.05). The one chronic exercise study included for this age group showed a moderate effect size of 0.69. These results are promising, although the number of studies is small and the studies themselves tend to have small samples. Wider conclusions from this meta-analysis were combined across all three age groups, which is a weakness given the stages of brain development seen across these ages.

The inconsistent findings reported in Etnier *et al.*'s (1997) global meta-analysis suggests that more focused analyses, such as with certain age groups or cognitive tasks, may lead to clearer conclusions. Indeed, inconsistent findings may be moderated by the type of cognitive functioning being assessed, such as simple reaction time tests or tasks requiring higher levels of executive functioning. To this end, Colcombe and Kramer (2003) argued in favour of theories of cognitive functioning being used to organise cognitive outcomes. They provided four types of theoretically driven cognitive functioning measures and then tested whether these differed in their effects from exercise. Specifically, they conducted a meta-analysis of RCTs of exercise training in adults aged 55 to 80 years. The four types of cognitive tasks tested were as follows:

- *Speed tasks*, such as reaction time and requiring low levels of cognitive processing.
- *Visuospatial tasks*, which are thought to be more susceptible to ageing than verbal tasks.

Table 5.3   Definitions of different types of executive functioning

Construct	Definition
Inhibition	The holding back or overriding of a psychological process, such as stopping, slowing down or reducing the chance of a behaviour occurring. In contrast to inhibition is impulsivity.
Working memory	Ability or capacity to keep information in your head that allows for this information to be used for current actions or responses.
Contextual memory	Recall of context such as time and place. Errors may be due to distractions or poor information-processing skills.
Set-shifting	The ability to think flexibly so that different situations may be responded to appropriately.
Cognitive flexibility	Ability to switch between different concepts and to think about several concepts simultaneously.
Planning	The ability to manage tasks, including organising thoughts and actions and anticipating consequences.

- *Controlled processing tasks*, such as tasks involving controlled and effortful processing of information but which, through learning, become more automatic over time.
- *Executive control tasks*, requiring higher levels of cognitive processing, such as coordination and working memory where mediation by the central executor is required, and they do not become automatic over time.

In their meta-analysis of RCTs, an overall effect size for experimental participants was 0.48 (calculated from the mean of pre- and post-intervention scores), showing a half-standard deviation effect from exercise on cognitive functioning. The largest effect was for executive control tasks, as predicted, although gains were seen in other categories. Results are illustrated in Figure 5.3.

> Key point: Physical fitness training in older adults is associated with superior cognitive functioning, especially for more difficult cognitive tasks.

Colcombe and Kramer (2003) tested other moderator variables and found that combining strength and aerobic exercise seemed to work best (ES = 0.59), although aerobic exercise alone was also effective (ES = 0.41). Other moderators included exercise session duration, with weaker effects for sessions of 15 to 30 minutes (ES = 0.18) compared to those of 31 to 45 minutes (ES = 0.61) and 46 to 60 minutes (ES = 0.47). The strongest effects, when looking at data by age groups, was for the 'mid-old' group aged 66 to 70 years (ES = 0.69). Those in the 'old-old' group, aged 71 to 80 years, also showed a positive effect (ES = 0.55), but was weaker for 'young-old' adults aged 55 to 65 years (ES = 0.30).

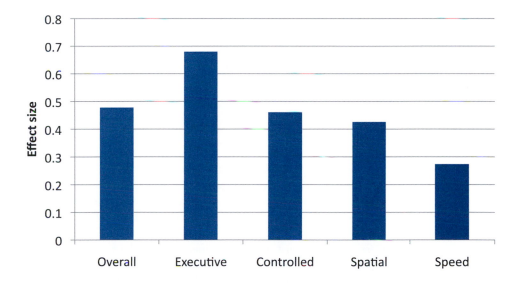

Figure 5.3 Mean effect sizes for exercising groups in RCTs of older adults. Graph shows the overall effect size and for the four types of cognitive functioning hypothesis.

Source: Colcombe and Kramer (2003).

These findings support the role of exercise and physical fitness in enhancing cognitive functioning in older adults. That the effects were moderated by the type of cognitive task assessed is particularly important as it suggests that tasks requiring higher levels of cognitive processing and involvement (executive function tasks) seem to benefit the most (Hall *et al.*, 2001). This might explain the somewhat disparate and confusing results from other reviews when such differentiation has not been made.

Unfortunately, although it was stated in the meta-analysis by Colcombe and Kramer (2003) that studies were coded on the basis of how much aerobic fitness improved during studies, this was not reported in the results. This is a pity, since improvement in fitness may be one mechanism, such as through the link to enhanced cerebral blood flow. Subsequently, Angevaren and colleagues (2008) followed up on this issue and conducted their own meta-analysis testing the hypothesis that improvements in cardiovascular fitness will account for changes in cognitive functioning in older adults without cognitive impairments.

This meta-analysis synthesised data from 11 RCTs. Effect sizes were calculated by comparing outcomes in aerobic exercise with other interventions (e.g. no treatment, strength or balance training, social activity) or no intervention. There were significant effect sizes for aerobic exercise when compared to other interventions for cognitive speed (ES = 0.26) and visual attention (ES = 0.26), and for auditory attention (ES = 0.52) and motor function (e.g. finger-tapping task) (ES = 1.17) when compared to no intervention. No other significant effects were found. However, only eight of 11 studies showed improvements in aerobic fitness and no mediation analysis was reported. That is, there was no reported test of whether changes in fitness actually accounted for changes in cognitive functioning.

Etnier *et al.* (2006) reported a meta-analysis of the relationship between aerobic fitness and cognitive functioning. They confirmed findings from earlier reviews that exercise was associated with better cognitive functioning, but could not support the view that this was due to superior physical fitness.

The findings summarised in this section of the chapter thus far refer to essentially healthy adults without existing cognitive impairment. However, in addition to taking this approach, it is also important to address the following two groups of adults concerning physical activity and cognitive functioning or decline:

•   those at risk of cognitive impairment;
•   patients with existing cognitive impairment.

Physical activity and cognitive impairment

The prevalence of cognitive impairment is rapidly increasing as the population ages. There are about 820,000 people with dementia in the UK, with 98 per cent of these cases being over the age of 65 years. Dementia is a clinical diagnosis based on a set of symptoms and history of cognitive decline, in particular of memory. However, it can also involve mood changes, and problems with communication and reasoning. There are several types of dementia, the most common being Alzheimer's disease and vascular dementia. Alzheimer's disease was first described by the German neurologist Alois Alzheimer early in the twentieth century, although reference to cognitive decline goes back to ancient times (Berchtold and Cotman, 1998). The disease involves protein plaques and tangles developing in the structure of the brain which lead to brain cells dying. Chemical changes in the brain also affect neurotransmission. Vascular dementia develops due to stroke and reduced blood supply, and often affects the ability to undertake mental planning. 'Alzheimer and other dementias' are predicted in high-income countries to become the seventh leading cause of death and the third leading cause of morbidity (disability adjusted life years) by 2030 (Mathers and Loncar, 2006).

Heyn and colleagues (2004) reported a meta-analysis on 30 RCTs concerning the effects of exercise on older adults with cognitive impairment. Participants were aged 66 to 91 years with an average age of 80 years; 72 per cent were women. Although most results concerned the physical effects of exercise, and how much patients could gain from exercise in fitness terms, they also reported positive cognitive effects, as shown in Figure 5.4.

Clifford and colleagues (2009) reviewed studies concerning exercise and the risk of developing dementia. Results from 13 studies may be summarised as follows:

- five studies showed reduced risk for dementia by 31 to 88 per cent for greater exercise frequency;
- four studies showed reduced risk of certain types of dementia;
- four studies showed no reduced risk of dementia.

The US Physical Activity Guidelines report (Physical Activity Guidelines Advisory Committee, 2008) cited 11 studies concerning the effects of physical activity on risk of dementia. The reduced risk was quantified by an odds ratio of 0.63, and nine comparisons out of 16 were significant (see Dishman *et al.*, 2013). This led to the conclusion that 'the weight of the available evidence from prospective cohort studies supports the conclusion that physical activity delays the incidence of dementia and the onset of cognitive decline associated with aging' (p. 467).

Hamer and Chida (2009) conducted a meta-analysis of prospective studies whereby baseline measures of physical activity were shown to predict the risk of overall dementia and Alzheimer's. Specifically, they analysed the most versus least active groups in each study and showed pooled relative risk to be 0.72 for dementia (i.e. 28 per cent risk reduction) and 0.55 for Alzheimer (45 per cent risk reduction). They concluded that their results suggested that

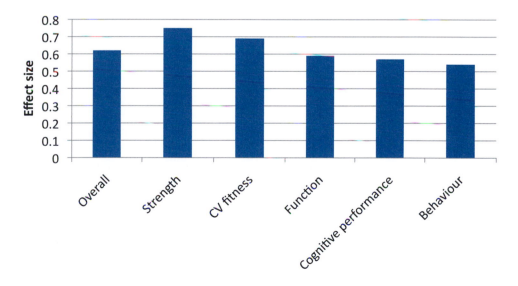

Figure 5.4 Fitness, cognitive and behavioural effects of exercise in older adults with cognitive impairment, as reported from the meta-analysis Heyn et al. (2004).

'physical activity is protective against future risk of dementia and Alzheimer's disease' (p. 9) but were unable to conclude about optimal doses of physical activity to achieve such effects.

Dishman and colleagues (2013) assessed whether it is possible to conclude that there is a causal link between physical activity and cognitive decline. They used the five epidemiologic criteria of temporal sequencing, strength of association, consistency, dose–response and plausibility. Conclusions based on comments by Dishman *et al.*, as well as other evidence from this chapter, are summarised in Table 5.4. From this evaluation, it may be concluded that there is increasing evidence suggestive of a causal link between physical activity and reduced risk of cognitive decline, at least based on the five criteria assessed. However, there is a great deal of research still needed to increase our confidence that this conclusion is robust.

> Key point: There is evidence suggesting a causal link between physical activity and a reduced risk of cognitive decline in older adults.

Physical activity and cognitive functioning in young adults: an illustrative study

Although it is more usual to select intervention evidence or prospective cohort studies when illustrating 'effects' of physical activity, here we consider a particularly interesting

Table 5.4   Judging whether physical activity is causally linked to cognitive decline (see Dishman *et al.*, 2013)

Criterion	Key question	Summary of evidence	Support
Temporal sequencing	Do low levels of PA precede cognitive decline?	Hamer and Chida (2009) showed prospective evidence of PA levels predicting future dementia.	Yes
Strength of association	How strong is the association between PA and cognitive decline?	Evidence of up to 45% lower risk of Alzheimer's from prospective PA studies, which is a meaningful effect (Hamer and Chida, 2009).	Yes
Consistency	Do studies consistently show an association and across different settings or populations?	Majority of prospective studies show effects (Dishman *et al.*, 2013).	Yes
Dose–response	Do higher levels of PA or fitness show better cognitive outcomes?	Some evidence for effects of elevated fitness on reduced risk of cognitive decline, but evidence is largely inconclusive. Limited studies have tested dose–response (Angevaren et al., 2008; Dishman et al., 2013; Heyn et al., 2004).	No
Plausibility	Are there plausible mechanisms that can explain an association between PA and cognitive decline?	There are plausible mechanisms that could explain effects of PA on cognitive impairment and decline, including increased cerebral blood flow, enhanced neural circuits, and plasticity and survival of brain neurons (Dishman *et al.*, 2013).	Yes

Note:
PA: physical activity.

observational study. Åberg and colleagues (2009) matched data from a very large cohort of Swedish males who were enlisted into national military service, with a sample size of over 1.2 million. Data from tests of cardiovascular fitness and muscular strength were analysed with linked data from a national database, including information on school achievement and socio-demographics. Data were also available on twin pairs and hence analyses could be performed estimating genetic effects. Cross-sectional and longitudinal analyses were undertaken. Key findings were as follows:

- Across nine categories of cardiovascular fitness there was a clear dose–response relationship with global intelligence and five other measures of intelligence (males aged 18 years).
- There was no association between global intelligence and muscular strength beyond the third stanine (males aged 18 years).
- Associations were largely unaffected when controlling for socio-demographic confounders.
- When testing effects for brother pairs as well as dizygous (DZ) and monozygous (MZ) twin pairs, results showed that effects were mainly associated with environmental, not genetic, factors.
- Increases in fitness between the ages of 15 and 18 years were associated with higher scores on intelligence.

The size of this study and the use of twin data are clearly strengths. However, it is not known how precise the measures were of fitness, and cognitive tests only reflected 'intelligence' rather than executive function. Nevertheless, this study provides quite convincing data that, for young men, fitness is associated with better cognitive outcomes.

Chapter summary

The association between physical activity and cognitive functioning is complex. Nevertheless, there is increasing evidence supportive of this link and, for cognitive impairment in later life, one might argue that this is showing a trend towards support for a causal connection.

In summary, therefore, we conclude the following:

- That there is evidence linking physical activity with cognitive functioning in young people, including measures of academic achievement. However, the research designs are often weak and open to bias.
- There is evidence showing an association between physical activity and cognitive functioning in adults and older adults.
- Evidence concerning the role of physical activity in reducing the risk of cognitive decline in older adults is getting stronger and is suggestive of a causal association.

While studies show that such links are evident and plausible, there are many problems with this field that require further attention. These are as follows:

1. Differentiating effects for types of physical activity and physical fitness.
2. Clarifying effects across different outcome measures for cognitive function, such as simple reaction time versus executive function tasks.

3.   Examining the physical environment and social context of physical activity and whether this is important for cognitive outcomes.
4.   Studying the association between physical activity and different cognitive indicators and disease state, such as in those asymptomatic of cognitive impairment, those at risk of impairment, and those with diagnosed cognitive impairment.
5.   Investigating neuro-biological, physiological, psychological and social mechanisms underpinning changes in cognitive function following physical activity.

References

Åberg, M.A.I., Pedersen, N.L., Toren, K., Svartengren, M., Backstrand, B., Johnsson, T. and Kuhn, H.G. (2009). Cardiovascular fitness is associated with cognition in young adulthood. *Proceedings of the National Academy of Sciences, 106*(49), 20906–20911.
Angevaren, M., Aufdemkampe, G., Verhaar, H., Aleman, A. and Vanhees, L. (2008). Physical activity and enhanced fitness to improve cognitive function in older people without known cognitive impairment. *Cochrane Database of Systematic Reviews, Issue 3* (Art. No.: CD005381). doi: 10.1002/14651858.CD005381.pub3.
Berchtold, N.C. and Cotman, C.W. (1998). Evolution in the conceptualization of dementia and Alzheimer's disease: Greco-Roman period to the 1960s. *Neurobiology of Aging, 19*(3), 173–189.
Best, J.R. (2010). Effects of physical activity on children's executive function: Contributions of experimental research on aerobic exercise. *Developmental Review, 30*, 331–351.
Biddle, S.J.H. and Asare, M. (2011). Physical activity and mental health in children and adolescents: A review of reviews. *British Journal of Sports Medicine, 45*, 886–895. doi: 10.1136/bjsports-2011-090185.
Centers for Disease Control and Prevention. (2010). *The Association Between School Based Physical Activity, Including Physical Education, and Academic Performance*. Atlanta, GA: US Department of Health and Human Services.
Clifford, A., Bandelow, S. and Hogervorst, E. (2009). The effects of physical exercise on cognitive function in the elderly: A review. In Q. Gariepy and R. Menard (eds), *Handbook of Cognitive Aging: Causes, Processes and Effects* (pp. 143–184). Hauppauge, NY: Nova Science Publishers.
Colcombe, S. and Kramer, A.F. (2003). Fitness effects on the cognitive function of older adults: A meta-analytic study. *Psychological Science, 14*(2), 125–130.
Davis, C.L., Tomporowski, P.D., McDowell, J.E., Austin, B.P., Miller, P.H., Yanasak, N.E. and Naglieri, J.A. (2011). Exercise improves executive function and achievement and alters brain activation in overweight children: A randomized, controlled trial. *Health Psychology, 30*(1), 91–98.
Dishman, R.K., Heath, G.W. and Lee, I-M. (2013). *Physical Activity Epidemiology* (2nd edn). Champaign, IL: Human Kinetics.
Etnier, J.L., Salazar, W., Landers, D.M., Petruzzello, S.J., Han, M. and Nowell, P. (1997). The influence of physical fitness and exercise upon cognitive functioning: A meta-analysis. *Journal of Sport and Exercise Psychology, 19*, 249–277.
Etnier, J.L., Nowell, P.M., Landers, D.M. and Sibley, B.A. (2006). A meta-regression to examine the relationship between aerobic fitness and cognitive performance. *Brain Research Reviews, 52*, 119–130.
Fedewa, A.L. and Ahn, S. (2011). The effects of physical activity and physical fitness on children's achievement and cognitive outcomes: A meta-analysis. *Research Quarterly for Exercise and Sport, 82*(3), 521–535.
Hall, C.D., Smith, A.L. and Keele, S.W. (2001). The impact of aerobic activity on cognitive function in older adults: A new synthesis based on the concept of executive control. *European Journal of Cognitive Psychology, 13*(1/2), 279–300. doi: 10.1080/09541440042000313.
Hamer, M. and Chida, Y. (2009). Physical activity and risk of neurodegenerative disease: A systematic review of prospective evidence. *Psychological Medicine, 39*, 3–11. doi: 10.1017/S0033291708003681.
Heyn, P., Abreu, B.C. and Ottenbacher, K.J. (2004). The effects of exercise training on elderly

persons with cognitive impairment and dementia: A meta-analysis. *Archives of Physical Medicine and Rehabilitation, 85*, 1694–1704.

Hogervorst, E., Clifford, A., Stock, J., Xin, X. and Bandelow, S. (2012). Exercise to prevent cognitive decline and Alzheimer's disease: For whom, when, what, and (most importantly) how much? (Editorial). *Journal of Alzheimer's Disease & Parkinsonism, 2*(3). doi: 10.4172/2161-0460.1000e117.

Howie, E.K. and Pate, R.R. (2012). Physical activity and academic achievement in children: A historical perspective. *Journal of Sport and Health Science, 1*, 160–169.

Kavale, K. and Mattson, P.D. (1983). 'One jumped off the balance beam': Meta-analysis of perceptual-motor training. *Journal of Learning Disabilities, 16*, 165–173.

Keeley, T.J.H. and Fox, K.R. (2009). The impact of physical activity and fitness on academic achievement and cognitive performance in children. *International Review of Sport and Exercise Psychology, 2*(2), 198–214.

Kirkendall, D.R. (1986). Effects of physical activity on intellectual development and academic performance. In G.A. Stull and H.M. Eckert (eds), *Effects of Physical Activity on Children* (pp. 49–63). Champaign, IL: Human Kinetics & American Academy of Physical Education.

Mathers, C.D. and Loncar, D. (2006). Projections of global mortality and burden of disease from 2002 to 2030. *PLoS Medicine, 3*(11), e442. doi: 10.1371/journal.pmed.0030442.

Physical Activity Guidelines Advisory Committee. (2008). *Physical Activity Guidelines Advisory Committee Report*. Washington, DC: Department of Health and Human Services.

Rasberry, C.N., Lee, S.M., Robin, L., Laris, B.A., Russell, L.A., Coyle, K.K. and Nihiser, A.J. (2011). The association between school-based physical activity, including physical education, and academic performance: A systematic review of the literature. *Preventive Medicine, 52*, S10–S20.

Sibley, B.A. and Etnier, J.L. (2003). The relationship between physical activity and cognition in children: A meta-analysis. *Pediatric Exercise Science, 15*, 243–256.

Singh, A.S., Uijtdewilligen, L., Twisk, J.W.R., van Mechelen, W. and Chinapaw, M.J.M. (2012). Physical activity and performance at school: A systematic review of the literature including a methodological quality assessment. *Archives of Pediatric and Adolescent Medicine, 166*(1), 49–55.

Slavin, R.E. (1995). Best evidence synthesis: An intelligent alternative to meta-analysis. *Journal of Clinical Epidemiology, 48*(1), 9–18.

Tomporowski, P.D. (2003). Cognitive and behavioral responses to acute exercise in youths: A review. *Pediatric Exercise Science, 15*, 348–359.

Tomporowski, P.D., Davis, C.L., Miller, P.H. and Naglieri, J.A. (2008). Exercise and children's intelligence, cognition, and academic achievement. *Educational Psychology Review, 20*, 111–131.

Trudeau, F. and Shephard, R.J. (2008). Physical education, school physical activity, school sports and academic performance. *International Journal of Behavioral Nutrition and Physical Activity, 5*(10), http://www.ijbnpa.org/content/5/1/10. doi: 10.1186/1479-5868-5-10.

Verburgh, L., Konigs, M., Scherder, E.J.A. and Oosterlaan, J. (2013). Physical exercise and executive functions in preadolescent children, adolescents and young adults: A meta-analysis. *British Journal of Sports Medicine, online first*. doi: 10.1136/bjsports-2012-091441.

Williams, H.G. (1986). The development of sensory-motor function in young children. In V. Seefeldt (ed.), *Physical Activity and Well-being* (pp. 106–122). Reston, VA: American Alliance for Health, Physical Education, Recreation, and Dance.

6 Physical activity and self-esteem

Does physical activity make you feel better about yourself?

Self-esteem is a topic that is widely spoken about by specialists and non-specialists alike. It crops up in general conversations among parents, teachers, co-workers, managers, and many more. Indeed, it is often regarded as a key part of one's mental health and well-being. Moreover, there is a widespread assumption that physical activity is a positive influence on self-esteem. For example, in her 2012 annual report, the Chief Medical Officer (CMO) for England stated that 'physical activity … can enable children and adolescents to … help to build positive personal attributes such as self-esteem and self-confidence' (https:// www.gov.uk/government/organisations/department-of-health). Yet if one thinks about this assumption more carefully, it is logical that not all physical activity experiences will enhance self-esteem. Some could undermine it! Indeed, the CMO's statement is properly circumspect in saying that physical activity can enable self-esteem development. This suggests that certain circumstances may have to be present for this to happen. In short, the association between physical activity and self-esteem is likely to be a little more complex than one might first think.

Specifically, in this chapter, we aim to:

- Define self-esteem and related components, including physical self-worth.
- Outline how self-esteem might be an antecedent as well as an outcome of physical activity.
- Comment on the different measures of self-esteem and related constructs, particularly in the physical domain.
- Appraise the evidence linking self-esteem and physical self-worth to involvement in physical activity for both young people and adults.

Self-esteem defined

Self-esteem is often seen as a key indicator of psychological well-being (Fox, 2000). The potential to enhance self-esteem is frequently used as a rationale for promoting participation, including in exercise and sport, and is a common justification for the teaching of physical education to children, and indeed for education more widely. Yet little is said about exactly what self-esteem is, how it is made up, or how different experiences might affect it.

Self-esteem reflects the degree to which individuals appraise and value themselves. It is concerned with feelings of 'good', however that is perceived. It is not the same, but is an extension of, the construct of 'self-concept'. Incorrectly, many researchers use the terms interchangeably. However, self-concept simply *describes* aspects of the self (e.g. I am a runner). Self-esteem, though, attaches a *value* to such descriptors (e.g. being a runner is important to me).

Key point: Self-concept simply *describes* aspects of the self (e.g. I am a runner) while self-esteem attaches a *value* to such descriptors (e.g. being a runner is important to me).

Self-esteem theory proposes that our global view of ourselves (global self-esteem) is underpinned by perceptions of ourselves in specific domains in our lives, such as social, academic and physical domains, and each of these domains is constructed from perceptions in relevant further sub-domains (Shavelson *et al.*, 1976). This is illustrated in Figure 6.1 whereby self-esteem is hypothesised to have a multidimensional and hierarchical structure. That is, there are many domains comprising self-esteem and there is a hierarchy going from general to more specific perceptions that we have. This means that the constructs lower down the hierarchy are more open to change but, consequently, those higher up will require more intensive or prolonged experiences to have an influence.

Self-esteem: antecedent or consequence of physical activity?

Before we appraise the evidence concerning whether physical activity is associated with self-esteem, we will outline two approaches that suggest that self-esteem could be an outcome as well as an antecedent of physical activity. In what is sometimes referred to as the 'motivational approach' or 'personal development hypothesis' (Sonstroem, 1997a, 1997b) self-esteem is

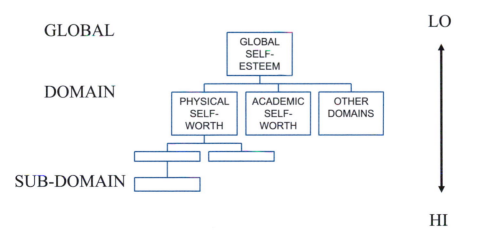

Figure 6.1   A hierarchical and multidimensional model of self-esteem

seen to act as a motivational drive or determinant of physical activity (see Figure 6.2). Here individuals high in self-esteem, or more likely in physical self-worth and related physical self-perceptions, are more likely to approach physical activity contexts because this is an area where competence and self-worth can be maintained or enhanced. It is highly improbable that people will freely choose areas where incompetence is demonstrated.

In addition, there is the 'skill development' ('personal development') hypothesis (Sonstroem, 1997a, 1997b) (see Figure 6.3). This proposes that self-esteem can be changed through experience, either positive or negative, through development in skills, task mastery, success, etc. This refers to self-esteem as an outcome of involvement in physical activity, in contrast to the motivational emphasis of the self-enhancement hypothesis. The skill development hypothesis underpins many physical education programmes for children. Of course, in reality, the two approaches are not mutually exclusive as initial involvement in physical activity, which may be externally motivated, may lead to enhanced self-perceptions of esteem and worth which, in turn, become motivators of subsequent activity. This could lead to a physical activity–self-esteem cycle (see Figure 6.4).

Measurement of self-esteem and physical self-perceptions

There are many measures of global self-esteem (Bowling, 1997). Two of the most common are the Tennessee Self-Concept Scale (Fitts, 1965) and Rosenberg's Self-Esteem Scale (Rosenberg, 1965). The Tennessee Self-Concept Scale is multifaceted with items including those assessing self-identity and self-acceptance, four domains of the moral-ethical self, personal self, family self and the physical self (e.g. 'I have a healthy body'). It is a long scale comprising 100 items in which participants state the degree of agreement that items reflect for them.

Rosenberg's Self-Esteem Scale has been used alongside measures of the physical self in the exercise psychology literature (Elavsky, 2010). Comprising only 10 items it is easy to use, and includes items such as 'I feel that I have a number of good qualities', 'on the whole, I feel satisfied with myself', and 'I feel I do not have much to be proud of'.

More contemporary and comprehensive measures have been clearly oriented towards a competence-based model of assessment of self-perceptions. Attempts at explaining human behaviour through an individual's desire to seek situations where they can display competence is not new in psychology. A comprehensive interpretation of competence motivation has been made by American developmental psychologist Susan Harter (Harter, 1978; Harter and

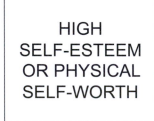

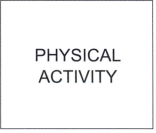

Figure 6.2   The motivational approach to physical activity and self-esteem

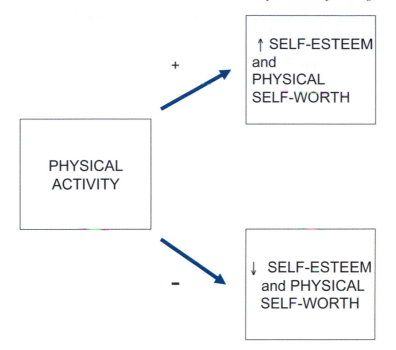

Figure 6.3   The personal development approach to physical activity and self-esteem

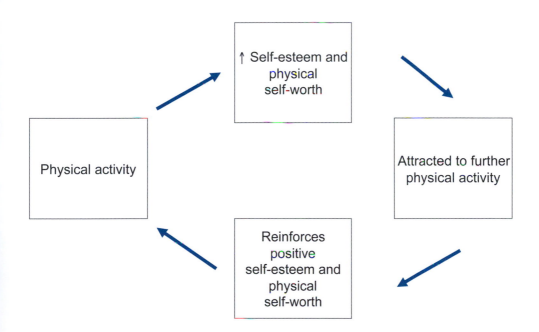

Figure 6.4   A positive physical activity and self-esteem cycle

Connell, 1984). She conceptualised competence as multidimensional by specifying domains of competence perceptions, such as scholastic and athletic competence. These domains are likely to become more differentiated with age (see Table 6.1). Second, she related self-perceptions of competence to motivational orientations and perceptions of control. Finally, she developed measuring instruments for the assessment of domains of competence and self-perceptions of adequacy.

Harter's theory suggests that individuals are motivated where their competence can be demonstrated, particularly if they also feel intrinsically oriented in that area and see themselves as having a perception of personal control. Successful mastery attempts under such conditions are associated with positive emotion and low anxiety. Harter's theory predicts that those high in perceived physical competence would be more likely to participate in physical activity. An over-reliance on perceptions of competence through traditional achievement settings (e.g. competitive sport) may make this approach less relevant to the health-related context (e.g. recreational walking) with which we are mainly concerned in this book, but nevertheless, the strength and attraction of Harter's theory centres on the development of psychometrically sound and developmentally based instruments for the testing of her model. It is also true that very low levels of perceived competence are not likely to attract people to certain behaviours. So even apparently 'competence-free' settings, such as fitness clubs, can evoke clear feelings related to competence and self-presentation that could impact upon self-esteem domains (see later in chapter).

The hierarchical structure of self-esteem has implications for research, especially when considering measurement. Many of the early studies measured only global self-esteem (GSE) but it is likely that physical activity participation will impact initially upon a sub-domain below GSE in the hierarchy which then may or may not affect GSE. In addition, although all dimensions contribute to global self-esteem, physical self-worth may be particularly important because of the position it occupies as the interface between the individual and the external world (Fox, 2000), and therefore changes in physical self-worth may be a meaningful

Table 6.1   Competence perception/adequacy sub-domains as represented in measures by Harter and colleagues

Children <8[1]	Children[2]	Students[3]	Adults[4]
Cognitive competence	Scholastic competence	Creativity	Sociability
Physical competence	Social acceptance	Intellectual ability	Job competence
Peer acceptance	Athletic competence	Scholastic competence	Nurturance
Maternal acceptance	Physical appearance	Job competence	Athletic abilities
	Behavioural conduct	Athletic competence	Physical appearance
		Appearance	Adequate provider
		Romantic relationships	Morality
		Social acceptance	Household management
		Close friendships	Intimate relationships
		Parent relationships	Intelligence
		Humour	Sense of humour
		Morality	

Sources:
1. Harter and Pike (1983).
2. Harter (1985).
3. Neeman and Harter (1986).
4. Messer and Harter (1986).

and important assessment endpoint in their own right. This is a point often missed when physical activity and self-esteem are mentioned in policy documents and in wider physical activity research.

Based on this approach, Ken Fox developed an operational measure of physical self-perceptions in which psychometrically sound scales assess the higher order construct of 'physical self-worth' (PSW) and its sub-domains of sport competence, perceived strength, physical condition and attractive body (Fox and Corbin, 1989). Figure 6.5 shows Fox's physical self-perception model based on this approach. Sub-domains are considered to be more transient and therefore less stable. For example, it is proposed that certain events are likely to affect more specific perceptions of self, such as the belief that one can jog the two miles to work, which, if reinforced over time, may eventually contribute to enhanced self-perceptions of physical condition or even physical self-worth. To this end, it is proposed that the four 'lower order' sub-domains will affect GSE only though PSW, rather than directly.

Fox and Corbin's (1989) Physical Self-Perception Profile (PSPP), therefore, measures physical self-worth and the four sub-domains of this construct just discussed and shown in Figure 6.5. Although these factors were derived initially from research on an American student population they seem to hold reasonably well with younger populations (Whitehead, 1995) and in different countries (Hagger *et al.*, 2003).

> Key point: Fox and Corbin's (1989) physical self-perception profile measures physical self-worth and the four sub-domains of sport competence, perceived strength, physical condition and attractive body.

Fox (1990) states that he uses three orientations in assessing self-perceptions: ability, learning and confidence. For the sport competence subscale, for example, he assesses perceptions of sport/athletic *ability* (e.g. '[some people] feel that they are really good at just about every sport'), ability to *learn* sport skills (e.g. '[some people] always seem to be among the quickest when it comes to learning new sports skills'), and *confidence* in the sports environment (e.g.

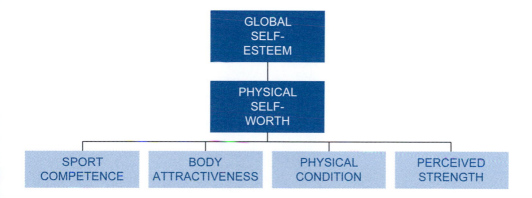

Figure 6.5 A model of physical self-perceptions proposed by Fox and Corbin
Source: Fox and Corbin (1989).

'[some people] are among the most confident when it comes to taking part in sports activities'). Comparative elements inevitably creep in, such as with reference to 'among the most confident …', even though the subject of the statement is mastery (participation) oriented. In addition, based on Harter's work, the PSPP adopts a forced-choice format whereby participants read two states, meant to be equally viable, and then choose which one reflects them. They then rate whether it is 'sort of true' or 'really true' for them. This is thought to reduce socially desirable responses, but it does add a layer of complexity that younger participants sometimes find difficult, leading to quite a large number of incorrect completed questionnaires (e.g. they tick both sides of the question). This format is shown in Figure 6.6.

What the PSPP, and other similar instruments, such as Marsh's 'Physical Self-Description Questionnaire' (PSDQ) (Marsh *et al.*, 1994), enable is for the investigation of how physical activity might affect differential aspects of self-perceptions, such as sports competence, and how these might impact upon physical self-worth and even global self-esteem. For example, participation in exercise may increase positive feelings about physical condition that may, in turn, affect physical self-worth and self-esteem. These relationships are thought to be more likely if the domain in question is seen to be important to the individual (Fox, 1998). However, Marsh and Sonstroem (1995) raise the issue of the function and specificity of importance ratings. For example, someone who perceives themselves to have low body attractiveness, but attaches high importance to attractiveness, may act in a similar way to another individual who has strong positive self-perceptions of their attractiveness and also high importance for the domain. The first person could be motivated for improvement (e.g. weight loss), whereas the second seems to demonstrate the effect of competence on

Really true for me	Sort of true for me				Sort of true for me	Really true for me
1	□ □	Some kids do very well at all kinds of sports	BUT	Other kids don't feel they are very good when it comes to sports.	□ □
2	□ □	Some kids feel uneasy when it comes to doing vigorous physical exercise	BUT	Other kids feel confident when it comes to doing vigorous physical exercise.	□ □
3	□ □	Some kids feel that they have a good-looking (fit-looking) body compared to other kids	BUT	Other kids feel that compared to most, their body doesn't look so good.	□ □
4	□ □	Some kids feel that they lack strength compared to other kids of their age	BUT	Other kids feel that they are stronger than other kids of their age.	□ □

Figure 6.6 Example items and format used in the Physical Self-Perception Profile for Adolescents

behaviour – they are motivated because they are competent or look good in, say, the Zumba class context. In other words, 'although self-concept researchers have often asked subjects to rate the importance of different self-concept domains, they may need to ask why a particular domain is important or in what situations it is important' (Marsh and Sonstroem, 1995, p. 101). That said, it is logical for self-perceptions to have greater impact when they are seen as important to the individual.

Evidence of a relationship between physical activity and self-esteem

Based on the proposals offered through the hierarchical and multidimensional model, as well as narrative reviews of the literature (e.g. Fox, 2000), it is widely thought that physical activity can enhance either physical self-worth or self-esteem, or both. However, the strength of the effect remains an important issue to identify. In this section we examine evidence, often using systematic reviews, to explore the strength of this effect in adults and young people.

Adults

McDonald and Hodgdon (1991) investigated the link between aerobic fitness training and 'self-concept' by conducting a meta-analysis of experimental training studies. This term included most standard measures of self-perceptions, including self-esteem, but also measures of body image. This weakens the ability of the study to isolate effects for more global measures of self-esteem. McDonald and Hodgdon reported an overall effect size (ES) of 0.56 from 41 studies, showing that fitness training is associated with improved ratings of the 'self'.

McDonald and Hodgdon (1991) included self-related measures from personality tests to form a 'self-esteem cluster'. This involved all measures from the 'self-concept' studies above, plus the self-sufficiency (scale Q2) and insecurity (scale O) subscales from the 16PF inventory. The ES was a 'moderate' 0.35 for the cluster.

In a more recent meta-analysis, Spence *et al.* (2005) focused specifically on studies examining self-esteem and physical activity in adults. They included 113 studies in their review, of which 71 were unpublished. The overall effect size was 0.23, showing that participation in physical activity resulted in a small, though significant, positive effect on self-esteem in adults. When Spence *et al.* explored possible moderators of this relationship they found that both fitness changes and type of programme influenced the size of the effect. Specifically, they found that a stronger effect (d = 0.32) on global self-esteem was observed in studies where there was a significant change in physical fitness compared to those where no change in fitness occurred (d = 0.15). In fact, this effect size for studies where no fitness change occurred was not significantly different from zero, suggesting that fitness change may be necessary to achieve changes in global self-esteem. In addition, compared to skills training activities (d = -0.03) larger effects were noted for exercise programmes (d = 0.26) or 'lifestyle-enrichment' programmes that included other activities alongside exercise, such as nutrition advice and relaxation (d = 0.36). Although initial fitness levels and initial levels of global self-esteem did not significantly moderate the relationship, the direction of influence was as expected, with those with lower initial fitness (d = 0.29) or lower initial self-esteem (d = 0.28) showing larger changes in global self-esteem than those reporting moderate initial fitness (d = 0.20) or self-esteem (d = 0.22). Other exercise-related variables, such as intensity, frequency, duration and length of programme, did not moderate the observed relationship. The overall effect size was also independent of sample variables, including age, gender, health status, and measurement (e.g. publication status, scale used and study quality). Results are shown in Figure 6.7.

Spence *et al.* raise an interesting point about power and sample size with respect to the studies included in the meta-analysis. As the overall effect size suggests a small treatment effect for physical activity on global self-esteem, then, in order for this effect to be detected at $\alpha = 0.05$ and power $= 0.80$ the sample size would need to be between 200 and 235. However, in 95 per cent of the studies included in the meta-analysis the sample size was less than 200. This means that some small treatment effects will be undetected and classed as non-significant.

Spence and colleagues concluded that while there is an effect for exercise on self-esteem in adults, the overall effect appears to be smaller than previously thought, and smaller than that reported by McDonald and Hodgdon (1991). If this is true, why might this be the case? First, many of the assumptions concerning an association between physical activity and self-esteem have not been based on strong data. It has often been just that – an assumption. Another possible reason for the disparity in results could relate to the constructs included under the heading of 'self-esteem' within the two meta-analyses. McDonald and Hodgdon included domain-specific self-perceptions alongside global constructs such as self-concept and self-esteem, whereas Spence *et al.* only included studies with global self-esteem as an outcome. Given that it is hypothesised that it is easier to change domain-level constructs, it is likely that the effect size reported by McDonald and Hodgdon is inflated as a result of combining results for global and sub-domain outcomes. With the development of hierarchical and multi-dimensional models, we now know that global self-esteem is affected by many life domains. Single-domain experiences, therefore, unless hugely powerful, are unlikely to affect GSE in a large way. On this basis, an effect size of around 0.2, as reported by Spence *et al.*, seems about

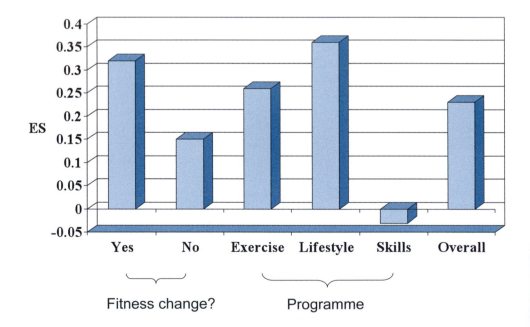

Figure 6.7 Summary effect sizes from the meta-analysis conducted by Spence *et al.*

Source: Spence *et al.* (2005).

right. Of course, if we were to meta-analyse studies investigating physical activity and *physical self-perceptions*, we would expect a higher effect. To this extent, we may well be measuring the wrong thing in GSE, or at least only part of the picture and a part least likely to change.

Spence *et al.* found that larger effects were observed for studies where participants improved their physical fitness, and this is more akin to the studies included in the meta-analysis by McDonald and Hodgdon. However, the conclusion concerning physical fitness is in contrast to earlier notions where the effects on self-esteem were thought to result from physical activity per se rather than rely on fitness gains (Sonstroem, 1984). Further work exploring fitness changes and perceptions of fitness changes is required.

> Key point: There is a small but significant effect of physical activity on self-esteem for adults.

Physical activity and self-esteem in adults: an illustrative study

A good example of a study examining the link between physical activity and the structure of self-esteem in adults is described here. Elavsky (2010) examined the hierarchical and multidimensional structure of self-esteem by exploring how physical activity in middle-aged women was related to global self-esteem and physical self-worth sub-components over a two-year period. The study participants were 143 women who had previously participated in a four-month RCT promoting exercise. The women completed physical activity and self-esteem questionnaires at the start and end of the RCT, and again two years after the RCT concluded. Physical activity was assessed by self-report using the Aerobics Center Longitudinal Study Physical Activity Survey (Kohl *et al.*, 1988) which allows for the calculation of weekly energy expenditure in leisure-time physical activity. Global self-esteem was assessed using the Rosenberg Self-Esteem Scale (Rosenberg, 1965) and the physical sub-domain was measured using the physical condition, strength and body attractiveness subscales of the Physical Self-Perception Profile (Fox and Corbin, 1989). In addition, self-efficacy and BMI were also assessed. A two-step analysis was performed. Step one examined the cross-sectional relationships between physical activity, BMI and self-efficacy and self-esteem measures using the post-intervention data and controlling for pre-intervention scores. Step two explored the longitudinal relationships between variables over the two-year follow-up period. The cross-sectional analysis showed significant ($p < 0.05$) direct effects of physical activity ($\beta = 0.14$), exercise self-efficacy ($\beta = 0.49$) and BMI ($\beta = -0.27$) on the physical condition self-domain, and BMI ($\beta = -0.61$) on the body attractiveness sub-domain. The sub-domains of physical condition ($\beta = 0.40$), attractiveness ($\beta = 0.43$) and strength ($\beta = 0.15$) were all significantly associated with physical self-worth which, in turn, had a direct effect on global self-esteem ($\beta = 0.40$).

These cross-sectional results offer some support for the hierarchical and multidimensional structure of self-esteem but stronger evidence comes from examining relationships over time, and seeing how changes in physical activity are related to changes in global self-esteem and its sub-components. In the second part of the analysis, Elavsky looked at how changes over two years in physical activity, exercise self-efficacy and BMI related to changes in self-esteem. Results showed that increases in physical activity ($\beta = 0.29$) and self-efficacy ($\beta = 0.34$), and decreases in BMI ($\beta = -0.19$), were associated with improvements in perceptions of physical condition ($p < 0.05$). Decreases in BMI were also related to increases in perceptions of body attractiveness ($\beta = -0.31$; $p < 0.05$). In addition, there were weak associations between decreases in BMI and increases in strength self-perceptions ($\beta = -0.12$; $p < 0.10$). At the sub-domain level, the increases in physical condition ($\beta = 0.21$) and body attractiveness self-perceptions ($\beta = 0.48$) were significantly associated with increases in physical self-worth which were, in turn, associated with increases in global self-esteem ($\beta = 0.25$). This second analysis offers stronger support for the hierarchical structure of self-esteem and demonstrates that physical activity participation can lead to long-term positive effects on self-esteem in middle-aged women.

Young people

Early reviews concluded that physical activity is associated with the development of self-esteem in young people (Calfas and Taylor, 1994; Gruber, 1986; Mutrie and Parfitt, 1998). For example, in a very early meta-analysis of play and physical education programmes for children, Gruber (1986) calculated an overall ES of 0.41 for self-esteem from 27 studies. Over 60 per cent of the studies produced positive effects on self-esteem. These results support a positive effect for physical activity on the self-esteem of youngsters. A more recent meta-analysis examined whether exercise interventions improved global self-esteem among children and young people aged 3 to 20 years (Ekeland *et al.*, 2004, 2005). This included eight trials that compared an exercise-alone intervention to a no-intervention control and found a moderate effect in favour of the intervention group (ES = 0.49). The relationship did not appear to be affected by type of exercise (although seven of the eight studies were based on aerobic exercise) or duration of the intervention (<10 weeks vs. >10 weeks). When the authors compared interventions with healthy children to interventions with children at risk of defined health problems they found significant findings only for this latter group (ES = 0.49). The trials were criticised for being mostly small scale, of short duration, and with no follow-up, meaning that sustainability of changes could not be assessed. A further four trials were identified that compared the effects of exercise as part of a comprehensive intervention package against no-intervention control groups and again a moderate positive effect on self-esteem in favour of the intervention was found (ES = 0.51). The size of this effect increased when the only study with healthy participants was excluded (ES = 0.64). It was suggested that the effects of exercise may have been underestimated in both sections of the review because all the studies used 'usual activity' as the control treatment and therefore comparisons are not between exercise and complete physical inactivity. Ekelund *et al.* concluded that exercise can lead to improvements in self-esteem in young people, at least in the short term and among those considered at risk.

Attempting to bring together the reviews on physical activity and mental health in young people, Biddle and Asare (2011, p. 889) conducted a 'review of reviews', including self-esteem. They concluded that:

> physical activity can lead to improvements in self-esteem, at least in the short term. However, there is a paucity of good quality research. Moreover, global measures of self-esteem can be affected by many factors beyond physical activity. Hence, measures of physical aspects of the self ... might be better targets for intervention.

Key point: Physical activity can lead to small improvements in self-esteem for young people.

Physical activity and self-esteem in young people: an illustrative study

A good example of a study examining the link between physical activity and self-esteem in young people is described here. Schmalz and colleagues (2007) were interested in exploring the links between participation in physical activity and global self-esteem among girls as they moved from late childhood into early adolescence. Specifically, the physical activity and global self-esteem of 197 non-Hispanic white girls were assessed at 9, 11 and 13 years of age. The strength of this longitudinal design is that it allows the direction of the relationship to be examined. That is, by following the same children over time the researchers were able to explore to what extent physical activity participation influenced future global self-esteem and, conversely, to what extent global self-esteem influenced future physical activity participation. Physical activity was assessed by a composite of three measures: self-reported inclination towards physical activity, self-reported participation in team sports and organised activities, and physical fitness measured using a shuttle run test (the Progressive Aerobic Cardiovascular Endurance Run) (Leger and Lambert, 1982). The use of a composite score including fitness as an indirect measure of physical activity was to try to overcome some of the limitations associated with a self-reported physical activity measure. Global self-esteem was measured using Harter's (1985) Self-Perception Profile for Children.

When the researchers analysed their data they found that self-esteem did not predict future physical activity participation, but higher physical activity participation at ages 9 and 11 years predicted higher self-esteem at 11 and 13 years respectively. However, these effects were influenced by age and BMI. For example, although there was always a significant effect of physical activity on future self-esteem, the effect was stronger between the ages of 9 and 11 years compared to between the ages of 11 and 13 years. Likewise, the positive effect of physical activity on self-esteem was greater in girls with above-average BMI. The researchers noted that as the girls in the study generally reported high levels of self-esteem, this may have masked the extent of the relationship between physical activity and self-esteem, meaning that the results may underestimate the benefits of physical activity in a general population of adolescent girls. The study concluded that physical activity promotes positive self-esteem among girls, particularly for younger, pre-adolescent girls and those with higher BMI.

> Key point: The belief that physical activity improves self-esteem is too simplistic. Physical activity can enhance self-esteem, and this is likely due to changes in physical self-perceptions.

Older adults

The physical health benefits of regular physical activity in older adults are well established, and there is evidence for improved mood and psychological well-being (see Chapter 2) and a reduction in depression (see Chapter 3). However, despite the importance of self-esteem to psychological well-being and evidence that self-esteem declines with age (Robins *et al.*, 2002), researchers have paid less attention to the effect of physical activity on the self-perceptions of older adults (Moore *et al.*, 2012; Opdendacker *et al.*, 2009; Taylor *et al.*, 2004). Systematic reviews and meta-analyses looking at physical activity and self-esteem have all focused on younger populations. In the one meta-analysis focused on physical activity and psychological well-being in older age (defined as mean age of 54 years and older), Netz *et al.* (2005) combined studies examining different aspects of self-perceptions into a cluster they called 'view of self'. This included studies examining self-efficacy, self-worth, self-esteem, self-concept, body image and perceived physical fitness. They found a small positive effect of physical activity on older adults' 'view of self', suggesting that physical activity may influence the self-perceptions of older adults, but unfortunately this study does not allow us to isolate the effect of physical activity on self-esteem. Several exemplar studies will be presented below to look more closely at this relationship.

Li *et al.* (2002) used an RCT to examine whether a six-month Tai Chi exercise intervention influenced global self-esteem and physical self-worth in older adults (mean age 73.2 years). Intervention participants took part in a 60-minute Tai Chi exercise class two times per week. Control participants continued their usual daily activities. Global self-esteem was assessed with the Rosenberg Self-Esteem Scale and domain-specific self-esteem was assessed with the Physical Self-Perception Profile. The sport competence subscale was not included because it was not thought relevant to the intervention activity or this age group. Assessments took place at baseline, in the middle of the intervention (three months) and at the end of the intervention (six months). Participants in the Tai Chi group showed improved levels of global self-esteem, physical self-worth and in the sub-domains of attractive body, strength and physical condition. The authors concluded that Tai Chi has the potential to positively influence facets of physical self-worth and self-esteem in older adults, which may lead to improvements in perceived quality of life. They also concluded that the results offered support for the hierarchical and multidimensional structure of self-esteem. While this study provided some insight into the relationship between physical activity and self-esteem in older adults, it only examined the effects within the intervention period and did not evaluate the long-term effect of the intervention.

McAuley *et al.* (2000) conducted a randomised controlled trial in inactive adults aged 60 to 75 years. Participants were randomised to either a walking intervention (n = 85) or a stretching/toning intervention (n = 89). The intervention lasted six months, and each group met for 50 minutes three times per week. The researchers were interested in examining the effects of the two different types of exercise on self-esteem, and whether the multidimensional hierarchical structure of self-esteem was supported. Self-esteem was assessed via the Rosenberg Self-Esteem Scale and domain-specific self-esteem was assessed via the physical self-worth, physical condition, attractive body and strength subscales of the Physical Self-Perception Profile. The sport competence subscale was not included owing to the nature of the sample (inactive older adults) and the modes of activity emphasised in the intervention. Assessments took place at baseline, at the end of the intervention (six months) and after a six-month follow-up (12 months). Results showed that both groups showed increases in all self-esteem measures during the intervention, followed by small but significant decreases during the follow-up. The only difference between the two groups was for strength esteem, with the toning group showing significantly greater increases during the trial and smaller decreases during follow-up.

These results demonstrate that physical activity can enhance self-esteem in older adults and that different types of physical activity could potentially be used to promote self-esteem. However, any gains in self-esteem are likely to only be maintained if physical activity participation is sustained.

The data in this study were also used to examine the hierarchical structure of self-esteem and results showed that, as predicted, changes in physical activity were related to changes in the body condition, body attractiveness and strength esteem subscales in both groups. The changes in body attractiveness and physical condition were then related to changes in physical self-worth. These results broadly support the hierarchical and multidimensional nature of self-esteem. Four years later the authors followed up the participants from this study and showed that these structural relationships were consistent across time, with older adults who reported the greatest reductions in physical activity also reporting the greatest reductions in sub-domain esteem (McAuley *et al.*, 2005).

A similar pattern of results was reported in a non-randomised control trial with older adults living in Belgium (Opdenacker *et al.*, 2009). Participants (mean age 67 years) were randomised to either a lifestyle physical activity intervention (n = 60) or a structured exercise intervention (n = 60). A control group (n = 66) was recruited separately for a 'checkup of fitness/health status'. The lifestyle group received an individualised physical activity programme, designed to be done at home. This group also received 16 booster phone calls during the intervention. The structured exercise intervention consisted of three sessions of 60 to 90 minutes each week in a fitness centre. Participants completed their own individualised exercise programme during each session. Self-esteem was assessed via the Rosenberg Self-Esteem Scale, and domain-specific self-esteem was assessed via the Physical Self-Perception Profile. Unlike the previous two studies, the sport competence subscale was included in this study. Assessments were made at baseline, post-intervention (11 months) and follow-up (23 months). Results showed that both interventions led to positive effects on the self-perceptions and self-esteem in both the short and long term. During the intervention the lifestyle group showed improvements in physical condition, sport competence, body attractiveness and physical self-worth. However, only the increase in body attractiveness remained significant at follow-up. In the structured exercise group during the intervention there were improvements in physical condition and sport competence, and these changes remained at follow-up. The effect sizes for these changes were in the range of 0.40 to 0.66, which is comparable to studies with other age groups (Spence *et al.*, 2005).

These three studies provide evidence of the potential for physical activity to influence the self-perceptions of older adults and that the structure of self-esteem is similar across different ages. The influence of physical activity does not appear limited to a specific type of activity, with positive results demonstrated for walking programmes, gym-based activities, lifestyle activities and Tai Chi. However, continued participation seems important to the maintenance of these effects.

Key point: Physical activity can influence the self-perceptions of older adults and is not limited to a specific type of activity, with positive results demonstrated for walking programmes, gym-based activities, lifestyle activities and Tai Chi.

Physical activity and self-esteem: further issues

It is our impression that the literature on physical activity and self-esteem has not developed greatly since the publication of our previous edition of this book. To encourage a wider view of this field, we discuss briefly the following topics:

- self-enhancement;
- self-presentation;
- unconditional self-worth;
- true vs. contingent self-esteem.

Self-enhancement and self-presentational concerns

We have known for a long time in psychology that people are attracted to areas that yield positive outcomes and withdraw or discount areas where possible negative outcomes may occur. This has important implications for physical activity interventions and self-esteem. We need to promote physical activities that are likely to be seen as positive and where threats to self-esteem are low or minimal. Given that self-esteem perceptions are often comparative (i.e. involve some perception of competence relative to others), we need to be cautious about promoting physical activities where this type of environment dominates. Many people's perceptions of their physical competence are based on views they developed in school physical education contexts, and much of this is still dominated by sport. To this end, people need greater exposure to non-competitive physical activities (e.g. fitness, recreational activity) to hopefully gain psychological well-being without threats to self-esteem. If sport is the medium of physical activity, the environment must allow for inclusive experiences where self-improvement and effort are rewarded.

Related to this is the notion of self-presentation. Physical appearance, gestures and movement, public self-consciousness, weight, appearance and physique anxiety, and modesty are all constructs listed in the contents page of Leary's (1995) book on 'Self-presentation'. Clearly, there is great potential for using such constructs in furthering our understanding of physical activity and self-perceptions in physical activity contexts.

Self-presentational concerns may affect physical activity choice, such as when one perceives the activity to be incompatible with one's image (e.g. in aerobic dance or lifting weights), or where anxiety is felt in displaying low levels of physical competence. As Leary (1992) says, 'people are unlikely to devote themselves to activities that convey impressions that are inconsistent with their roles, others' values, or social norms' (p. 342).

Hart and colleagues (1989), for example, have studied the construct of 'social physique anxiety'. Specifically, they propose that people high in such anxiety, in comparison to those who are not anxious, 'are likely to avoid situations in which their physique is under scrutiny of others (e.g. swimming in public) … avoid activities that accentuate their physiques (including aerobic activities that might be beneficial to them) … and attempt to improve their physiques through a variety of means, some of which may be harmful (e.g., fasting)' (p. 96). The National Fitness Survey in England in the early 1990s showed that concerns about lack of sports competence were major barriers to participation in physical activity (Sports Council and Health Education Authority, 1992). How generalisable such feelings are remains to be seen. For some individuals, feelings of 'not being the sporty type' may generalise across many different physical activities, whereas for others they may only affect one or two specific activities. Indeed, most physical activities, such as sports, occur in such public settings that self-presentational issues are hard to ignore. Coupled with this is the widespread social acceptance and admiration of physical expertise. This means that social anxiety in physical activity contexts is likely to be common. People are more likely to experience social anxiety when they are motivated to make desirable impressions on others but have low feelings of self-efficacy in being able to do so. In summary, future work on physical activity and self-esteem may need to account for the issues of self-enhancement and self-presentational concerns.

Unconditional self-worth and true vs. contingent self-esteem

It is most common to judge our feelings of self-esteem and self-worth relative to other people. It is actually hard not to do so. But to have self-esteem based solely on 'achievements', performance and behaviours is limiting and may not always be psychologically healthy. Parents are often advised that their love and regard for their own children should be unconditional and not based on some external comparative standard. This is rarely reflected in models of self-esteem or measurement and should be something we take more account of.

Related to this is the notion of 'true' vs. 'contingent' self-esteem. As Deci and Ryan (1995) propose, true self-esteem develops as one acts in accordance with one's own volition (meeting the need for autonomy), experiences a sense of efficacy (meeting the need for competence), and is loved or regarded based on who they are and not what they have achieved (need for social relatedness). As such, true self-esteem is 'more stable, more securely based in a solid sense of self' (Deci and Ryan, 1995, p. 32). In contrast, a contingent self-esteem is 'feelings about oneself that … are dependent on matching some external standard of excellence or living up to some interpersonal or intrapsychic expectations' (p. 32). This means that it is more reliant on social comparison, which can be a more fragile basis for self-perceptions. The notions of true or contingent self are rarely discussed in the literature concerning physical activity and self-esteem, yet the underlying theoretical perspectives of Self-Determination Theory, offered by Deci and Ryan (2002), are well known in exercise psychology.

Chapter summary

Self-esteem is often seen as a key component of mental health and well-being. The potential for physical activity to improve self-esteem is often used as a rationale for the promotion of physical activity programmes. This chapter has examined evidence for this relationship. Based on this evidence we conclude the following:

- There is evidence supporting the multidimensional, hierarchical structure of self-esteem.
- Physical activity has a small to moderate effect on self-perceptions.
- The effects of physical activity are greatest at the physical sub-domain level (e.g. sport competence, body attractiveness, physical strength and physical condition), but changes at this lower level lead to favourable changes in physical self-worth, which can then lead to changes in global self-esteem.
- The relationship between physical activity and self-esteem may be observed, regardless of the age of participants.
- Self-esteem benefits can be gained from a variety of physical activities.

References

Biddle, S.J.H. and Asare, M. (2011). Physical activity and mental health in children and adolescents: A review of reviews. *British Journal of Sports Medicine*, 45, 886–895. doi: 10.1136/bjsports-2011-090185.

Bowling, A. (1997). *Measuring Health: A review of quality of life measurement scales* (2nd edn). Buckingham: Open University Press.

Calfas, K.J. and Taylor, W.C. (1994). Effects of physical activity on psychological variables in adolescents. *Pediatric Exercise Science, 6*, 406–423.

Deci, E.L. and Ryan, R.M. (1995). Human autonomy: The basis for true self-esteem. In M. Kernis (ed.), *Efficacy, Agency and Self-esteem* (pp. 31–49). New York: Plenum Press.

—— (eds). (2002). *Handbook of Self-determination Research*. Rochester: The University of Rochester Press.

Ekeland, E., Heian, F., Hagen, K.B., Abbott, J. and Nordheim, L.V. (2004). Exercise to improve self-esteem in children and young people. *The Cochrane Database of Systematic Reviews*, Issue 1. Art. No.:CD003683. doi:003610.001002/14651858. CD14003683.pub14651852.

Ekeland, E., Heian, F. and Hagen, K.B. (2005). Can exercise improve self esteem in children and young people? A systematic review of randomised controlled trials. *British Journal of Sports Medicine, 39,* 792–798.

Elavsky, S. (2010). Longitudinal examination of the exercise and self-esteem model in middle-aged women. *Journal of Sport and Exercise Psychology, 32,* 862–880.

Fitts, W.H. (1965). *Tennessee Self-concept Scale Manual.* Nashville, TN: Counselor Recordings and Tests.

Fox, K.R. (1990). *The Physical Self-perception Profile Manual.* DeKalb, IL: Office of Health Promotion, Northern Illinois University.

Fox, K.R. (1998). Advances in the measurement of the physical self. In J. L. Duda (Ed.), *Advances in sport and exercise psychology measurement* (pp. 295–310). Morgantown, WV: Fitness Information Technology.

———. (2000). The effects of exercise on self-perceptions and self-esteem. In S.J.H. Biddle, K.R. Fox and S.H. Boutcher (eds), *Physical Activity and Psychological Well-being* (pp. 88–117). London: Routledge.

Fox, K.R. and Corbin, C.B. (1989). The Physical Self Perception Profile: Development and preliminary validation. *Journal of Sport and Exercise Psychology, 11,* 408–430.

Gruber, J.J. (1986). Physical activity and self-esteem development in children: A meta-analysis. In G.A. Stull and H.M. Eckert (eds), *Effects of Physical Activity on Children* (pp. 30–48). Champaign, IL: Human Kinetics.

Hagger, M.S., Biddle, S.J.H., Chow, E.W., Stambulova, N. and Kavussanu, M. (2003). Physical self-perceptions in adolescence: Generalizability of a hierarchical multidimensional model across three cultures. *Journal of Cross-Cultural Psychology, 34,* 611–628.

Hart, E.A., Leary, M.R. and Rejeski, W.J. (1989). The measurement of social physique anxiety. *Journal of Sport and Exercise Psychology, 11,* 94–104.

Harter, S. (1978). Effectance motivation reconsidered: Toward a developmental model. *Human Development, 21,* 34–64.

———. (1985). *Manual for the Self-Perception Profile for Children.* Denver, CO: University of Denver.

Harter, S. and Connell, J.P. (1984). A model of children's achievement and related self perceptions of competence, control and motivational orientations. In J.G. Nicholls (ed.), *Advances in Motivation and Achievement. III. The development of achievement motivation* (pp. 219–250). Greenwich, CT: JAI Press.

Harter, S. and Pike, R. (1983). *Procedural Manual to Accompany the Pictorial Scale of Perceived Competence and Social Acceptance for Young Children.* Denver, CO: University of Denver.

Kohl, H.W., Blair, S.N., Paffenbarger, R.S., Macera, C.A. and Kronenfeld, J.J. (1988). A mail survey of physical activity habits as related to measured physical fitness. *American Journal of Epidemiology, 127,* 1228–1239.

Leary, M.R. (1992). Self presentational processes in exercise and sport. *Journal of Sport and Exercise Psychology, 14,* 339–351.

———. (1995). *Self-presentation: Impression management and interpersonal behavior.* Dubuque, IO: Wm C. Brown.

Leger, L.A. and Lambert, J. (1982). A multistage 20-m shuttle run test to predict VO2max. *European Journal of Applied Physiology, 49,* 1–12.

Li, F., Harmer, P., Chaumeton, N.R., Duncan, T.E. and Duncan, S. (2002). Tai chi as a means to enhance self-esteem: A randomized controlled trial. *Journal of Applied Gerontology, 21,* 70–89.

Marsh, H.W. and Sonstroem, R.J. (1995). Importance ratings and specific components of physical self-concept: Relevance to predicting global components of self-concept and exercise. *Journal of Sport and Exercise Psychology, 17,* 84–104.

Marsh, H.W., Richards, G.E., Johnson, S., Roche, L. and Tremayne, P. (1994). Physical Self-Description Questionnaire: Psychometric properties and the multitrait-multimethod analysis of relations to existing instruments. *Journal of Sport and Exercise Psychology, 16,* 270–305.

McAuley, E., Blissmer, B., Katula, J., Duncan, T.E. and Mihalko, S.L. (2000). Physical activity, self-esteem, and self-efficacy relationships in older adults: A randomized controlled trial. *Annals of Behavioral Medicine, 22*(2), 131–139.

McAuley, E., Elavsky, S., Motl, R., Konopack, J.F., Hu, L. and Marquez, D.X. (2005). Physical activity, self-efficacy, and self-esteem: Longitudinal relationships in older adults. *Journal of Gerontology: Psychological Sciences, 60B*, 268–275.

McDonald, D.G. and Hodgdon, J.A. (1991). *Psychological Effects of Aerobic Fitness Training: Research and theory*. New York: Springer-Verlag.

Messer, B. and Harter, S. (1986). *Manual for the Adult Self-Perception Profile*. Denver, CO: University of Denver.

Moore, J.B., Mitchell, N.G., Beets, M.W. and Bartholomew, J.B. (2012). Physical self-esteem in older adults: A test of the indirect effect of physical activity. *Sport, Exercise and Performance Psychology, 1*, 231–241.

Mutrie, N. and Parfitt, G. (1998). Physical activity and its link with mental, social and moral health in young people. In S.J.H. Biddle, J.F. Sallis and N. Cavill (eds), *Young and Active? Young people and health-enhancing physical activity: Evidence and implications* (pp. 49–68). London: Health Education Authority.

Neeman, J. and Harter, S. (1986). *Manual for the Self-Perception Profile for College Students*. Denver, CO: University of Denver.

Netz, Y., Wu, M-J., Becker, B.J. and Tenebaum, G. (2005). Physical activity and psychological well-being in advanced age: A meta-analysis of intervention studies. *Psychology and Aging, 20*(2), 272–284.

Opdendacker, J., Dececluse, C. and Boen, F. (2009). The longitudinal effects of a lifestyle physical activity intervention and a structured exercise intervention on physical self-perceptions and self-esteem in older adults. *Journal of Sport and Exercise Psychology, 31*, 743–760.

Robins, R.W., Trzesniewski, K.H., Tracy, J.L., Gosling, S.D. and Potter, J. (2002). Global self-esteem across the lifespan. *Psychology and Aging, 17*, 423–434.

Rosenberg, M. (1965). *Society and the Adolescent Self-image*. Princeton, NJ: Princeton University Press.

Schmalz, D.L., Deane, G.D., Birch, L.L. and Davison, K.K. (2007). A longitudinal assessment of the links between physical activity and self-esteem in early adolescent non-hispanic females. *Journal of Adolescent Health, 41*(6), 559–565.

Shavelson, R.J., Hubner, J.J. and Stanton, G.C. (1976). Self-concept: Validation of construct interpretations. *Review of Educational Research, 46*, 407–441.

Sonstroem, R.J. (1984). Exercise and self-esteem. *Exercise and Sport Sciences Reviews, 12*, 123–155.

——. (1997a). Physical activity and self-esteem. In W.P. Morgan (ed.), *Physical Activity and Mental Health* (pp. 127–143). Washington, DC: Taylor & Francis.

——. (1997b). The physical self-system: A mediator of exercise and self-esteem. In K.R. Fox (ed.), *The Physical Self: From motivation to well-being* (pp. 3–26). Champaign, IL: Human Kinetics.

Spence, J.C., McGannon, K.R. and Poon, P. (2005). The effect of exercise on global self-esteem: A quantitative review. *Journal of Sport and Exercise Psychology, 27*, 311–334.

Sports Council and Health Education Authority. (1992). *Allied Dunbar National Fitness Survey: Main findings*. London: Author.

Taylor, A., Cable, N., Faulkner, G., Hillsdon, M., Narici, M. and van der Bij, A. (2004). Physical activity and older adults: A review of health benefits and the effectiveness of interventions. *Journal of Sports Sciences, 22*, 703–725.

Whitehead, J.R. (1995). A study of children's physical self-perceptions using an adapted physical self-perception profile questionnaire. *Pediatric Exercise Science, 7*, 132–151.

Part III

Physical activity correlates and theories

7 Physical activity correlates and barriers

Factors related to being active

What factors seem to be related to higher or lower levels of physical activity? The behavioural epidemiology framework shows that interventions designed to change behaviour need to be underpinned by evidence on the key factors thought to be associated with the behaviour. These factors are 'correlates' or 'determinants'. These may include barriers to the behaviour.

Purpose of the chapter

The purpose of this chapter is to summarise the evidence concerning the correlates of physical activity, including barriers to participation. This is a fundamental aspect of the psychology of physical activity, although it includes more than just psychological constructs. Specifically, in this chapter we aim to:

- summarise the evidence concerning the correlates of physical activity for young people, adults and older adults;
- discuss the key enablers and barriers to physical activity;
- consider the literature dealing with descriptive approaches to motivation, such as that addressing children's and adult's participation motives.

It is often not easy to start, maintain or resume some health behaviours. Physical activity is certainly no exception to this. The complex psychological, social, environmental and biological influences on involvement in physical activity merely highlight the difficulty of singling out one perspective, theory or approach in attempting to understand the field. Nevertheless, discussion concerning physical activity inevitably covers the topics of 'influences' and 'barriers'. In introducing his report on physical activity and health in 2004, the Chief Medical Officer for England at the time, Professor Sir Liam Donaldson, said that 'we now need a culture shift' to achieve national physical activity goals and that 'current levels of physical activity are a reflection of personal attitudes about time use and of cultural and societal values' (Department of Health, 2004, pp. iii–iv). Understanding personal 'enablers' or 'drivers', as well as barriers – individual, social, cultural and environmental – represents our own challenge as researchers. These are the 'correlates' of physical activity – factors thought to be associated with participation in physical activity. It reflects phase 3 of the behavioural epidemiology framework. It is important to identify factors that may be associated with the adoption and maintenance of behaviour so that such factors can be targeted in interventions. However, it is not always easy to identify correlates or barriers for some sectors of the population, as much of the research has focused on only a few industrialised countries. More research is needed on low- and middle-income countries and across different domains of physical activity, such as travel, work, recreation and sport (Bauman *et al.*, 2012). Moreover, those with disabilities are often under-researched (Jaarsma *et al.*, 2014; Rimmer *et al.*, 2004).

How correlates might function in behaviour change

Correlates research represents an important step in the design of effective interventions for at least two reasons: (1) correlates of physical activity which cannot be changed (e.g. sex, age; often referred to as 'moderators') may be used to identify target groups who may be at particular risk of low levels of physical activity; and (2) correlates which can be changed become the focus of intervention strategies ('mediators' of change). This is because it is hypothesised that changes in these correlates will lead to changes in physical activity. For example, interventions may identify individuals who perceive a key barrier to be 'lack of time' (time thereby being a correlate of physical activity), and then to seek ways to overcome such perceptions. The correlate of 'time' acts as a mediator of physical activity behaviour change. This mediating variable model has been put forward as a way of understanding behaviour change, and how correlates need to be changed for behaviour to change (Baranowski *et al.*, 1998; Rhodes and Pfaeffli, 2010).

The meditating variable model is represented in its simplest form in Figure 7.1. For physical activity interventions the framework suggests that changes in physical activity are the result of changes in mediating variables such as barriers, and these changes in mediating variables are the result of interventions that were designed to induce change in these variables (Baranowski and Jago, 2005). During evaluation of interventions it is important that these hypothesised mediator pathways are assessed, as this allows critical components of interventions to be identified (MacKinnon *et al.*, 2000), and provides evidence of 'what works' for changing behaviour (Lubans *et al.*, 2008). Correlates identified as mediators may then be

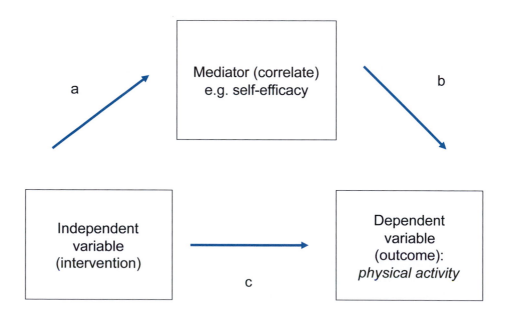

Figure 7.1   The role of correlates as mediators of physical activity behaviour change

employed in subsequent interventions and those demonstrated to not mediate behaviour change discarded. Mediation analysis also helps to improve theories of behaviour change. For example, if an intervention results in physical activity behaviour change, but this change is not explained by the hypothesised mediating variables within the underlying theoretical models, this indicates that the theory is incomplete and needs further development (Baranowski *et al.*, 1998).

According to Baron and Kenny (1986), to demonstrate that a variable functions as a mediator, certain conditions must be met. First, the intervention must result in changes in the hypothesised mediator (for example, the intervention results in decreases in perceived barriers or increases in a correlate such as self-efficacy – Path 'a' in Figure 7.1). Second, variations in the proposed mediator are significantly related to variations in the dependent variable (for example, changes in barriers to physical activity are significantly related to changes in actual physical activity behaviour – Path 'b'). Finally, when paths 'a' and 'b' are statistically controlled, a previously significant relation between the independent and dependent variables (e.g. between the intervention and physical activity behaviour) is reduced, with the strongest demonstration of mediation occurring when Path 'c' is zero (Cerin and MacKinnon, 2008).

What are the key correlates of physical activity?

Correlates of physical activity are best organised into six major categories:

- socio-demographic correlates, such socio-economic status, gender and age;
- biological correlates, such as fitness or body fatness;
- psychological correlates, such as confidence and attitude;
- behavioural correlates; these are other behaviours associated with physical activity, such as smoking or diet;
- social correlates, such as social support and family interactions;
- environmental correlates, such as cycle paths and weather conditions.

In this chapter, we will summarise evidence concerning correlates of physical activity for the three groups of young people, adults and older adults.

Correlates of physical activity for young people

A great deal of literature exists on the correlates of physical activity for young people (children and adolescents). Indeed, there are now many reviews of evidence, including a 'review of reviews' (Biddle *et al.*, 2011). Most of the reviews summarise cross-sectional evidence. Recent reviews of prospective studies (Uijtdewilligen *et al.*, 2011) and determinants of change (Craggs *et al.*, 2011) show that rather fewer studies have used these designs.

Socio-demographic correlates

Age and gender have been thought to be consistent socio-demographic correlates of physical activity in youth. Males and children usually report more physical activity than females and adolescents. Particularly in girls, participation falls quite rapidly in the teenage years. Age differences in activity in the early pre-school years, however, are not evident (Hinkley *et al.*, 2008). In contrast, recent data from two prospective studies showed that older adolescents had higher physical activity levels than their younger counterparts (Uijtdewilligen *et al.*,

2011). Given the paucity of prospective studies in this field, confirmation of this finding is required.

Data on ethnicity are less comprehensive and may differ between and within countries. Trends suggest greater physical activity for 'white' ethnic groups, but clearly this distinction is likely to mask many other possible differences and similarities. In the UK, for example, physical activity is particularly low in some south Asian ethnic groups, such as those from Bangladesh, India and Pakistan origins (Townsend *et al.*, 2012). A small number of prospective studies show a negative association between ethnicity expressed as African-American and adolescent physical activity (Uijtdewilligen *et al.*, 2011).

Socio-economic status (SES) is frequently assumed to be associated with physical activity levels. However, the data often show variable findings, dependent on the nature of the physical activity under investigation. A summary of the evidence on adolescents by Stalsberg and Pedersen (2010) showed that of 60 studies, 37 showed a positive association between SES and physical activity, but only six showed a negative association. There was no association in 20 studies. While this shows a tendency for adolescents in higher SES groups to be more active, the variability is noteworthy. Some forms of physical activity will be more dependent on financial resources than others, and some will be more encouraged in some cultures than others.

Biological correlates

The most frequently studied biological correlate for young people is weight status (e.g. body fat or BMI). This has been shown to be negatively related to physical activity but usually in a small way or, often, rather inconsistently (Biddle *et al.*, 2011; Sallis *et al.*, 2000). Associations in childhood can be difficult to detect due to measurement issues such as maturity and measurement error, particularly for self-reported physical activity.

Psychological correlates

Several reviews have addressed psychological correlates, although the data are too few to draw conclusions on pre-school children (Biddle *et al.*, 2011; Hinkley *et al.*, 2008). For pre-adolescent school-age children, Sallis *et al.* (2000) reported that physical activity is positively associated with intentions and 'preferences', although the latter was not defined. The finding on intentions was supported by two prospective studies on children and two on adolescents reviewed by Uijtdewilligen *et al.* (2011). The same review concluded that perceived behavioural control is also associated with greater physical activity for adolescents when using prospective designs, and Craggs *et al.* (2011) supported this finding when reviewing physical activity change studies (see Chapter 8 for more on the construct of perceived behavioural control).

For adolescents, reviews found that higher levels of perceived competence were associated with greater physical activity, with Biddle *et al.* (2005) reporting the strength of the association to be small for adolescent girls. For children, Sallis *et al.* (2000) reported that perceived competence had an indeterminate relationship with physical activity from seven studies. 'Achievement orientation' was identified by Sallis *et al.* as being positively associated with physical activity in adolescents, although no further information is provided in the review as to the exact nature of this variable. This finding was confirmed by van der Horst *et al.* (2007) and appears to be best reflected by a mastery (task) goal orientation prominent in literature on young people's achievement motivation (see Roberts *et al.*, 2007).

Surprisingly, self-efficacy (confidence) and enjoyment have not been consistently associated with higher levels of activity across some of the reviews of cross-sectional evidence. While Biddle *et al*. (2005) report a positive association for physical activity for adolescent girls with self-efficacy and enjoyment, Sallis *et al*. report that self-efficacy is inconsistently associated with activity in both children (nine studies) and adolescents (13 studies), while enjoyment of PE for adolescents was found to be unrelated to activity across five studies. Van der Horst *et al*. (2007) confirm this. However, Craggs *et al*. (2011) did report a positive and consistent association for self-efficacy on *changes* in physical activity for children aged 10 to 13 years and adolescents aged 14 years and above. This is more convincing evidence because it reviews only studies where physical activity levels changed and the correlate/determinant of interest was also assessed.

It is clear that the intuitive logic of an association between enjoyment and physical activity is not supported by the available evidence. Moreover, as discussed in Chapter 2, the construct of enjoyment and related positive affect is complex. Simple associations between physical activity and self-reported enjoyment may mask more subtle feelings of satisfaction, importance and value attached to physical activity. Some physical activities, particularly during participation, may not elicit pure 'fun' or 'enjoyment' per se, but could be associated with feelings of satisfaction or pleasure. The small but significant effect size between 'affective judgement' and physical activity reported by Nasuti and Rhodes (2013) may reflect this.

Issues of body image and appearance seem to be important for adolescent girls and are negatively associated with physical activity. Specifically, the correlates of perceived body attractiveness, importance of appearance and physical self-worth were all small to moderate in their strength of association with physical activity in adolescent girls (Biddle *et al*., 2005). However, Sallis *et al*. (2000) reported that associations with perceived physical appearance and body image for adolescents were inconclusive, while van der Horst *et al*. (2007) found no association with physical activity for 'self-perception'. Global feelings of self-esteem were unrelated to physical activity in Sallis *et al*.'s review across all six studies. Associations between these types of correlates and physical activity may be dependent on the self-perception construct being assessed, age and gender (see Chapter 6).

Behavioural correlates

Previous physical activity (Craggs *et al*., 2011) and healthy diet have been associated with physical activity in youth (Biddle *et al*., 2011). These are considered to be 'behavioural' correlates. The variable of 'previous physical activity' suggests that some measure of 'tracking' takes place; that is, the more active children remain so as they age. Evidence for tracking, however, is not as strong as we sometimes might think. Statistical associations for activity patterns between different ages are, at best, 'moderate' and sometimes 'small'. Of course, this will depend on the periods of the life course being studied, the type of physical activity or sedentary behaviour being assessed, and the length of time between assessments. Tracking from childhood into adolescence is small for self-reported measures of physical activity and even smaller when objective assessments are conducted. Unsurprisingly, tracking from childhood to adulthood is almost non-existent while from adolescence into adulthood it is small to moderate (Telama, 2009). Associations decline as the length of assessment period increases (Telama *et al*., 2005), and this is true for sedentary behaviours (Biddle *et al*., 2010).

Sedentary behaviour during the after-school and weekend periods is associated with less physical activity in youth (Atkin *et al*., 2008). The key issue here is the temporal aspect of the potentially competing behaviour; that is, sedentary behaviour. Some sedentary behaviours, such as TV viewing, are unlikely to detract from physical activity at certain time periods (e.g. late evening) but could at other times, as suggested here for the after-school period.

> Key point: Sedentary behaviours are only likely to compete with opportunities to be physically active at certain times of the day or week.

For adolescents, Sallis *et al.* (2000) found that previous physical activity was a correlate, alongside community sports participation. Taking part in physical education and school sports also predicted higher activity levels for adolescents in the review by van der Horst *et al.*, while Biddle *et al.* found that competitive sports participation was a correlate of physical activity in adolescent girls. No such relation was found for pre-school children in just two studies (Biddle *et al.*, 2011).

Socio-cultural correlates

These correlates typically centre on different forms of parental, sibling and peer behaviour and support, and reviews by Gustafson and Rhodes (2006), Edwardson and Gorely (2010), and Pugliese and Tinsley (2007) have focused on parental correlates of physical activity only. This provides a growing evidence base for the potential influence of parents on young people's physical activity. The studies on parental correlates may best be summarised into those that address the association between parental 'support' and those assessing the association between parental physical activity and child physical activity.

Initially, and somewhat surprisingly, Sallis *et al.* (2000) and Ferriera *et al.* (2007) reported no consistent social/cultural correlates of physical activity in pre-adolescent children. Parental support was associated with adolescent physical activity by Sallis *et al.* (2000) and Biddle *et al.* (2005). Similarly, parental interaction with the child during physical activity was associated with more activity in pre-school children (Hinkley *et al.*, 2008). The most comprehensive reviews in this area are by Gustafson and Rhodes (2006), Pugliese and Tinsley (2007), and Edwardson and Gorely (2010).

Gustafson and Rhodes (2006) located 19 studies examining parental support of physical activity for young people from 1992 to 2003, with 16 being cross-sectional and three longitudinal. A strong positive association was reported in all but one of the studies reflecting parental encouragement, involvement and facilitation.

Edwardson and Gorely (2010) also reviewed parental influence but they analysed their 96 studies by intensities and types of physical activity. They found that for children, parental involvement (overall physical activity and leisure-time physical activity), and overall support (organised physical activity) were associated with types of activity, whereas for adolescents, the main associations were for parental support (MVPA, vigorous physical activity, overall physical activity), attitudes/beliefs (MVPA, overall physical activity), transport (MVPA, organised physical activity) and encouragement (physical activity frequency).

Pugliese and Tinsley (2007) conducted the only meta-analysis in this area by aggregating associations across 30 studies between parental socialisation factors and child or adolescent physical activity. They reported significant but small associations between young people's physical activity and parental encouragement and instrumental behaviour (e.g. transporting the child to physical activity). When all parent socialisation factors were considered together, including parental physical activity, the association with child and adolescent physical activity was statistically small (r = 0.17) but significant.

A common assumption in this area is that active parents will have active children. However, the evidence supporting this is rather mixed. Biddle *et al.* (2005) found a small to moderate positive association between physical activity of adolescent girls and the physical activity level of the father, and Hinkley *et al.* (2008), for pre-school children, found an association with parental physical activity. Edwardson and Gorely's comprehensive coverage of parental influences did show some associations for children with parental modelling (perceived parental physical activity) but actual physical activity levels of parents only associated with the physical activity of adolescents, and more at higher levels of intensity. The father's activity seemed more clearly associated than that of the mother. Edwardson and Gorely also reviewed longitudinal studies and found that overall physical activity of adolescents was associated with the father's own activity levels. Pugliese and Tinsley (2007) reported a significant but small effect size for young people's physical activity and parental activity. The studies reviewed by Craggs *et al.* (2011) showed no association with changes in physical activity for children with the variables of parental role modelling and parental physical activity.

In reviewing 24 studies where measures of both parental and child physical activity existed, Gustafson and Rhodes (2006) concluded that there is 'much uncertainty' (p. 88) about the relationship between parental and child activity levels. This conclusion appears to still be valid, although the small trends that exist seem to favour associations between young people's physical activity and that of their fathers. Figure 7.2 summarises the likely strength of association between parental correlates and their child's physical activity. It shows that the association between parental and child physical activity (route a) is, at best, small whereas the association between parental support and the child's physical activity (route c) is much stronger. One would expect physically active parents to be supportive and encouraging.

Key point: The physical activity levels of children are likely to be influenced by the support and encouragement of their parents more than by how active the parents are.

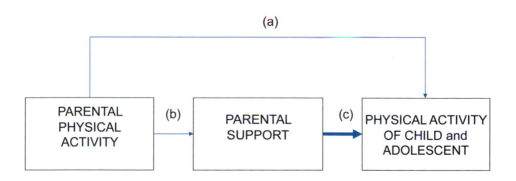

Figure 7.2   Associations between parental physical activity and support, and physical activity levels of young people, suggesting that the strongest association is between parental support and physical activity

Environmental correlates

Environmental correlates of physical activity have gained increasing momentum in research over the past decade (Bauman *et al.*, 2012). For example, positive associations with the physical activity of children were reported by Sallis *et al.* (2000) for time spent outside and facility/programme access. Time outside was also a correlate for pre-school children's activity levels (Hinkley *et al.*, 2008). The season of the year and an urban/rural distinction were inconsistently associated with activity.

For adolescents, Sallis *et al.* found only three variables studied at least three times: equipment, opportunities to exercise and sports media influence. Only 'opportunities to exercise' was consistently and positively associated with physical activity. Unfortunately, we have no further information on the nature of these opportunities, although Sallis *et al.* did find that the availability of equipment was unrelated to physical activity in this age group.

Biddle *et al.* (2005) identified 18 environmental variables studied as correlates of physical activity in adolescent girls. These included local facilities, crime, access, the school PE environment and seasonal factors. None were studied more than twice and thus did not meet their inclusion criterion.

Ferreira *et al.*'s (2007) review of children's environmental correlates found that time spent outside was a consistent correlate of activity, supporting the finding from Sallis *et al.* (2000). In addition, Ferreira and colleagues found that school physical activity policy was also associated with greater activity. Such policies addressed time allowed for free play, time spent outdoors at school, and number of field trips. For adolescents, in contrast to Sallis *et al.*, Ferreira *et al.* found no association between activity and 'access to community physical activity facilities'. Davison and Lawson (2006), on the other hand, did find a positive association for 'availability of recreation facilities', including permanent play structures, in schools, when analysing data across children and adolescents. In addition, they reported that higher levels of physical activity were associated with living closer to school.

Ferreira *et al.* found that objectively assessed neighbourhood crime incidence was negatively associated with physical activity, but adolescent perceptions of safety were not. Similarly, Davison and Lawson found a negative association between physical activity and objective measures of area deprivation and crime, but not for perceived safety.

Environmental factors can be important, but not invariably so. The greater likelihood of time inside, precipitated by busy roads, fear of safety for children, and availability of attractive home-based sedentary entertainment, almost certainly contributes to lower than optimal levels of physical activity for children and adolescents.

> Key point: Correlates of physical activity for young people include socio-demographic, biological, psychological, behavioural, socio-cultural and environmental factors.

Correlates of physical activity for adults and older adults

As for young people, there are numerous reviews of correlates of physical activity for adults. Some focus on 'older' adults, but, given the variation in demarcating such age limits, we have combined adults and older adults in this section of the chapter.

Sallis and Owen (1999) summarised the evidence on the correlates of physical activity for adults. Trost *et al.* (2002) provided an update on this, and Bauman *et al.* have briefly summarised most of the key reviews (Bauman *et al.*, 2012). Subsequently, there have been further reviews on personality (Rhodes and Smith, 2006), occupational correlates (Kirk and Rhodes, 2011), life events (Allender *et al.*, 2008; Koeneman *et al.*, 2011), the role of parenthood (Bellows-Riecken and Rhodes, 2008), transition into retirement (Barnett *et al.*, 2012), environmental factors (Duncan *et al.*, 2005; Humpel *et al.*, 2002), walking (Owen *et al.*, 2004; Saelens and Handy, 2008), and correlates in older age (Koeneman *et al.*, 2011; van Stralen *et al.*, 2009). These topics suggest that the influences on physical activity may be more complex in adults due to varied and changing life events and circumstances, with likely strong effects for age.

Socio-demographic correlates

Physical activity is typically inversely associated with age in adulthood, although retirement can be associated with an increase in recreational physical activity (Barnett *et al.*, 2012) as shown in the Longitudinal Aging Study Amsterdam (Koeneman *et al.*, 2012). Reviews show males to be more active than females. Education and related socio-economic status markers show that lower levels of these indicators were associated with less physical activity (Bauman *et al.*, 2012). For example, Kirk and Rhodes' (2011) review of occupational correlates of physical activity showed that those in white-collar/professional occupations had higher leisure-time physical activity than those in blue-collar occupations.

Biological correlates

An inverse association is evident between obesity and physical activity. However, some argue that obesity is a precursor of low levels of physical activity as well as an outcome (Bauman *et al.*, 2012). Health status is also a correlate, and this is consistent with Allender *et al.*'s (2008) conclusion that changes to physical status influence participation.

Psychological correlates

For psychological correlates of physical activity, Trost *et al.* reported that there was evidence for a consistent positive association with physical activity for enjoyment, expected benefits, intention, perceived health, self-motivation, self-efficacy, stage of behaviour change and self-schemata for exercise, and negative associations for barriers and mood disturbance. The strongest evidence appeared to be for self-efficacy (Bauman *et al.*, 2012), and this is likely to be more important for behaviours that require effort, such as structured fitness programmes. Looking across the summary of evidence of reviews provided by Bauman *et al.*, there is great inconsistency as to the extent of association between psychological variables and adult physical activity, except for self-efficacy.

Key point: A key psychological correlate of physical activity for adults is self-efficacy.

Behavioural correlates

Trost *et al.* (2002) reported that physical activity history in childhood/youth was not associated with adult activity, whereas an association was found for activity history in adulthood. This might reflect the fact that adulthood could either be a more stable period of life or that physical activity measures are made closer together. Other studies of tracking show that the further apart the measures, the weaker the association between the two. As stated earlier, tracking from childhood to adulthood is almost non-existent while from adolescence into adulthood it is small to moderate (Telama, 2009). Other behavioural factors associated with physical activity for adults include smoking (negative) and healthy diet (positive).

Socio-cultural correlates

There is some evidence to suggest that the provision of social support is associated with higher levels of physical activity (Trost *et al.*, 2002), although Bauman *et al.*'s (2012) review of reviews showed very mixed evidence. On the other hand, Allender and colleagues (2006) reviewed qualitative studies and found that social networks appeared to be important factors in whether adults were involved in physical activity or not.

Interestingly, it appears that parenthood may also be associated with lower levels of physical activity (Allender *et al.*, 2008). Review-level evidence presented by Bellows-Riecken and Rhodes (2008) showed a clear negative association of physical activity levels for parents compared to non-parents, with a meta-analytic effect size between 0.4 and 0.5, and mothers being less active than fathers.

Environmental correlates

For environmental factors, Bauman *et al.*'s (2012) summary of nine reviews suggested considerable variability in the extent to which environmental factors were associated with different forms of physical activity. This is summarised in Table 7.1 and shows that the best evidence is for recreational facilities and locations and the transport environment for total and leisure-time physical activity. But the table also shows that a great deal of the evidence is largely inconclusive.

> Key point: Environmental correlates of physical activity for adults are largely inconclusive, although there are positive trends for facilities and transport environment.

Commentary on older adults

Although data on older adults have been included in the section on adults, we feel that this population is too important not to provide additional comments. As stated, it is not always easy to filter the findings for older adults from other studies of adults as the age groups selected for studies overlap. Nevertheless, we can say that the knowledge concerning the potential correlates of physical activity in older adults is relatively understudied (King, 2001; van Stralen *et al.*, 2009). The review by van Stralen *et al.* (2009) provided evidence for correlates of physical activity initiation and maintenance in adults aged 50 years and over. Key to their review is that they only included longitudinal and experimental studies. They rated the evidence for potential correlates as 'convincing' if more than 66 per cent of the studies for that correlate reported a significant result in the same direction, 'probable' if between 50 and 66 per cent of the studies were in the same direction, and 'weak' if fewer than 50 per cent of the studies were in the same direction. Although many potential correlates emerged, few

Table 7.1 Summary conclusions from reviews on environmental correlates of physical activity reported by Bauman *et al.* (2012) (figures refer to the number of reviews concluding the degree of support for the named correlate)

Environmental correlate	Correlate supported	Inconclusive evidence	Not correlated
Active transport			
Neighbourhood design	2	3	1
Transport environment	0	6	0
Social environment	0	2	1
Aesthetics	0	3	2
Leisure-time PA			
Recreational facilities and locations	1	4	1
Transport environment	2	3	1
Social environment	0	2	2
Aesthetics	2	1	2
Total physical activity			
Neighbourhood design	1	5	1
Recreational facilities and locations	5	3	0
Transport environment	4	4	0
Social environment	1	6	1
Aesthetics	3	3	1

Table 7.2 Convincing (bold) and probable correlates of physical activity initiation and maintenance in older adults (adapted from van Stralen *et al.*, 2009)

Correlates	Initiation	Maintenance
Biological	Physical health status (+)	**Physical health status (+)** Physical fitness (+)
Psychological	**Self-efficacy (+)** **Intention (+)** **Motivational readiness to change (+)** **Action planning (+)** Outcome expectations (+)	**Intention (+)** **Enjoyment (+)** **Motivational readiness to change (+)** **Realisation of outcome expectations (+)** **Perceived benefits (+)** Self-efficacy (+) Perceived barriers (−) Mood status (+) Stress (−)
Behavioural	**Physical activity level at baseline (+)** Smoking (−)	**Exercise habits (+)** **Physical activity level at baseline (+)** Smoking (−)
Social	Social support from significant others (+) Social norms (+)	
Environmental	**Perceived access (+)** **Crime (safety) (+)** **Programme format (Home)(+)**	**Programme format (Home)(+)**

of these had been studied frequently enough to enable meaningful conclusions to be drawn. Using the data provided by van Stralen *et al.*, and applying a further criterion used by Sallis *et al.* (2000) of a correlate having been examined within at least three separate studies, Table 7.2 summarises the correlates for which there is convincing and probable evidence during physical activity initiation and maintenance in older adults. Some similarities in correlates in initiation and maintenance may be seen, but there are also some differences. For example, outcome expectations are probably important during the initiation phase but realisation of these outcomes is probably important for maintenance. Sources of social support from family and friends are probably important during initiation of physical activity but not during maintenance. These findings support the potential importance of distinguishing between adopting and maintaining physical activity; something rarely done in this area of research.

It is clear from Table 7.2 that there are significant gaps in our understanding of influences on physical activity behaviour in older adults. An acknowledged limitation of the review by van Stralen *et al.* was that the studies often included only healthy volunteers and it is possible that those living with chronic illness, disability or frailty may have different correlates for physical activity. Moreover, many adults in the age range covered (50-plus) are not considered 'old' by many standards and may be in better health and fitter than many of their younger counterparts. For example, the UK guidelines for physical activity differentiate guidelines for adults from older adults at the age of 65 years (Chief Medical Officers of England, Scotland, Wales and Northern Ireland, 2011). Moreover, physical functioning will determine, to some extent, what physical activity may be appropriate and feasible, and hence will determine what correlates are more important. As stated in the Chief Medical Officers' Report for the UK guidelines,

> this population has sometimes been separated into the 'younger old', 'old' and 'older old'. However, chronological age has quite limited value when describing differences in health, physical function and disease status. Many people in their late 80s do as well as those in their late 60s while some in their early 70s have functional status more expected of a 90 year old.
>
> (Chief Medical Officers of England, Scotland, Wales and Northern Ireland, 2011, p. 41)

Key point: Correlates of physical activity for older adults may depend on the functional status of the individual.

Physical activity motives and barriers

In addition to the study of wider correlates of physical activity, exercise psychologists and others interested in physical activity participation have investigated people's stated reasons or motives for involvement, facilitators of participation and perceived barriers. This has adopted a descriptive approach using self-reported perceived reasons for starting, maintaining or ceasing involvement, or factors that might inhibit participation. This area of research lacks some precision, as constructs are often used interchangeably, such as those shown in Table 7.3.

This is largely an 'atheoretical' approach but provides a useful starting point for understanding people's 'surface' motivation and perceived barriers. It does not, of course, help explain physical activity involvement in more detailed or theoretical ways, but may still be

Table 7.3 Defining and clarifying the constructs of motives, facilitators, expected outcomes and barriers for physical activity

Construct	Definition	Comment
Motive	Stated reason for participation in physical activity	Could be stated as reason to start or maintain involvement; these may be different
Facilitator	Factor expressed as possible enabler of physical activity	May not be the same as motive or simply the opposite of stated barrier
Expected outcome	Perceived outcome from involvement in physical activity	Sometimes referred to as 'outcome expectancies' – what people perceive, or want, from their physical activity involvement; also need to account for how important such outcomes are to the individual
Barrier	Factor thought to discourage or prevent physical activity	Could be stated as barrier to any involvement or barrier to increasing current levels of physical activity

informative. To this end, research mainly started in the 1980s on motives and barriers has not been updated much, and one might argue that it may not need to be. We have basic information on how people view physical activity motives and barriers.

Motives and barriers stated by young people

Much of the early research on children's participation motivation tended to focus on competitive sport rather than more diverse aspects of physical activity. However, this is not surprising, as children are less likely to participate in fitness pursuits currently favoured by adults, at least not until mid- to late adolescence. Nevertheless, it is important that we understand more fully the reasons children give for participation or non-participation in recreational play or, for example, in active travel.

Interviews with young people and their parents in England (Mulvihill *et al.*, 2000) have shown that children aged 5 to 11 years are often physically active and are enthusiastic about activity. They appear to be motivated by enjoyment and social elements of participation, while for those aged 11 to 15 years enjoyment was stated as important (and this was enhanced when an element of choice was evident), and feelings of well-being. Motives for weight control started to emerge in girls at this age.

Early research on this topic came from Finland (Telama and Silvennoinen, 1979) with a survey of over 3,000 11- to 19-year-olds. This showed clear changes in motivation for physical activity as a function of age and gender. Boys and younger adolescents were more interested in achieving success in competition but by late adolescence very few showed interest in this factor. This trend was reversed for motives associated with relaxation and recreation. Fitness motivation was strongest among those who often thought about sport and took part in sports club activities. This fitness motive was unimportant for 18- to 19-year-olds, or for those uninterested or inactive in sport.

Data from the English Sports Council's survey of young people and sport (Mason, 1995) showed that from a sample of over 4,000 6- to 16-year-olds motives are diverse, ranging from general enjoyment to fitness and friendships. Similar results have been reported in North American research such as the Canada Fitness Survey (1983) which sampled over 4,500 young people aged 10 to 19 years of age, as well as a recent survey in Northern Ireland

(Carmichael, 2010). As shown in Table 7.3, some of these motives may actually be perceived or expected outcomes of participation. For example, in the Northern Ireland survey, 60 to 80 per cent of young people reported fun, keeping fit, learning skills and improving health as their main 'benefits' of participation in sport and physical activity (Carmichael, 2010).

More recently, in addition to identifying motives for participation, researchers and policy-makers have become interested in what factors might be seen to facilitate involvement. These could sometimes be similar to correlates of physical activity but also differ. Two key areas of facilitators emerged from qualitative work with youth in the US (Moore et al., 2010). Both urban and rural youth stated that social and facility issues were important insofar as their friends needed to be involved and they required access to space and facilities.

Although developing, rather less has been written about motives and barriers for physical activity for young people with disabilities. Using systematic review methods, Shields et al. (2012) found that facilitators of physical activity for such youth included peer involvement, family support, accessible facilities, proximity of location to be active, better opportunities and skilled staff. Moreover, social contacts, fun and relaxation have been identified as facilitators of sport involvement for young people with disabilities (Jaarsma et al., 2014).

In summary, young people are motivated for diverse reasons, including fun and enjoyment, learning and improving skills, being with friends, success and winning, and physical fitness and health. The latter factor may also include weight control and appearance for older youth. Facilitators are oriented towards social and access/facility concerns.

As with motives for participation, there appear to be numerous barriers to physical activity in children and adolescents. For example, Coakley and White (1992) conducted 60 in-depth interviews with 13- to 23-year-olds, half of whom had decided to participate in one of five different sports initiatives in their local town. The others had either ceased involvement or had decided not to participate at all. The decision to participate or not appeared to be influenced by perceptions of competence, by external constraints, such as money and opposite-sex friends, degree of support from significant others, and past experiences, including school PE. Negative memories of school PE included feelings of boredom and incompetence, lack of choice, and negative evaluation from peers. Feelings of embarrassment in sport settings, mainly due to perceived incompetence or concerns over self-presentation associated with their physique during puberty, are common (Mason, 1995). Overall, these findings appear to be unchanged over the past few decades. Indeed, more recent Northern Ireland data support this as factors 'putting off' young people taking part in sport and physical activity involved competence-based barriers ('I'm not fit'; 'I'm not good at sport or physical activity'); 'I find it embarrassing to exercise in front of others') (Carmichael, 2010). Those with disabilities have mentioned the disability itself to be a barrier (Jaarsma et al., 2014).

A highly cited barrier is that of 'lack of time', and this has even been reported as a barrier for 5- to 11-year-olds (Mulvihill et al., 2000), perhaps reflecting less discretionary time being allowed by parents (Sturm, 2004). It is also a barrier for those with disabilities (Jaarsma et al., 2014). Environmental barriers, such as road traffic and fear of safety, may be interrelated with such barriers. Indeed, evidence is clear that parents have markedly reduced the ability of children to roam far from the home in recent decades and this has been associated with fears of safety (Shaw et al., 2013). This undoubtedly reduces physical activity and increases in-home sedentary behaviour. For example, parents in the qualitative study by Moore et al. (2010) expressed the view that TV viewing was a barrier to greater physical activity of children.

The common barrier of lack of time, however, may mask several underlying barriers and perceptions. While it is accepted that we all have to budget our time, we have a great deal of discretion as to how we allocate that time. For example, in a Northern Ireland survey, 25 per cent of girls but only 17 per cent of boys stated that not having enough time, or having a preference to do other things, were factors 'putting them off' taking part in sport or physical activity. Moreover, 25 per cent of girls but only 15 per cent of boys stated that a barrier was having too much homework. Both boys and girls are likely to have comparable discretionary time and demands; hence these statements on barriers are really likely to be statements about the value and interest they attach to being physically active. This point is rarely acknowledged in the interpretation of national survey data on barriers.

Motives and barriers stated by adults

Several population surveys have addressed issues associated with participation motivation. With some exceptions, such as the Campbell's Survey of Well-Being (Wankel and Mummery, 1993), the breadth of data collection attempted has precluded questions being close to theoretical frameworks. Consequently, most such surveys provide just descriptive data on beliefs, attitudes and motives. Nevertheless, given the large samples often included in these works, these can provide valuable information.

In 1992, the results of the Allied Dunbar National Fitness Survey (ADNFS) in England (Sports Council and Health Education Authority, 1992) were published. This was an ambitious project involving over 4,000 16- to 74-year-olds from 30 regions of England. Home interviews took place on 1,840 men and 2,109 women for up to 1.5 hours, with subsequent physical measures conducted in the home and in mobile laboratories.

The home interview involved questions on involvement in physical activities as well as health, lifestyle and health-related behaviours, barriers and motivation for exercise, social background, personal attributes and general attitudes. The most important motivational factors for physical activity were 'to feel in good shape physically', 'to improve or maintain health' and 'to feel a sense of achievement'. Motives associated with weight control and physical appearance were also important for women. Motives of 'fun' were more likely to be reported by younger people whereas older respondents reported the factor of 'independence' higher than others.

A study of over 15,000 people from 15 countries in the European Union found that the most likely reason given for physical activity participation was to maintain good health, whereas weight control were less likely to be endorsed (see results for the EU alongside the UK in Figure 7.3) (Zunft *et al.*, 1999).

It has often been stated that 'dropping out' of physical activity should not be seen as an 'all-or-none' phenomenon but as an ongoing process of change. For example, Sallis and Hovell's (1990) 'Natural History Model' of physical activity has at least two different routes that could be taken by adults who cease participation. One route is to become physically inactive, while the other is to cease participation temporarily but to return at a later date, or even switch to a new activity. Motivational factors affecting these routes may be different. Indeed, why some adults resume participation after a period of inactivity continues to be poorly understood.

Perceived lack of time is frequently cited as the major barrier to physical activity for adults. Owen and Bauman (1992) reported on just over 5,000 inactive Australians and found that the reason 'no time to exercise' was much more likely to be reported by those in the 25 to 54 age group compared with those over 55 years, data confirmed in a subsequent study in Australia (Booth *et al.*, 1997), as well as the ADNFS.

In the ADNFS, reported barriers to preventing adults from taking more 'exercise' were classified into five main types: physical, emotional, motivational, time and availability. This is

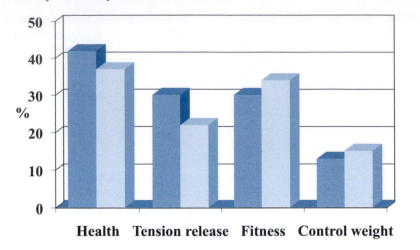

Figure 7.3   Responses (%) for four motives for physical activity from the EU (an average of 15 countries, including the UK), and the UK

Source: Data from Zunft *et al.* (1999).

a useful way of analysing barriers for large population surveys, as it gives a wider picture of barriers and some information for possible interventions. Time barriers appeared to be the most important for both men and women, although women were likely to report emotional barriers to exercise (e.g. 'I'm not the sporty type') more than men. This is likely to be related to perceptions of competence and the perceived effort required to be sufficiently physically active for health. Based on these data, it is important to note that participation in something as simple as cycling or jogging might be avoided on the basis of self-presentational concerns. It makes one wonder how people developed such self-presentations and whether early experiences of 'exercise' in school were not as appropriate as perhaps they should have been. Certainly one can understand the self-presentational concerns in sport where competence levels are so clearly displayed. Interestingly, Australian data show that where the cost of physical activity was seen as a barrier to participation, participants were more likely to adopt walking, showing the potential ease of involvement in this form of activity (Salmon *et al.*, 2003). Predictably, in the ADNFS, the physical and emotional barriers increased across the age groups, while, as reported, time barriers decreased, at least for those over 55 years of age.

For those with disabilities, interview data have shown that barriers to physical activity include the built and natural environment, costs, equipment, emotional and psychological barriers, perceptions and attitudes of others, and policies (Rimmer *et al.*, 2004). Similarly, a qualitative study with adults with mild to moderate learning disabilities living in hostel accommodation showed that barriers included unclear policy guidelines for day service provision, financial constraints, geographical location in respect of local facilities and open space, and limited options for local physically active leisure (Messent *et al.*, 1999).

Useful though the approach used in surveys is, including the ADNFS, replicable instruments that are psychometrically validated are rarely used. In attempting to address this inconsistency in measurement, both Sechrist and colleagues (1987) and Steinhardt and Dishman (1989) developed scales for the assessment of exercise barriers, as well as perceived benefits. Initial psychometric work by Steinhardt and Dishman revealed the barriers of time, effort, obstacles and 'limiting health'. Sechrist *et al.* identified barriers labelled exercise milieu, time expenditure, physical exertion and family encouragement. Little research has been done to further validate the scales, although they do appear to reflect the barriers reported in population surveys.

There is also a measure for physical activity motives. Ryan and colleagues (1997) developed the Motivation for Physical Activity Measure (MPAM-R) which comprises five 7-point subscales: fitness (e.g. 'to have more energy'), appearance (e.g. 'to be attractive to others'), competence (e.g. 'to obtain new skills'), enjoyment (e.g. 'because I enjoy this activity') and social motives (e.g. 'want to be with my friends'). It was used in a recent mixed-methods study summarised below.

> Key point: Correlates of physical activity can involve simple reasons (motives) for getting involved as well as facilitators and barriers. These are useful but sometimes superficial constructs that may not fully explain participation.

Barriers and facilitators: an illustrative study

Withall *et al.* (2011) conducted an interesting mixed-methods study with low-income people in the UK city of Bristol. The sample was mainly adult, with 16 per cent under 18 and 59 per cent over 54 years of age. Three sets of data were analysed. First, participation motives were assessed using the MPAM-R for those taking part in local physical activity sessions. Second, the researchers interviewed local residents who did not take part in physical activity, and finally they interviewed physical activity session leaders. The main purpose was to examine barriers and facilitators for both adoption and retention of physical activity in a group low in SES.

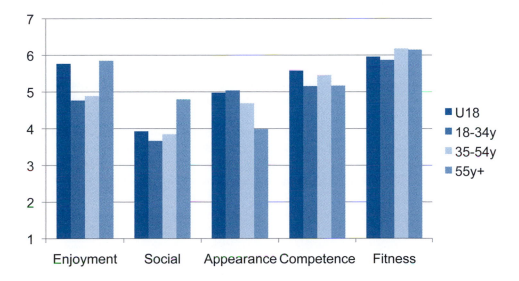

Figure 7.4   Data on motives for physical activity

Source: Withall *et al.* (2011).

Results from the MPAM-R showed that those taking part in physical activity sessions did so primarily for fitness, but also expressed reasonably strong motives for competence and enjoyment, with some age differences. Social aspects were rated lowest, but were still around the scale mid-point, with older adults more strongly endorsing this motive. Data are shown in Figure 7.4. In addition, the authors analysed motives across different types of physical activities (aerobics, strength and flexibility, dance, and sport) and, not surprisingly, this made a difference. For example, those taking part in aerobics and strength activities supported the motive of fitness above others, whereas those in dance and sport seemed motivated by enjoyment and fitness.

The interviews with those not taking part in physical activity revealed barriers associated with attitudes (e.g. some feelings of exercise being irrelevant), motivations (e.g. weight issues; physical and mental health), barriers (e.g. lack of confidence, cost), enablers (e.g. attend with a friend, good availability), and awareness (e.g. patchy awareness of available sessions). Motivating factors identified by session leaders included weight and health issues for older adults, and socialising and enjoyment. Barriers included lack of confidence and perceived competence, and cost.

Chapter summary

This chapter has been necessarily broad to allow for a more focused discussion in the subsequent chapters on physical activity correlates from a more theoretical perspective. In summary, therefore, we conclude the following:

- Correlates are factors associated with participating in physical activity.
- Correlates may best be described under the headings of socio-demographic, biological, psychological, behavioural, social/cultural and environmental. All categories include correlates that appear to be associated with involvement and could be used in behaviour change studies. Not all correlates will be causally related to physical activity.
- Correlates of physical activity for young people include age, gender, intentions, self-efficacy, sedentary behaviour after school and at weekends, parental support, and time outside.
- Common motives for physical activity for young people are fun, skill development, affiliation, fitness, success and challenge.
- Correlates of physical activity for adults include gender, self-efficacy, activity history, social support, access to recreational facilities and locations, and the local transport environment
- Common motives for physical activity for adults change across stages of the life cycle. Younger adults are motivated more by challenge, skill development and fitness, whereas older adults are more interested in participation for reasons of health and enjoyment.
- Key perceived barriers are lack of time and access, as well as issues of safety and feelings of incompetence.

References

Allender, S., Cowburn, G. and Foster, C. (2006). Understanding participation in sport and physical activity among children and adults: A review of qualitative studies. *Health Education Research: Theory and Practice, 21*(6), 826–835. doi: 10.1093/her/cyl063.

Allender, S., Hutchinson, L. and Foster, C. (2008). Life-change events and participation in physical activity: A systematic review. *Health Promotion International, 23*, 160–172.

Atkin, A.J., Gorely, T., Biddle, S.J.H., Marshall, S.J. and Cameron, N. (2008). Critical hours: Physical activity and sedentary behavior of adolescents after school. *Pediatric Exercise Science, 20*, 446–456.

Baranowski, T. and Jago, R. (2005). Understanding mechanisms of change in children's physical activity programs. *Exercise and Sport Sciences Reviews, 33*(4), 163–168.

Baranowski, T., Anderson, C. and Carmack, C. (1998). Mediating variable framework in physical activity interventions: How are we doing? How might we do better? *American Journal of Preventive Medicine, 15*(4), 266–297.

Barnett, I., Guell, C. and Ogilvie, D. (2012). The experience of physical activity and the transition to retirement: A systematic review and integrative synthesis of qualitative and quantitative evidence. *International Journal of Behavioral Nutrition and Physical Activity, 9*(1), 97. doi: 10.1186/1479-5868-9-97.

Baron, R.M. and Kenny, D.A. (1986). The moderator–mediator variable distinction in social psychological research: Conceptual, strategic, and statistical considerations. *Journal of Personality and Social Psychology, 51*, 1173–1182.

Bauman, A.E., Reis, R.S., Sallis, J.F., Wells, J.C., Loos, R.J.F., Martin, B.W. and The Lancet Physical Activity Series Working Group. (2012). Correlates of physical activity: Why are some people physically active and others not? *The Lancet, July*, 31–44.

Bellows-Riecken, K.H. and Rhodes, R.E. (2008). A birth of inactivity: A review of physical activity and parenthood. *Preventive Medicine, 46*(2), 99–110. doi: 10.1016/j.ypmed.2007.08.003.

Biddle, S.J.H., Whitehead, S.H., O'Donovan, T.M. and Nevill, M.E. (2005). Correlates of participation in physical activity for adolescent girls: A systematic review of recent literature. *Journal of Physical Activity and Health, 2*, 423–434.

Biddle, S.J.H., Pearson, N., Ross, G.M. and Braithwaite, R. (2010). Tracking of sedentary behaviours of young people: A systematic review. *Preventive Medicine, 51*, 345–351. doi: 10.1016/j. ypmed.2010.07.018.

Biddle, S.J.H., Atkin, A., Cavill, N. and Foster, C. (2011). Correlates of physical activity in youth: A review of quantitative systematic reviews. *International Review of Sport and Exercise Psychology, 4*(1), 25–49.

Booth, M.L., Bauman, A., Owen, N. and Gore, C.J. (1997). Physical activity preferences, preferred sources of assistance, and perceived barriers to increased activity among physically inactive Australians. *Preventive Medicine, 26*, 131–137.

Canada Fitness Survey. (1983). *Canadian Youth and Physical Activity*. Ottawa: Author.

Carmichael, M. (2010). Young people and sport 2010: Findings from the Young Persons' Behaviour and Attitudes Survey. Belfast: Department of Culture, Arts and Leisure.

Cerin, E. and MacKinnon, D.P. (2008). A commentary on current practice in mediating variable analyses in behavioural nutrition and physical activity. *Public Health Nutrition, 12*(8), 1182–1188.

Chief Medical Officers of England, Scotland, Wales and Northern Ireland. (2011). *Start Active, Stay Active: A report on physical activity from the four home countries' Chief Medical Officers*. London: Department of Health (http://www.dh.gov.uk/en/Publicationsandstatistics/Publications/PublicationsPolicyAndGuidance/DH_128209).

Coakley, J. and White, A. (1992). Making decisions: Gender and sport participation among British adolescents. *Sociology of Sport Journal, 9*, 20–35.

Craggs, C., Corder, K., van Sluijs, E.M.F. and Griffin, S.J. (2011). Determinants of change in physical activity in children and adolescents: A systematic review. *American Journal of Preventive Medicine, 40*(6), 645–658. doi: 10.1016/j.amepre.2011.02.025.

Davison, K.K. and Lawson, C.T. (2006). Do attributes in the physical environment influence children's physical activity? A review of the literature. *International Journal of Behavioral Nutrition and Physical Activity, 3*, 19.

Department of Health. (2004). *At Least Five a Week: Evidence on the impact of physical activity and its relationship to health. A report from the Chief Medical Officer*. London: Author.

Duncan, M., Spence, J. and Mummery, W.K. (2005). Perceived environment and physical activity: A meta-analysis of selected environmental characteristics. *International Journal of Behavioral Nutrition and Physical Activity, 2*(1), 11. doi: 10.1186/1479-5868-2-11.

Edwardson, C.L. and Gorely, T. (2010). Parental influences on different types and intensities of physical activity in youth: A systematic review. *Psychology of Sport and Exercise, 11*(6), 522–535.

Ferreira, I., van der Horst, K., Wendel-Vos, W., Kremers, S., van Lenthe, F.J. and Brug, J. (2007). Environmental correlates of physical activity in youth – A review and update. *Obesity Reviews, 8*(2), 129–154.

Gustafson, S.L. and Rhodes, R.E. (2006). Parental correlates of physical activity in children and early adolescents. *Sports Medicine, 36*(1), 79–97.

Hinkley, T., Crawford, D., Salmon, J., Okely, A.D. and Hesketh, K. (2008). Preschool children and physical activity: A review of correlates. *American Journal of Preventive Medicine, 34*(5), 435–441.

Humpel, N., Owen, N. and Leslie, E. (2002). Environmental factors associated with adults' participation in physical activity: A review. *American Journal of Preventive Medicine, 22*(3), 188–199.

Jaarsma, E.A., Dijkstra, P.U., Geertzen, J.H.B. and Dekker, R. (2014). Barriers to and facilitators of sports participation for people with physical disabilities: A systematic review. *Scandinavian Journal of Medicine and Science in Sports,* Published online: 15 April 2014. doi: 10.1111/sms.12218.

King, A.C. (2001). Interventions to promote physical activity by older adults. *Journals of Gerontology Series A – Biological Sciences and Medical Sciences, 56* Spec No 2(2), 36–46.

Kirk, M.A. and Rhodes, R.E. (2011). Occupation correlates of adults' participation in leisure-time physical activity: A systematic review. *American Journal of Preventive Medicine, 40*(4), 476–485. doi: 10.1016/j.amepre.2010.12.015.

Koeneman, M., Verheijden, M., Chinapaw, M. and Hopman-Rock, M. (2011). Determinants of physical activity and exercise in healthy older adults: A systematic review. *International Journal of Behavioral Nutrition and Physical Activity, 8*(1), 142. doi: 10.1186/1479-5868-8-142.

Koeneman, M., Chinapaw, M.J., Verheijden, M., van Tilburg, T., Visser, M., Deeg, D.J. and Hopman-Rock, M. (2012). Do major life events influence physical activity among older adults: The Longitudinal Aging Study Amsterdam. *International Journal of Behavioral Nutrition and Physical Activity, 9*(1), 147. doi: 10.1186/1479-5868-9-147.

Lubans, D.R., Foster, C. and Biddle, S.J.H. (2008). A review of mediators of behavior in interventions to promote physical activity among children and adolescents. *Preventive Medicine, 47*, 463–470.

MacKinnon, D., Krull, J. and Lockwood, C. (2000). Equivalence of the mediation, confounding and suppression effect. *Prevention Science, 1*, 173–181.

Mason, V. (1995). *Young People and Sport in England, 1994.* London: Sports Council.

Messent, P.R., Cooke, C.B. and Long, J. (1999). Primary and secondary barriers to physically active healthy lifestyles for adults with learning disabilities. *Disability and Rehabilitation, 21*, 409–419.

Moore, J.B., Jilcott, S.B., Shores, K.A., Evenson, K.R., Brownson, R.C. and Novick, L.F. (2010). A qualitative examination of perceived barriers and facilitators of physical activity for urban and rural youth. *Health Education Research, 25*(2), 355–367. doi: 10.1093/her/cyq004.

Mulvihill, C., Rivers, K. and Aggleton, P. (2000). *Physical Activity 'At Our Time': Qualitative research among young people aged 5 to 15 years and parents.* London: Health Education Authority.

Nasuti, G. and Rhodes, R.E. (2013). Affective judgment and physical activity in youth: Review and meta-analyses. *Annals of Behavioral Medicine, 45*(3), 357–376. doi: 10.1007/s12160-012-9462-6.

Owen, N. and Bauman, A. (1992). The descriptive epidemiology of a sedentary lifestyle in adult Australians. *International Journal of Epidemiology, 21*, 305–310.

Owen, N., Humpel, N., Leslie, E., Bauman, A. and Sallis, J.F. (2004). Understanding environmental influences on walking: Review and research agenda. *American Journal of Preventive Medicine, 27*(1), 67–76.

Pugliese, J. and Tinsley, B. (2007). Parental socialization of child and adolescent physical activity: A meta-analysis. *Journal of Family Psychology, 21*(3), 331–343.

Rhodes, R.E. and Pfaeffli, L. (2010). Mediators of physical activity behaviour change among adult non-clinical populations: A review update. *International Journal of Behavioral Nutrition and Physical Activity, 7*(1), 37.

Rhodes, R.E. and Smith, N.E.I. (2006). Personality correlates of physical activity: A review and meta-analysis. *British Journal of Sports Medicine, 40*(12), 958–965. doi: 10.1136/bjsm.2006.028860.

Rimmer, J.H., Riley, B., Wang, E., Rauworth, A. and Jurkowski, J. (2004). Physical activity participation among persons with disabilities: Barriers and facilitators. *American Journal of Preventive Medicine, 26*(5), 419–425.

Roberts, G.C., Treasure, D.C. and Conroy, D.E. (2007). Understanding the dynamics of motivation in sport and physical activity: An achievement goal interpretation. In G. Tenenbaum and R.C. Eklund (eds), *Handbook of Sport Psychology* (3rd edn) (pp. 3–30). Hoboken, NJ: John Wiley & Sons.

Ryan, R.M., Frederick, C.M., Lepes, D., Rubio, N. and Sheldon, K.M. (1997). Intrinsic motivation and exercise adherence. *International Journal of Sport Psychology, 28*, 335–354.

Saelens, B.E. and Handy, S.L. (2008). Built environment correlates of walking: A review. *Medicine and Science in Sports and Exercise, 40*, S550–S566.

Sallis, J.F. and Hovell, M. (1990). Determinants of exercise behavior. *Exercise and Sport Sciences Reviews, 18*, 307–330.

Sallis, J.F. and Owen, N. (1999). *Physical Activity and Behavioral Medicine.* Thousand Oaks, CA: Sage.

Sallis, J.F., Prochaska, J.J. and Taylor, W.C. (2000). A review of correlates of physical activity of children and adolescents. *Medicine and Science in Sports and Exercise, 32*, 963–975.

Salmon, J., Owen, N., Crawford, D., Bauman, A. and Sallis, J.F. (2003). Physical activity and sedentary behavior: A population-based study of barriers, enjoyment, and preference. *Health Psychology, 22*, 178–188.

Sechrist, K.R., Walker, S.N. and Pender, N.J. (1987). Development and psychometric evaluation of the exercise benefits/barriers scale. *Research in Nursing and Health, 10*, 357–365.

Shaw, B., Watson, B., Frauendienst, B., Redecker, A., Jones, T. and Hillman, M. (2013). *Children's Independent Mobility: A comparative study in England and Germany (1971–2010).* London: Policy Studies Institute.

Shields, N., Synnot, A.J. and Barr, M. (2012). Perceived barriers and facilitators to physical activity for children with disability: A systematic review. *British Journal of Sports Medicine, 46*, 989–997. doi:910.1136/bjsports-2012-090236.

Sports Council and Health Education Authority. (1992). *Allied Dunbar National Fitness Survey: Main findings.* London: Author.

Stalsberg, R. and Pedersen, A.V. (2010). Effects of socioeconomic status on the physical activity in adolescents: A systematic review of the evidence. *Scandinavian Journal of Medicine and Science in Sports, 20*, 368–383.

Steinhardt, M.A. and Dishman, R.K. (1989). Reliability and validity of expected outcomes and barriers for habitual physical activity. *Journal of Occupational Medicine, 31*, 536–546.

Sturm, R. (2004). The economics of physical activity: Societal trends and rationales for interventions. *American Journal of Preventive Medicine, 27*(Supplement 1), 126–135.

Telama, R. (2009). Tracking of physical activity from childhood to adulthood: A review. *Obesity Facts: The European Journal of Obesity, 3*, 187–195. doi: 10.1159/000222244

Telama, R. and Silvennoinen, M. (1979). Structure and development of 11 to 19 year olds' motivation for physical activity. *Scandinavian Journal of Sports Sciences, 1*, 23–31.

Telama, R., Yang, X., Viikari, J., Valimaki, I., Wanne, O. and Raitakari, O. (2005). Physical activity from childhood to adulthood: A 21-year tracking study. *American Journal of Preventive Medicine, 28*(3), 267–273.

Townsend, N., Bhatnagar, P., Wickramasinghe, K., Scarborough, P., Foster, C. and Rayner, M. (2012). *Physical Activity Statistics 2012.* London: British Heart Foundation.

Trost, S.G., Owen, N., Bauman, A.E., Sallis, J.F. and Brown, W. (2002). Correlates of adults' participation in physical activity: Review and update. *Medicine and Science in Sports and Exercise, 34*, 1996–2001.

Uijtdewilligen, L., Nauta, J., Singh, A., van Mechelen, W., Twisk, J.W.R., van der Horst, K. and

Chinapaw, M.J.M. (2011). Determinants of physical activity and sedentary behaviour in young people: A review and quality synthesis of prospective studies. *British Journal of Sports Medicine, 45*, 896–905. doi: 10.1136/bjsports-2011-090197.

van der Horst, K., Chin, A. Paw, M.J., Twisk, J.W.R. and Van Mechelen, W. (2007). A brief review on correlates of physical activity and sedentariness in youth. *Medicine and Science in Sports and Exercise, 39*(8), 1241–1250.

van Stralen, M.M., De Vries, H., Mudde, A.N., Bolman, C. and Lechner, L. (2009). Determinants of initiation and maintenance of physical activity among older adults: A literature review. *Health Psychology Review, 3*(2), 147–207.

Wankel, L.M. and Mummery, K.W. (1993). Using national survey data incorporating the theory of planned behavior: Implications for social marketing strategies in physical activity. *Journal of Applied Sport Psychology, 5*, 158–177.

Withall, J., Jago, R. and Fox, K.R. (2011). Why some do but most don't. Barriers and enablers to engaging low-income groups in physical activity programmes: A mixed methods study. *BMC Public Health, 11*(1), 507. doi: 10.1186/1471-2458-11-507.

Zunft, H-J.F., Friebe, D., Seppelt, B., Widhalm, K., de Winter, A-M.R., de Almeida, M.D.V. and Gibney, M. (1999). Perceived benefits and barriers to physical activity in a nationally representative sample in the European Union. *Public Health Nutrition, 2*(1a), 153–160.

8   Physical activity and attitude
Active people have attitude!

Health promotion campaigns are often aimed at changing beliefs or knowledge on the assumption that such changes are necessary to bring about a change in behaviour. Unfortunately, changes in awareness, attitudes, beliefs and knowledge far from guarantee changes in behaviour, although they may be an important first step in such a process. Although any inference of a causal link between beliefs and behaviour cannot usually be sustained, it does seem reasonable to assume that beliefs and attitudes will have some influence on our actions. Indeed, such an assumption has occupied social psychologists for many years in health research (Conner and Norman, 1996; Stroebe and Stroebe, 1995).

A number of theoretical models have been proposed that attempt to explain the role of attitudes in human behaviour. This chapter, therefore, outlines the major integrating theories in health-related attitudes, and reports research findings that have a bearing on physical activity behaviours. Specifically, in this chapter we aim to:

- define and delimit the attitude construct;
- briefly overview the early descriptive approach to the study of physical activity attitudes;
- summarise the Health Belief Model – a foundational model on health beliefs and attitudes – and research findings from physical activity;
- review the theoretical foundations and contemporary physical activity research of the Theories of Reasoned Action and Planned Behaviour;
- investigate the intention–behaviour gap and ways of closing this gap.

Defining attitudes

Attitudes are about feelings and behaviour. The study of attitudes in social psychology has a long yet controversial history, particularly when attempting to predict behaviours from people's stated attitudes. Even so, Olson and Zanna (1993) report that 'attitude and attitude change remain among the most extensively researched topics by social psychologists' (p. 118). Yet the extensive use of the word 'attitude' in everyday speech has rendered it prone to misinterpretation, or to be used in a way that is ill defined or too vague. Rarely is it stated whether the 'attitudes' referred to are about beliefs or feelings, for example. A typical statement may be found in the introduction to the 2011 UK guidelines for physical activity. The four UK country Chief Medical Officers, in their joint opening statement, say that 'Our aim is that as many people as possible become aware of these guidelines. ... However, this report does not and indeed cannot set out the specific messages we need to reach communities across the UK with diverse needs, lifestyles and attitudes to activity' (Chief Medical Officers of England, Scotland, Wales and Northern Ireland, 2011, p.4). Instead of 'attitudes' they could equally have said 'motivations', 'beliefs' or 'feelings' and conveyed a broadly similar message.

Attitude has been defined as 'a psychological tendency that is expressed by evaluating a particular entity with some degree of favour or disfavour' (Eagly and Chaiken, 1993, p.1), suggesting that there is a key 'affective' (emotional) element of attitude. However, a three-component model of attitude (Hovland and Rosenberg, 1960) suggests that in addition to attitudes having an affective component, they can also have a belief (cognitive) and behavioural component (see Figure 8.1).

We can only really infer attitudes. Attitude, like personality, motivation and some other psychological constructs, is hypothetical and not open to direct observation. The responses often used to infer attitudes may be either verbal or non-verbal in each of the cognitive, affective and behavioural categories of the three-component model (Ajzen, 1988). These are illustrated in Table 8.1, with examples from physical activity.

Table 8.1   Examples of inferring physical activity attitudes from different responses (adapted from Ajzen, 1988)

	Response category		
Response mode	*Cognitive*	*Affective*	*Behavioural*
Verbal	Expressions of beliefs concerning physical activity	Expressions of likes and dislikes concerning physical activity	Expressions of intention to be physically active or inactive
Non-verbal	Thoughts of the benefits concerning physical activity	Anticipated regret (of missing a session of exercise)	Approach or avoidance of physical activity and related contexts

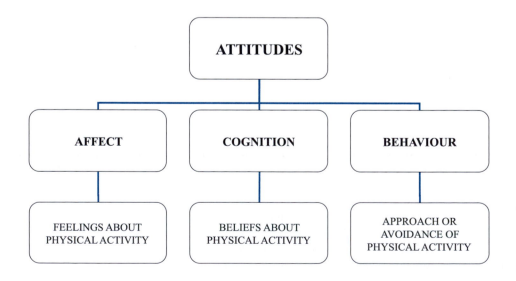

Figure 8.1   The three-component view of attitudes applied to physical activity

Early attitude-based research in health concerned the nature of beliefs. Indeed, the question of why people do, or do not, seek health care has been an important one for health psychologists over the past few decades. The field was initially typified by diverse findings and an apparently irreconcilable set of behavioural predictors. However, in the 1950s, a group of American social psychologists attempted to integrate the work on health behaviours by developing an attitude-based model of health decision-making – The Health Belief Model (HBM) (Becker *et al.*, 1977; Conner and Norman, 1994; Janz and Becker, 1984; Sheeran and Abraham, 1996).

Key point: Attitudes are about feelings, but will also involve beliefs and behaviour.

The Health Belief Model (HBM)

The HBM developed from Kurt Lewin's 'field theory' and an expectancy-value approach to motivation and behaviour. This means that people often make decisions about behaviours based on the expectations of what might happen if they do or do not act in that way (i.e. what will be the outcomes?) and also on what value (how important is it?) they place on such outcomes. Lewin's perspective advocated that behaviour is influenced by the individual's characteristics and the environment. His 'field theory' stated that we exist in a 'life space' of regions of both positive and negative value, and forces attract and repel us from these regions. Illness is a region of negative value and hence we are motivated to avoid it most of the time, and this formed a central tenet of the HBM.

The HBM was devised in an attempt to predict health behaviours, primarily in response to low rates of adoption and adherence of preventive health care behaviours. Becker *et al.* (1977) stated that the HBM was adopted as an organising framework for four main reasons:

- The model has potentially modifiable variables.
- The model is derived from sound psychological theory.
- Although the HBM was first developed to account for preventive health behaviours, it has also been employed successfully to account for 'sick-role' and 'illness' behaviours. 'Sick-role' behaviours are primarily associated with seeking treatment or a remedy for illness, whereas 'illness' behaviours are primarily associated with seeking advice or help on the nature and/or extent of the illness.
- The HBM is consistent with other health behaviour models.

The HBM has been applied to a wide variety of health behaviours, including physical activity, although the literature on physical activity is not extensive. The model hypothesises that people will not seek preventive health behaviours unless:

- they possess minimal levels of health motivation and knowledge;
- they view themselves as potentially vulnerable to the illness;
- they view the condition as threatening;
- they are convinced of the efficacy of the 'treatment';
- they see few difficulties in undertaking the action.

These factors can be modified by socio-economic and demographic factors, as well as prompts (referred to as 'cues to action' in the model), such as media campaigns or the illness of a close friend or relative. The HBM is illustrated in Figure 8.2.

The majority of the HBM research has involved illness, sick-role or preventive behaviours and has 'a clear-cut avoidance orientation' (Rosenstock, 1974, p.333) and has often involved the study of single 'one-off' behaviours such as clinic attendance. Its applicability to physical activity, therefore, is questionable, but it may apply to activity contexts that involve such one-off decisions, as discussed later.

In 1984, after a decade of systematic research using the HBM, a review was published (Janz and Becker, 1984). It was reported that 'the HBM has continued to be a major organising framework for explaining and predicting acceptance of health and medical care recommendations' (p. 1). They concluded that:

- there was substantial support for the model across more than 40 studies;
- the HBM is the most extensively researched model of health-related behaviours;
- 'perceived barriers', when studied, was the most consistently powerful predictor;
- beliefs associated with susceptibility appeared to be more important in preventive health behaviours;
- beliefs in the perceived benefits of action seemed more important in sick-role and illness behaviours;
- despite the variability of measuring instruments, the HBM has remained robust across a wide variety of settings and with a wide variety of research techniques.

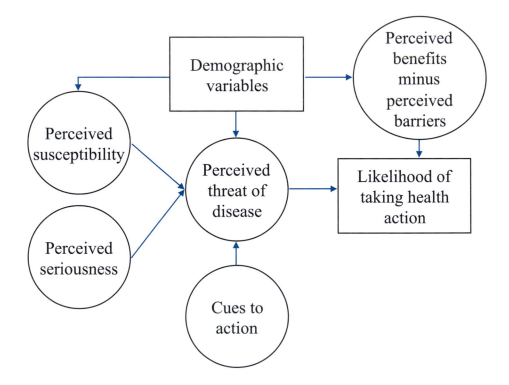

Figure 8.2   A simplified version of the Health Belief Model

Despite this optimistic view, Harrison and colleagues (1992) went further and tested the HBM with adults using meta-analysis but with much stricter criteria for inclusion of studies than by Janz and Becker (1984). From 147 research studies, Harrison *et al.* excluded all but 16 on various criteria, including lack of a behavioural dependent variable, did not measure susceptibility, severity, benefits and costs in the same study, and lack of information about scale reliability. Overall, small but significant effect sizes were found for all four dimensions of the model but effect sizes varied greatly across the dimensions. In addition, they reported that prospective studies had significantly smaller effect sizes than retrospective ones, thus further weakening the case in favour of the HBM.

From evidence on physical activity and the HBM (e.g. Biddle and Ashford, 1988; Lindsay-Reid and Osborn, 1980), it appears that the optimistic conclusions of Janz and Becker (1984) and, to a certain extent the low but significant effect sizes reported in Harrison *et al.*'s (1992) meta-analysis, do not necessarily hold true for physical activity. Although isolated variables, such as barriers, do relate to physical activity, the model as a whole has been relatively unsuccessful in predicting the adoption and/or maintenance of physical activity. Indeed, it could be argued that there is greater support for beliefs about health concerns and worries from the HBM predicting non-participation. For example, some people may believe that vigorous exercise will cause harm rather than good.

There is little doubt about the general heuristic appeal of the HBM. However, a number of points can be made in criticism of the model and associated research, and in particular in relation to its use in physical activity settings (Godin, 1994; Sonstroem, 1988; Stroebe and Stroebe, 1995; Wallston and Wallston, 1985).

First, one must question the holistic nature of the model. Is it one model or merely a collection of individual variables? Indeed, some have argued that because the list of potential variables is so large, the model is untestable (Wallston and Wallston, 1985). Similarly, what relationships exist between the variables and how should the model variables be tested?

Second, there has been a lack of consistency in the operationalising of variables and the measuring tools used. Psychometric developments have been made in the measurement of exercise benefits, outcomes and barriers (Sechrist *et al.*, 1987; Steinhardt and Dishman, 1989) but these instruments were not developed as tools for the direct assessment of the HBM.

The illness-avoidance orientation of the model is generally not appropriate for the explanation or prediction of physical activity. However, the increasing recognition of physical activity as a health behaviour, manifesting itself in promotion schemes such as family doctor-initiated 'exercise on prescription' schemes (Fox *et al.*, 1997; Taylor, 1999), may mean that the HBM is an appropriate framework for some physical activity contexts.

> Key point: The Health Belief Model has intuitive appeal, but its application to physical activity has not been clearly demonstrated.

Theoretical approaches to attitudes in physical activity

The study of attitudes has interested sport and exercise scientists for a long time, although the initial research efforts were primarily descriptive (Kenyon, 1968) and failed to specify clear behavioural targets for the attitudes. For example, it is unlikely that agreement with a general statement concerning one's 'liking' for physical activity will predict specific physical activity behaviours such as swimming or walking. Disaffection with such limitations led to the development of the Theory of Reasoned Action by American social psychologists Icek Ajzen (latterly changing the spelling of his name to Aizen) and Martin Fishbein (Ajzen and Fishbein, 1980; Fishbein and Ajzen, 1975). Ajzen's modification of this model – the Theory of Planned Behaviour – has been tested extensively in the physical activity and health literature and will be discussed later.

The descriptive approach to attitude measurement inevitably led researchers to question whether attitudes actually did predict behaviours at all – called the 'attitude–behaviour discrepancy'. Ajzen and Fishbein's approach sought to increase the strength of association between attitudes and behaviours by not only stating hypothesised antecedents of attitude, but also saying that attitude and behaviour measures must be compatible, thus having a degree of correspondence. For example, generalised attitudes towards physical activity will predict participation in jogging less well (if at all) than attitudes towards jogging. Correspondence between measures is a prudent approach to research in this area. In addition, attitudes were predicted to influence behaviour indirectly through intentions.

> Key point: Generalised statements concerning 'physical activity' will not predict participation in specific physical activities.

The Theory of Reasoned Action

Proposed by Ajzen and Fishbein (Ajzen and Fishbein, 1980; Fishbein and Ajzen, 1975), the Theory of Reasoned Action (TRA) is concerned with 'the causal antecedents of volitional behaviour' (Ajzen, 1988, p.117). It is based on the assumption that intention is an immediate determinant of behaviour, and that intention, in turn, is predicted from attitude and subjective (social) normative factors. The TRA, however, was proposed to predict 'volitional behaviour' – behaviour where essentially the motivation of the individual was paramount and no external barriers existed (Eagly & Chaiken, 1993). The TRA is illustrated in Figure 8.3, alongside the Theory of Planned Behaviour (TPB), and has been used extensively in early research on physical activity.

Ajzen and Fishbein suggested that the attitude component of the model is a function of the beliefs held about the specific behaviour, as well as the evaluation, or value, of the likely outcomes. The measurement of such variables, they suggest, should be highly specific to the behaviour in question in order to achieve correspondence, or compatibility, between assessed attitude/subjective norm questions and the behaviour being predicted. It is recommended that questionnaire item content for testing the TRA be derived from interview material gathered from the population to be studied. Three factors should be considered in terms of achieving correspondence:

- *Action and target*: Attitude and behaviour need to be assessed in relation to a specific action, such as taking part in an exercise class, rather than a general attitude object such as physical activity.
- *Context*: Reference should be made to the context in which the behaviour takes place (e.g. '… at this health club').
- *Time*: Time should be clearly specified (e.g. 'attending this exercise class three times a week over the next two months').

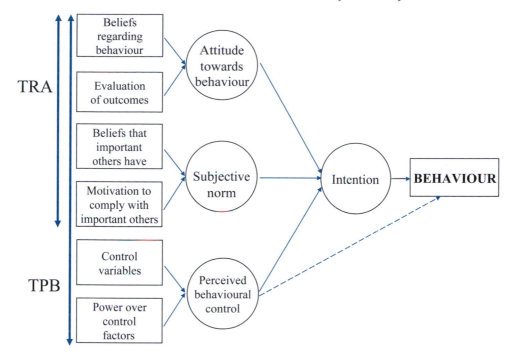

Figure 8.3 Theories of Reasoned Action (TRA) and Planned Behaviour (TPB)

Ajzen (1988) proposed that these factors should be assessed at the same level of generality/ specificity. Of course, very high correspondence, such as predicting attendance at the fitness club on Tuesdays from items that refer only to exercising at the club on Tuesdays, will have limited generalisability and, indeed, may appear trivial. Vague attitude measures about 'exercise' may be less than precise and be weak predictors, yet we also want to have the ability to generalise; thus some compromise between the two may sometimes be necessary. Kenyon's (1968) Attitude Toward Physical Activity scale, for example, assesses only the target (physical activity) and not the context or time. Perhaps this has led to some researchers being confused about the role of attitudes in physical activity. For example, Dishman and Sallis (1994) concluded, in their review of studies of supervised and unsupervised settings, that 'attitudes' are largely unrelated to physical activity. This is a surprising conclusion given the clear evidence showing that both intentions and attitudes are related to physical activity when appropriate theoretical models, such as the TRA, are used (Hagger *et al.*, 2002; Hausenblas *et al.*, 1997). Similarly, King *et al.* (1992) say that intentions do not predict actual behaviour in adult studies of exercise. This also is not correct and, indeed, intentions are even better predictors of physical activity than attitudes (Hagger *et al.*, 2002). Correlations between intention and physical activity are consistently positive and statistically significant. Indeed, Sallis and Owen (1999), in reference to meta-analytic evidence from Hausenblas *et al.* (1997), describe the correlations between intentions and exercise as 'substantial' (p. 118).

The subjective norm component of the TRA ('normative component') comprises the beliefs of significant others and the extent that one wishes or is motivated to comply with such beliefs or people. The relative importance of the attitudinal and normative components will depend on the situation under investigation. For example, one might hypothesise that adolescent health behaviours, in some contexts, will be more strongly influenced by the normative component (expressed through peer influence) than the attitudinal component, but this trend may be reversed with adults.

The Theory of Reasoned Action (TRA) and physical activity

The TRA has received a great deal of attention in social psychology generally (Ajzen, 1988) and in health contexts (Armitage and Conner, 2001). Although not without its critics, particularly in respect of the causal structure of the model and emphasis on volitional behaviour (Liska, 1984), it has also been recommended and used in physical activity research for many years (Godin, 1993, 1994; McAuley and Courneya, 1993).

The work of Gaston Godin and co-workers in Canada has provided the most extensive test of the TRA in exercise settings and he was the first to review the research on physical activity. Godin (1993) reported that about 30 per cent of the variance in intention is explained by the attitudinal and normative components of the TRA, although the attitudinal component is nearly always the stronger of the two predictors. Indeed, the normative component has been inconsistently associated with physical activity participation.

Subsequently, three meta-analyses have been conducted using the TRA and the Theory of Planned Behaviour in physical activity. The findings from the TRA constructs are summarised in Table 8.2. Hausenblas *et al.* (1997) analysed 31 exercise studies and they found that intention had a strong association with exercise behaviour, and attitude was associated strongly with intention. The same pattern of associations was noted by Hagger *et al.* (2002) when analysing effects from 44 to 70 studies. The more recent review of 111 studies by Symons Downs and Hausenblas (2005) reported effect sizes that showed a similar pattern to those of the previous reviews. As shown in Table 8.2, there were large effect sizes for the association of behaviour with both intention and attitude. In all reviews, it is clear that the strength of association for attitude on intention is twice that of subjective norm. Moreover, attitude is associated with intention to the same degree that intention is to behaviour.

The Theory of Reasoned Action: conclusion and critique

The TRA has received support in physical activity contexts, and Godin (1994) suggests that 'when attitude is measured within a proper theoretical framework, it seems an important determinant of exercise behavior' (p. 122). Based on the evidence presented, the TRA attitudinal component appears to be influential in predicting intentions to be physically active, and intentions predict behaviour to a certain extent. From a practical standpoint this suggests that interventions that attempt to alter beliefs and affective perceptions of the outcomes of physical activity may be useful.

Although the normative component of the TRA has not been such a strong predictor of intentions in physical activity studies, it is still important. Interventions that are possible include public health campaigns which persuade the public that exercise is 'normal' and not just for the young, fit and 'sporty'.

The TRA has not been without its critics. For example, the following points highlight issues for consideration:

• The TRA is a unidirectional model and fails to offer the possibility that variables in the model can act in a reciprocal manner.

Table 8.2   Summary of associations between constructs from the Theories of Reasoned Action and Planned Behaviour[1] reported across three meta-analytic reviews concerning physical activity

Association	Hausenblas *et al.* (1997)		Hagger *et al.* (2002)	Symons Downs and Hausenblas (2005)
	ES[2]	*Correlation*	*Correlation*[3]	*ES*
Intention –behaviour	1.09	0.47	0.51	1.01
Attitude – intention	1.22	0.52	0.60	1.07
Attitude – behaviour	0.84	0.39	0.35	
Subjective norm –intention	0.56	0.27	0.32	0.59
Subjective norm –behaviour	0.18	0.09	0.17	
PBC[4] –intention	0.97	0.43	0.57	0.51
PBC – behaviour	1.01	0.45	0.39	0.90

Notes:
1. PBC is unique to the TPB. Other variables also exist in the TRA and TPB.
2. ES: Effect size.
3. Corrected (reweighted) for sampling error and measurement error.
4. PBC: perceived behavioural control.

- The model relies solely on cognitions (beliefs) and omits other potentially important determinants of action, such as personality and environmental influences.
- The TRA predicts behaviour from measures of behavioural intention taken at one point in time. Similar attitudinal models of behaviour (Bentler and Speckart, 1981; Triandis, 1977) take into account prior behaviour. In the exercise context, 'habitual' physical activity is often the goal of public health initiatives and therefore research may usefully investigate the role of past behaviour in addition to other TRA variables, and this may include 'conscious' processing of the pros and cons of physical activity (as one might expect in a theory of *reasoned* action), as well as the less conscious modes of processing, such as the routine of walking to work when one does not possess a car or have access to public transport. In other words, little or no conscious decision-making is required – it's automatic or a 'habit' (Gardner *et al.*, 2011). As it stands, the TRA may only predict new behaviours rather than habitual ones. The distinction between activity adoption and maintenance is important. However, the role of past behaviour is a difficult one to judge at times. It can appear rather obvious, and even unhelpful if we wish to identify behavioural determinants, to state that past behaviour is the best predictor of current or intended behaviour. However, it does suggest that prior activity habits are important.
- The distinction between intentions and expectations may be important (Olson and Zanna, 1993). We could decide (intention) to exercise but realise that it is rather too difficult (expectation).
- The TRA was developed to account for behaviours that are under volitional control (Ajzen, 1988). Consequently, the theory may not predict behaviours where other factors may be influential. In the case of physical activity, there may be a number of behavioural barriers preventing the behaviour from being totally volitional (e.g. responsibilities to others, job, distance from facilities, etc.). A revised TRA – the 'Theory of Planned Behaviour' (TPB; see later in this chapter) – is an attempt to account for behaviour under 'incomplete' volitional control.

- Insufficient attention has been paid to the measurement of behaviour within the TRA. Without an accurate measure of the behaviour, the principle of correspondence cannot be applied satisfactorily. This casts some doubt on several studies, such as when assessment relies on unvalidated self-reports or uses inappropriate 'objective' measures, such as pedometers for people who get their physical activity predominantly through cycling or swimming.
- The TRA allows the investigation of the interrelationships between attitudes, subjective norms, intentions and a single behaviour. It does not account for alternative behaviours. For example, although many people intend to be more physically active, few see this through to action in a sustained way. This could be due to physical activity being of lower priority than other behaviours, and so just does not get to the top of the list of 'things to do'.
- Intention should predict behaviour quite well when both intention and behaviour are measured in close proximity or, in the case of measurement, take place some time apart; the prediction will be affected by how intentions change during this time interval (Ajzen and Fishbein, 1980). This is the issue of 'intentional stability' and is one that has largely been ignored in physical activity research. Recent evidence suggests that while attitude–intention links are stable over time (at least over six weeks), behaviour–intention relationships weaken over time (Chatzisarantis et al., 2005). This is supported by the meta-analysis by Symons Downs and Hausenblas (2005) where they showed larger effects for stability up to one month (ESs = 1.19–1.20) but weaker effect sizes for time intervals greater than one month (ES = 0.76).
- Finally, there appears to be a potential discrepancy between the inconsistent role of subjective norms in using the TRA and the belief that social support is a determinant of physical activity (Dishman and Sallis, 1994). Although social support may not be exactly the same as social influence/subjective norm (Taylor et al., 1994), the similarities are such that we should expect the social normative component of the TRA to be more closely linked to exercise behaviour than has typically been the case. Two explanations are possible. First, we may not be assessing subjective norms appropriately in TRA studies and this may be forcing respondents to misinterpret the meaning behind the statements. A second possibility is that some people may be reluctant to admit that they require motivation from others and certainly do not want to admit that they wish 'to comply' with these people (e.g. adolescents with parents).

In summary, the TRA has been at the forefront of re-establishing attitude research as a powerful force in social psychology, and both health and exercise psychology have been quick to utilise such an approach. The TRA has proved to be a viable unifying theoretical framework that has been successful in furthering our understanding of exercise intentions and behaviours. It has also been instrumental in moving research on physical activity correlates from being largely atheoretical to theoretical.

The Theory of Planned Behaviour (TPB)

The TRA has provided a model that has been successful in predicting behaviour and intentions for actions that are primarily volitional and controllable. However, in the case of physical activity, volitional control is likely to be 'incomplete' (Ajzen, 1988), although Godin (1993) suggests that different types of physical activity may differ from each other in this respect.

Ajzen's theorising and research (Ajzen, 1985, 1988, 1996; Ajzen and Madden, 1986; Schifter and Ajzen, 1985) suggests that the TRA is insufficient for behaviours where volitional control is incomplete; in other words, where resources and skills are required (Eagly and Chaiken, 1993). Consequently, Ajzen proposed an extension of the TRA for such behaviours and called this the Theory of Planned Behaviour (TPB). The TPB is the same as the TRA but with the additional variable of 'perceived behavioural control', as illustrated in Figure 8.3. Perceived behavioural control (PBC) is defined by Ajzen (1988) as 'the perceived ease or difficulty of performing the behaviour' (p. 132) and is assumed 'to reflect past experience as well as anticipated impediments and obstacles' (p. 132). Figure 8.3 links perceived control with both intentions and behaviour. This suggests that the variable has a motivational effect on intentions, such that individuals wishing to be physically active, but with little or no chance of being so (because of largely insurmountable behavioural barriers at the time), are unlikely to do so regardless of their attitudes towards activity or the social factors operating. This overcomes one of the problems of the TRA alluded to earlier when a distinction was made between intentions and expectations.

For Ajzen (1991), the construct of perceived behavioural control refers to general perceptions of control. He compared it overtly with Bandura's (1977) construct of self-efficacy that captures judgements of one's ability to execute volitional behaviours required to produce important outcomes (see Chapter 10). The construct of PBC is also underpinned by a set of control beliefs and the perceived power of these beliefs (Ajzen and Fishbein, 1980). Control beliefs refer to the perceived presence of factors that may facilitate or impede performance of behaviour. Perceived power refers to the perceived impact that facilitative or inhibiting factors may have on the performance of behaviour (Ajzen, 1991). In the same way that an expectancy-value model is used to form indirect antecedents of attitudes and subjective norm, an indirect measure of PBC may be formed from each control belief multiplied by its corresponding perceived power rating (Ajzen, 1991).

The inclusion of perceived behavioural control in the TPB is important because it reveals the personal and environmental factors that affect behaviour (Ajzen, 1985). To the extent that PBC influences intentions and behaviour, the researcher can evaluate which behaviours are under the volitional control of the individual and the degree to which the behaviour is impeded by personal and/or environmental factors. Ajzen (1991) hypothesised that when control over the behaviour was problematic, perceived behavioural control would exert two types of effects within the TPB. First, PBC would influence intentions alongside attitudes and subjective norms. This additive effect reflects the *motivational* influence of perceived control on decisions to exercise. Second, perceived behavioural control may predict behaviour directly, especially when perceptions of behavioural control are realistic. This direct effect reflects the actual, real constraints or barriers for the behaviour. In this case PBC is a proxy measure of *actual* control over the behaviour (Ajzen, 1991).

Ajzen (1988) argues that perceived behavioural control will accurately predict behaviour under circumstances only when perceived control closely approximates actual control (hence the use of a broken line in Figure 8.3). For example, whereas some people may have a strong perception of control over their body weight, the reality may be different since there are biological factors likely to affect weight gain and loss that are beyond personal control. In such situations one would not expect perceived control to be a strong predictor of weight change, although it is possible for it to predict to a lesser degree. Similarly, one would expect better predictions of exercise *behaviour* (e.g. frequency of exercise) from perceived control compared with exercise *performance* (e.g. a fitness test score), since the latter is less controllable due to factors such as heredity, practice and the test environment.

Evidence from the Theory of Planned Behaviour

The TPB is appropriate for use in the study of physical activity, particularly as it is a behaviour that has many barriers; thus it is only partly under volitional control. The testing of the TPB in physical activity is now extensive.

A comprehensive test of the TPB was conducted by Hagger and colleagues (2002). They meta-analysed 72 studies that allowed calculations of the relationships proposed in either the TRA or the TPB (see Table 8.2). In addition to reporting correlations between variables, they achieved three objectives:

1. By using the correlation matrix, they tested the TRA and the TPB through path analysis.
2. They tested the additional variance accounted for by adding variables to the TRA. This was done by first adding PBC (hence testing the TPB), then self-efficacy, and finally past behaviour.
3. They tested three moderator variables: age, attitude-intention strength, and the time between the assessment of past behaviour and present behaviour.

Results supported the TPB with intention being a direct predictor of behaviour, intention being predicted more strongly by attitudes than subjective norms (the latter showing a small contribution), and PBC being associated with behaviour through intention. Self-efficacy (a more internal aspect of PBC) added to the prediction of both intentions and behaviour, while past behaviour was associated with all TPB variables. Of most importance was the finding that by adding past behaviour to the model, the strength of other paths was reduced, suggesting that studies which do not assess past behaviour may be obtaining artificially high correlations.

Nevertheless, the relationship between attitude and intentions remained, even when past behaviour was included. Hagger *et al.* (2002, p. 23) concluded:

> [W]hile past behaviour had a significant and direct influence on intention, attitude, PBC, and self-efficacy, these cognitions are also necessary for translating past decisions about behavioural involvement into action. This is consistent with the notion that involvement in volitional behaviours such as regular physical activity involves both conscious and automatic influences.

Hagger *et al.*'s analysis also showed that intentions are more strongly associated with behaviour in older participants, possibly because of their greater experience. Young people may also have additional controls, such as parental influence, precluding full translation of intentions. In addition, results showed that the time between assessment of past behaviour and current behaviour did not affect the strength of relationships, unlike in the meta-analysis published three years later by Symons Downs and Hausenblas (2005).

Theory of Planned Behaviour: illustrative population-based studies

Most studies in this area are relatively small, yet both Wankel and Mummery (1993) and Plotnikoff *et al.* (2011) have managed to integrate TPB items into large population surveys. Wankel and Mummery analysed 'the Campbell Survey of Well-being'. This involved over 4,000 Canadians who had previously participated in the 1981 Canada Fitness Survey. In predicting physical activity intention, Wankel and Mummery (1993) found that across the different age and gender groups, intentions were associated with attitudes, social norm/ support and perceived behavioural control. For the total sample, 31 per cent of the variance in intentions was explained by the three TPB variables. This is a reasonable approximation of estimates from other studies.

A similar study, also in Canada, involved over 4,000 adolescents. Self-reported physical activity was assessed alongside the TPB variables (Plotnikoff *et al.*, 2011). The TPB model was supported. Both PBC and intention predicted physical activity levels, accounting for 43 per cent of the variance, and attitude, subjective norm and PBC predicted intention accounting for 59 per cent. Attitude was the strongest of the three variables in its association with intention.

While both of these studies have the strength of using large samples, they also have weaknesses. These include the use of mainly single-item measures, the use of only self-reported physical activity by Plotnikoff and colleagues, and no behavioural measure by Wankel and Mummery. Moreover, these studies are cross-sectional, thus precluding measures of future physical activity and any conclusion regarding temporal relations and causality.

The Theory of Planned Behaviour: conclusion and critique

Many of the criticisms of the TRA already discussed may be applied to the TPB, with the exception of the point concerning volition, since the inclusion of perceived behavioural control accounts for this. However, as Godin (1993) has suggested, it is unclear which physical activities are perceived to be volitionally controlled and which are not. It seems reasonable to suggest that walking will be seen by most people to be quite controllable, yet activities requiring facilities and high costs are likely to be seen to be much less controllable. This factor needs to be taken into account in future studies as we seek to predict participation in both structured and unstructured physical activities. However, Ajzen (1988, p. 127) warns that:

> [A]t first glance, the problem of behavioral control may appear to apply to a limited range of actions only. Closer scrutiny reveals, however, that even very mundane activities, which can usually be executed (or not executed) at will, are sometimes subject to the influence of factors beyond one's control.

One problem with the TPB is the lack of consistency in defining and assessing perceived behavioural control. Ajzen (1991) defines perceived behavioural control in terms of both perceived resources and opportunities as well as perceived power to overcome obstacles; thus the construct represents both control beliefs and perceived power. Studies incorporating self-efficacy and PBC often find that they make independent contributions to the prediction of intentions or behaviour. For example, Terry and O'Leary (1995) found items reflecting self-efficacy and PBC to be distinct. Moreover, they found that self-efficacy predicted intentions to be physically active, but not activity itself, whereas PBC predicted physical activity but not intention. PBC seems to include beliefs built on past experience as well as external barriers, whereas self-efficacy refers to beliefs concerning whether the individual feels that he or she can perform a behaviour without necessarily distinguishing types of constraints. Self-efficacy is more akin to internal control (Hagger *et al.*, 2002).

Perhaps a key point of criticism concerning the TPB is the lack of extensive experimental support. Most of the literature using the TPB has relied on observational methods, and rather few have been experimental studies of behaviour change. In an editorial, Sniehotta and colleagues (2014) are highly critical of the TPB for this reason and call for the theory to be retired. Certainly more intervention evidence is needed.

Interestingly, Hagger and Chatzisarantis (2014) use the TPB as a building block for a more comprehensive 'integrated behaviour change model', and include autonomous motivation as well as implicit (less conscious) attitudes and motivation. The model is shown in Figure 8.4.

Reasons for the success and popularity of the TPB may be attributed to its efficacy in predicting intention and behaviour, its relative parsimony, and its flexibility. Furthermore, the original constructs of the TPB have been shown to mediate the direct effect of other constructs on intentions and behaviour, suggesting that the belief systems that underpin the directly measured theory constructs are able to account for the effects of other variables that have previously accounted for unique variance in behaviour (Conner and Abraham, 2001). However, researchers have also indicated that the theory does not account for all of the variance in intention and behaviour, nor does it mediate the effects of certain 'external variables' (S.D. Rhodes *et al.*, 2003), personality and belief-based constructs on intentions and behaviour (Bagozzi and Kimmel, 1995; Conner and Abraham, 2001; Conner and Armitage, 1998; R.E. Rhodes *et al.*, 2002). Paradoxically, this 'weakness' has become the theory's greatest strength. Ajzen (1991) states that the theory should be viewed as a flexible framework into which other variables may be incorporated, provided that they make a meaningful and unique contribution to the prediction of intentions and there is a theoretical reason for the inclusion of such variables.

The theory has demonstrated considerable flexibility and has been adopted by researchers as a general framework to investigate the effect of a number of additional social cognitive constructs on intention and behaviour (Conner and Armitage, 1998). However, there are additional considerations regarding attitude constructs. These include affective versus

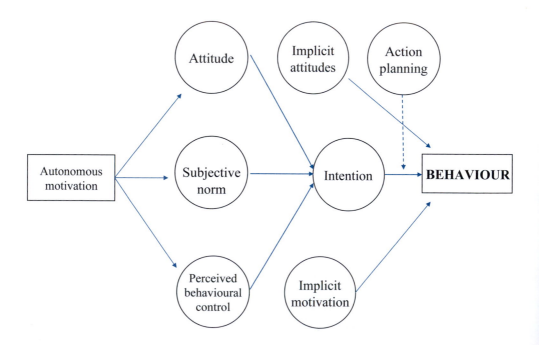

Figure 8.4   A proposed integrated behaviour change model

instrumental attitudinal judgements, the intention–behaviour gap, and the use of implementation intentions in closing this gap.

> Key point: The Theory of Planned Behaviour has been successful in developing our understanding of attitudes and physical activity – being active is mainly associated with more positive attitudes, having perceptions of control, and stronger intentions. However, experimental evidence is less convincing.

Affective versus instrumental attitudinal judgements

As shown in the opening section of this chapter, attitudes comprise affective, cognitive and behavioural components. However, some frameworks, such as the TPB, combine affective and cognitive elements, such as asking people to rate items concerning possible outcomes of physical activity and also how important these outcomes are. The separate effects of affective elements of attitudes need stating. For example, it is often assumed that we are more motivated by liking a behaviour, or enjoying it, than beliefs of its benefits for health. If this is true, then affective elements of attitude will be stronger predictors of intentions and behaviour than cognitive elements.

A systematic review was conducted by R.E. Rhodes and colleagues (2009) where they investigated 'affective judgements' and physical activity. They defined affective judgements as 'overall pleasure/displeasure, enjoyment, and feeling states expected from enacting physical activity' (p.181). Both correlational (n = 85 samples) and experimental (n = 20) studies were analysed. Correlational studies showed a summary effect size of r = 0.42. For 38 samples where there was also a measure of instrumental attitude, affective attitude had the larger effect (r = 0.42 vs. r = 0.25). Intervention studies were less effective in changing affective judgements; thus it was difficult for Rhodes *et al.* to conclude about affective attitude and physical activity from experimental designs. Nevertheless, Conner *et al.* (2011) have shown that targeting affective attitudes can change self-reported physical activity, and this is consistent with Lawton *et al.*'s (2009) prospective analysis. In summary, it is recommended that studies assess both affective and instrumental attitudes.

> Key point: Affective attitudes are likely to be stronger predictors of health intentions and behaviour than instrumental attitudes. Affective attitudes should be targeted in interventions.

Mind the gap! The intention–behaviour gap

Despite the theoretical and practical utility of the TPB, its fundamental weakness is that intentions only partly explain or predict behaviour. This is the so-called 'intention–behaviour gap' and is a fundamental premise in human psychology: we have good intentions but often fail to turn these into sustainable behaviour change.

The intention–behaviour gap is best exemplified by New Year resolutions. The good intentions for more physical activity, less food and alcohol intake, some weight loss, stopping smoking, and other desired health outcomes are, in the majority of cases, doomed to failure. Rhodes and de Bruijn (2013) suggest that while there are theoretically four main groups of people based on their intentions and behaviour (see Table 8.3), some 36 per cent will be classified as 'unsuccessful intenders', supporting the notion of an intention–behaviour gap.

There are many possible explanations for this, including lack of preparation for behaviour change (see Chapter 11) as well as factors that 'get in the way' of translating intentions into behaviour. Factors that may enhance or detract from good translation of intentions into behaviour are referred to as moderators of this link. These were reviewed by Rhodes and Dickau (2013). They analysed 38 potential moderators from 57 studies and found that the most consistent was intentional stability, while there was also evidence for the role for 'anticipated regret' and conscientiousness. Intentional stability refers to how stable people's ratings of intentions are over time. This may partly be a function of the length of time between stated intentions and actual behaviour, as typically intentions fluctuate over time. We can help maintain the level of intentions by using what are called 'implementation intentions' (see below).

'Anticipated regret' refers to the desire to avoid feeling guilt or regret about certain actions, such as not exercising or overeating. Anticipating such negative feelings is thought to assist in carrying out good intentions. For example, if I anticipate that not going to the gym today will lead to feelings of guilt later on, then I will be more motivated to find the time to go the gym, thus acting out my intentions. Sandberg and Conner (2008) conducted a meta-analysis of studies investigating the anticipated regret construct in the TPB framework across multiple behaviours. They found a clear effect on intention with a weighted correlation of 0.47 from 25 studies. The association with behaviour was smaller but still significant (0.32).

Conscientiousness was identified by Rhodes and Dickau (2013) as a moderator of the intention–behaviour relationship. Being conscientious is having a tendency to strive to achieve, to be self-disciplined and orderly. This may be a function of stable individual differences, or it may be developed over time. It is likely to be developed through planning of physical activity (e.g. specific exercise sessions), keeping a record of what you do (self-monitoring), setting clear and measurable goals, and getting feedback on progress.

According to Rhodes and Dickau's (2013) systematic review, therefore, the gap between physical activity intentions and behaviour is partly a function of the stability of intentions over time, the anticipation of regret or negative affect if the behaviour is missed, and being conscientious. From a practical point of view, these findings suggest that we need to keep intentions stable (see the following section on implementation intentions), anticipate how we will feel if not being physically active (but also anticipate positive affect from participation), and plan well to boost conscientiousness.

Table 8.3   Classification of people based on intentions and behaviour in physical activity (adapted from Rhodes and de Bruijn, 2013)

	Intention to be physically active		Actual physical activity	
Group	High	Low	High	Low
Non-intenders		x		x
Non-intenders who then become active		x	x	
Unsuccessful intenders	x			x
Successful intenders	x		x	

Implementation intentions

One approach that has been put forward to help close the intention–behaviour gap is 'implementation intentions' (Gollwitzer, 1999). These are self-regulatory strategies (goals and plans) that involve specifying when, how and where performance of the behaviour will take place. Implementation intentions were developed specifically from concerns about the intention–behaviour gap.

Experimental paradigms using implementation intention strategies require research participants to specify explicitly *when*, *where* and *how* they will engage in an intended behaviour. According to Gollwitzer (1999), implementation intentions help people move from a motivational (intentional) phase to a volitional (behavioural) phase ensuring that intentions are converted into action (see the HAPA model in Chapter 11). Research has indicated that forming implementation intentions decreases the probability of people failing to initiate their goal-directed intentions at the point of initiation (Orbell, 2000). This is because planning when and where to initiate a behaviour strengthens the mental association between representations of situations and representations of actions.

Motivational strategies focus on increasing intention levels but do not facilitate the enactment of intentions, while volitional strategies, such as implementation intentions, increase the probability that these strong intentions will be converted into action without necessarily changing intentions. Research has supported the use of these combined techniques in increasing exercise behaviour. For example, Prestwich *et al.* (2003) demonstrated that an intervention that had a combination of a rational decision-making strategy, or decisional balance sheet (weighing up the pros and cons), and implementation intentions was more effective in promoting physical activity behaviour than either of the strategies alone. These results support the existence of two distinct phases of motivation: a *motivational or pre-decisional* phase during which people decide whether or not to perform a behaviour, and a *volitional, post-decisional* or implemental phase during which people plan when and where they will convert their intentions into behaviour (Gollwitzer, 1999). As a consequence, interventions that combine motivational and volitional techniques are likely to be most effective in promoting physical activity behaviour. Implementation intentions regarding stair use in a hospital were also found to predict higher levels of stair use even though actual intentions to use the stairs were similar among intervention and control participants (Kwak *et al.*, 2007).

In an extensive meta-analysis of studies investigating implementation intentions, Gollwitzer and Sheeran (2006) reported a moderate to large effect size (0.65). Similar findings were reported for correlational and experimental studies, self-report and objective measures, and for published and unpublished studies.

Two main problems in physical activity adherence are behavioural adoption (getting started) and maintenance (keeping it going). Gollwitzer and Sheeran (2006) provide examples of implementation intentions for 'failing to get started' and 'getting derailed'. These may be applied to physical activity, as shown in Table 8.4.

Alternative attitude models for the study of physical activity

The majority – probably a very large majority – of the literature concerning intentions, beliefs and attitudes towards physical activity has adopted the framework of the TRA or TPB. This is why we have focused most of our attention on this model. However, we have raised a number of criticisms and concerns about this approach. Moreover, there are other theories and models that are either relevant to physical activity or have actually been used

Table 8.4   Example implementation intentions for physical activity contexts (adapted from Gollwitzer
and Sheeran, 2006)

Main Issue	Specific problem to focus on	Example implementation intention statement
Failure to become physically active	Remembering to do the behaviour	'And if the bus gets to the post office, I will get off to walk the rest'
	Seizing opportunities	'And if I see Chris in the office today, I will arrange the golf game'
	Overcoming initial reluctance	'And if it is Monday 12.30, it's gym time. It's in my diary'
Failure to maintain physical activity involvement	Suppressing unwanted attention responses	'And if I see the lift, I will ignore it and seek out the stairs'
	Suppressing unwanted behavioural responses	'If I feel I am tired, I will go for a walk'
	Blocking detrimental self-states	'And if I have driven the car to work, I will park it further away from my office'

in physical activity research. Two approaches that are relevant include The Health Action Process Approach (HAPA) and Protection Motivation Theory. The HAPA model is reviewed in Chapter 11.

Protection Motivation Theory (PMT)

A model that has some similarities with the Health Belief Model, as well as with the TRA/ TPB, is that of Rogers' 'Protection Motivation Theory' (PMT) (Floyd *et al.*, 2000; Rogers, 1983). This too is a cognitive model based on expectancy-value principles and was originally developed as an explanation for the effects of 'fear appeals' in health behaviour change. Some have argued that 'health threats' might be a better term, as the model is really one of health decision-making (Wurtele and Maddux, 1987). Health behaviour intentions ('protection motivation') are predicted from the cognitive appraisal mechanisms shown in Figure 8.5. Support has been found for the model using meta-analysis (Floyd *et al.*, 2000). Specifically, significant effect sizes ranging from small to large were found for all PMT variables, with the strongest effect for self-efficacy.

Prentice-Dunn and Rogers (1986) contrast the PMT with the HBM and suggest that the PMT has some distinct advantages. They say that the PMT has more of an organisational framework and is not open to the criticism of merely being a catalogue of variables. Second, the division of cognitive appraisals into threat and coping categories helps to clarify how people think about health decision-making. Third, PMT includes self-efficacy, a variable found to be a powerful mediator of behaviour change in other studies (see Chapter 10).

Only a few studies have directly tested PMT in a physical activity context, although other studies provide evidence indirectly (see Godin, 1994). Floyd and colleagues (2000) suggest that adherence to medical treatment regimens and exercise studies show large effect sizes, but the two types of studies were not reported separately. Stanley and Maddux (1986) tested PMT alongside self-efficacy in the prediction of exercise behaviour of American undergraduate students. Using an experimental design, they found that manipulations of perceived

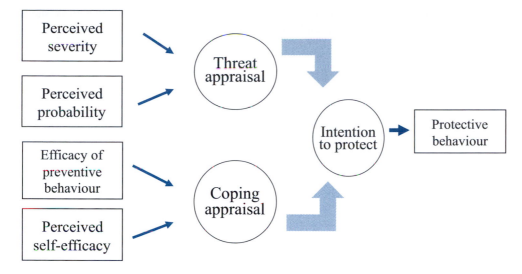

Figure 8.5   A simplified version of Protection Motivation Theory

response efficacy (outcome expectancy) and self-efficacy through written persuasive communications successfully predicted intentions to exercise.

Wurtele and Maddux (1987) asked 160 sedentary undergraduate women to read persuasive appeals for increasing their exercise levels. The appeals were varied along the four dimensions of severity, vulnerability, response efficacy and self-efficacy. PMT includes two types of efficacy. 'Response efficacy' refers to the belief that a response will produce the desired outcome, whereas 'self-efficacy' refers to the belief in one's ability to initiate and maintain the desired behaviour (see Prentice-Dunn and Rogers, 1986). Results showed that only vulnerability and self-efficacy predicted intentions to exercise which, in turn, were predictive of self-reported exercise. Those with high self-efficacy also had strong intentions to exercise even though they were not exposed to the vulnerability-enhancing or response efficacy-enhancing conditions in the study. This confirms the important role of self-efficacy in behaviour change. It was also found that the threat appeals were ineffective in changing exercise intentions.

Milne and colleagues (2002) provided a longitudinal test of PMT alongside the use of implementation intentions. While increases in threat, coping appraisal and intention were brought about through an intervention, exercise behaviour was unchanged. However, enhancement of the PMT-based intervention was achieved by the introduction of a condition that enhanced implementation intentions.

Consistent with Milne *et al.* (2002), Godin (1994) concluded that 'in general, messages conveying a persuasive threat seem effective in enhancing participants' intention to change their behaviors, but they are less effective in inducing and sustaining changes in behaviour'. However, he then went on to say that PMT 'has limited usefulness for the study of exercise behavior' (p. 117). This conclusion may be premature, certainly when combined with other interventions or looking at similar health behaviours (Floyd *et al.*, 2000).

Although one may not be comfortable with physical activity motivation based on fear or health threats, and also noting that the results of PMT research are more favourable towards the role of self-efficacy than health threats per se, research so far suggests that PMT sheds light on some important constructs and processes in physical activity decision-making.

Models of attitude change

An area of attitude theory relevant to this discussion is that of persuasion. Olson and Zanna (1993) say that 'the single largest topic within attitudes literature is persuasion: attitude change resulting from exposure to information from others' (p. 135). For example, McGuire's (1969) sequence of cognitive responses, or 'chain of persuasion', suggests that for a message to influence behaviour, it must involve the following:

- *Exposure*: the recipient must be exposed to the message.
- *Attention*: the message must be attended to.
- *Comprehension*: the message must be understood. It is thought that when the message is not clearly understood, attitudes may be more influenced by the credibility of the source, whereas this is thought not to be so important when the message is understood (Olson and Zanna, 1993).
- *Yielding*: the message must be persuasive; the recipient is persuaded by the content.
- *Retention*: the message must be retained, even in the face of competing messages and influences.
- *Retrieval*: the ability to retrieve the message from memory when needing to act.
- *Decision*: a decision to act in accord with the message, sometimes in the face of competing messages.
- *Behaviour*: acting in accordance with the message.

The approach to attitude change advocated by McGuire (1969) suggests that attitudes are formed and changed as a result of careful thought and consideration of the relevant issues. This is similar to the Ajzen/Fishbein approach already discussed in this chapter through the Theories of Reasoned Action and Planned Behaviour. Other attitude change theories suggest that the processing of information is not so logical (Eagly and Chaiken, 1993). For example, the 'heuristic-systematic' model, proposed by Chaiken (1980), says that such thoughtful processing of information only occurs when the person is motivated and able to do so. Persuasion may occur, however, if the person is unmotivated, but this will be temporary and may depend on other factors, such as environmental cues. When motivated, the strength of the argument is thought to determine the degree of persuasion, and attitude change is likely to be more permanent.

Similar to the heuristic-systematic approach is the 'elaboration-likelihood' model proposed by Petty and Cacioppo (1986). They proposed that the 'central' route to attitude change involves an elaboration of the message through conscious thought, as in the heuristic-systematic model. The 'peripheral' route to attitude change and persuasion includes other forms of attitude change that are not related to deliberation or much thought, such as being exposed to the message. The elaboration-likelihood approach advocates that people are motivated to hold 'correct' attitudes. 'Elaboration involves making relevant associations, scrutinising the arguments, inferring their value, and evaluating the overall message' (Fiske and Taylor, 1991, p.478). Important factors to consider in these approaches to attitude change include the following:

- The communicator of the message, such as attractiveness and expertise.

- The message itself, including difficulty, repetition and 'involvement' with the message or attitude object.
- Audience involvement: 'the respondent's amount and valence of cognitive response determines the type of effect that occurs. Because cognitive responses demand an actively thinking recipient, audience involvement has influenced each of the effects [communicator and message] discussed so far' (Fiske and Taylor, 1991, p. 487).

Such approaches to attitudes suggest that it is not just about conscious and logical decision-making when arriving at intentions and behaviour. There may be less conscious processes at work, and this approach is gaining impetus in health behaviour change (see Chapter 9). For example, the 'behaviour change wheel' (Michie *et al.*, 2011) suggests motivational elements of health behaviour change will involve both reflective (conscious, deliberative) and automatic (less conscious) processes (see Chapter 12). The TPB is an example of a reflective approach to attitudes and behaviour, and it is sometimes a criticism of the theory that it is too 'logical' and 'rational' (Sutton, 2004).

Chapter summary and conclusions

Most people would agree that an important area for better understanding the behaviour of physical activity is attitudes. However, such an all-embracing construct cannot explain all that we do, but it remains central to the psychology of physical activity determinants and behaviour change.

In this chapter, therefore, we have:

- defined attitude and components of the attitude construct;
- summarised the approach adopted through the Theories of Reasoned Action and Planned Behaviour, the two most commonly used theories in physical activity attitude research;
- discussed the important issues of the distinction between affective and instrumental attitudes, the intention–behaviour gap, and implementation intentions;
- described other approaches to the study of attitudes, including the Health Belief Model and Protection Motivation Theory.

In summary, therefore, we conclude the following:

- The early physical activity attitude research was mainly descriptive and assessed only the target of physical activity, and not the action, context or time elements of attitude believed to be critical in linking attitude with behaviour. This approach, therefore, has limited utility.
- The Health Belief Model has been shown to be a reasonably effective integrating social psychological framework for understanding health decision-making, although meta-analytic results suggest that small amounts of variance in health behaviours are accounted for by the major dimensions of the HBM.
- The utility of the HBM in physical activity settings has not been demonstrated clearly, probably due to the inappropriate emphasis of the HBM on illness avoidance.
- The TRA has consistently predicted exercise intentions and behaviour across diverse settings and samples; attitude is a strong predictor of intention, but subjective norm is less so.

- The TPB appears to add to the predictive utility of the TRA in physical activity; perceived behavioural control has been shown to be an accurate predictor of intentions and behaviour in observational research.
- Both TRA and TPB models are limited by their focus on conscious decision-making through cognitive processes; they are essentially static and uni-dimensional approaches, and the prediction of physical activity from intentions may depend on the proximity of measurement of these two variables.
- The TRA and TPB have, however, been the most successful approaches in exercise psychology linking attitudes and related variables to intentions and participation, but experimental evidence is less convincing.
- Affective attitudes are more strongly related to intentions and behaviour than instrumental expressions of attitude.
- There is a gap between stated intentions and actual behaviour. This gap can be closed by having stable intentions, operating implementation intentions and adopting conscientious strategies.
- Protection Motivation Theory may be useful in predicting exercise intentions, but current data are more supportive of the role of efficacy beliefs rather than health threats themselves.

References

Ajzen, I. (1985). From intentions to actions: A theory of planned behavior. In J. Kuhl and J. Beckmann (eds), *Action Control: From cognition to behavior* (pp. 11–39). New York: Springer-Verlag.

———. (1988). *Attitudes, Personality and Behaviour*. Milton Keynes: Open University Press.

———. (1991). The Theory of Planned Behavior. *Organizational Behavior and Human Decision Processes, 50*, 179–211.

———. (1996). The directive influence of attitudes on behavior. In P.M. Gollwitzer and J.A. Bargh (eds), *The Psychology of Action* (pp. 385–403). New York: Guilford Press.

Ajzen, I. and Fishbein, M. (1980). *Understanding Attitudes and Predicting Social Behaviour*. Englewood Cliffs, NJ: Prentice-Hall.

Ajzen, I. and Madden, T.J. (1986). Prediction of goal-directed behaviour: Attitudes, intentions, and perceived behavioural control. *Journal of Experimental Social Psychology, 22*, 453–474.

Armitage, C. and Conner, M. (2001). Efficacy of the Theory of Planned Behaviour: A meta-analytic review. *British Journal of Social Psychology, 40*(4), 471–499. doi: 10.1348/014466601164939.

Bagozzi, R.P. and Kimmel, S.K. (1995). A comparison of leading theories for the prediction of goal-directed behaviours. *British Journal of Social Psychology, 34*, 437–461.

Bandura, A. (1977). Self-efficacy: Toward a unifying theory of behavioral change. *Psychological Review, 84*, 191–215.

Becker, M.H., Haefner, D.P., Kasl, S.V., Kirscht, J.P., Maiman, L.A. and Rosenstock, I.M. (1977). Selected psychosocial models and correlates of individual health-related behaviours. *Medical Care, 15* (Supplement), 27–46.

Bentler, P. and Speckart, G. (1981). Attitudes 'cause' behaviours: A structural equation analysis. *Journal of Personality and Social Psychology, 40*, 226–238.

Biddle, S.J.H. and Ashford, B. (1988). Cognitions and perceptions of health and exercise. *British Journal of Sports Medicine, 22*, 135–140.

Chaiken, S. (1980). Heuristic versus systematic information processing and the use of source versus message cues in persuasion. *Journal of Personality and Social Psychology, 39*, 752–766.

Chatzisarantis, N.L.D., Hagger, M.S., Biddle, S.J.H. and Smith, B. (2005). The stability of the attitude–intention relationship in the context of physical activity. *Journal of Sports Sciences, 23*, 49–61.

Chief Medical Officers of England, Scotland, Wales and Northern Ireland. (2011). *Start Active, Stay Active: A report on physical activity from the four home countries' Chief Medical Officers*. London:

Department of Health (http://www.dh.gov.uk/en/Publicationsandstatistics/Publications/PublicationsPolicyAndGuidance/DH_128209).

Conner, M. and Abraham, C. (2001). Conscientiousness and the theory of planned behavior: Toward a more complete model of the antecedents of intentions and behavior. *Personality and Social Psychology Bulletin, 27*, 1547–1561.

Conner, M. and Armitage, C. (1998). Extending the theory of planned behavior: A review and avenues for further research. *Journal of Applied Social Psychology, 28*(15), 1429–1464.

Conner, M. and Norman, P. (1994). Comparing the Health Belief Model and the Theory of Planned Behaviour in health screening. In D.R. Rutter and L. Quine (eds), *Social Psychology and Health: European perspectives* (pp. 1–24). Aldershot: Avebury.

Conner, M. and Norman, P. (eds). (1996). *Predicting Health Behaviour*. Buckingham: Open University Press.

Conner, M., Rhodes, R.E., Morris, B., McEachan, R. and Lawton, R. (2011). Changing exercise through targeting affective or cognitive attitudes. *Psychology and Health, 26*(2), 133–149. doi: 10.1080/08870446.2011.531570.

Dishman, R.K. and Sallis, J.F. (1994). Determinants and interventions for physical activity and exercise. In C. Bouchard, R.J. Shephard and T. Stephens (eds), *Physical Activity, Fitness, and Health* (pp. 203–213). Champaign, IL.: Human Kinetics.

Eagly, A.H. and Chaiken, S. (1993). *The Psychology of Attitudes*. Fort Worth, TX: Harcourt Brace Jovanovich.

Fishbein, M. and Ajzen, I. (1975). *Belief, Attitude, Intention and Behaviour: An introduction to theory and research*. Reading, MA: Addison-Wesley.

Fiske, S.T. and Taylor, S.E. (1991). *Social Cognition*. New York: McGraw-Hill.

Floyd, D.L., Prentice-Dunn, S. and Rogers, R.W. (2000). A meta-analysis of research on protection motivation theory. *Journal of Applied Social Psychology, 30*(2), 407–429.

Fox, K.R., Biddle, S.J.H., Edmunds, L., Bowler, I. and Killoran, A. (1997). Physical activity promotion through primary health care in England. *British Journal of General Practice, 47*, 367–369.

Gardner, B., de Bruijn, G.J. and Lally, P. (2011). A systematic review and meta-analysis of applications of the Self-report Habit Index to nutrition and physical activity behaviours. *Annals of Behavioral Medicine, 42*, 174–187.

Godin, G. (1993). The theories of reasoned action and planned behavior: Overview of findings, emerging research problems and usefulness for exercise promotion. *Journal of Applied Sport Psychology, 5*, 141–157.

——. (1994). Social-cognitive models. In R.K. Dishman (ed.), *Advances in Exercise Adherence* (pp. 113–136). Champaign, IL: Human Kinetics.

Gollwitzer, P.M. (1999). Implementation intentions: Strong effects of simple plans. *American Psychologist, July*, 493–503.

Gollwitzer, P.M. and Sheeran, P. (2006). Implementation intentions and goal achievement: A meta-analysis of effects and processes. *Advances in Experimental Social Psychology, 38*, 69–119. doi: 10.1016/50065-2601(06).

Hagger, M.S. and Chatzisarantis, N.L.D. (2014). An integrated behavior change model for physical activity. *Exercise and Sport Sciences Reviews, 42*(2), 62–69. doi: 0091-6331/4202/62-69.

Hagger, M.S., Chatzisarantis, N.L.D. and Biddle, S.J.H. (2002). A meta-analytic review of the Theories of Reasoned Action and Planned Behaviour in physical activity: Predictive validity and the contribution of additional variables. *Journal of Sport and Exercise Psychology, 24*, 3–32.

Harrison, J.A., Mullen, P.D. and Green, L.W. (1992). A meta-analysis of studies of the Health Belief Model with adults. *Health Education Research: Theory and Practice, 7*, 107–116.

Hausenblas, H., Carron, A.V. and Mack, D.E. (1997). Application of the Theories of Reasoned Action and Planned Behavior to exercise behavior: A meta-analysis. *Journal of Sport and Exercise Psychology, 19*, 36–51.

Hovland, C.I. and Rosenberg, M.J. (eds). (1960). *Attitudes, Organisation and Change: An analysis of consistency among attitude components*. New Haven, CT: Yale University Press.

Janz, N.K. and Becker, M.H. (1984). The Health Belief Model: A decade later. *Health Education Quarterly, 11*, 1–47.

Kenyon, G.S. (1968). Six scales for assessing atitudes toward physical activity. *Research Quarterly, 39*, 566–574.

King, A.C., Blair, S.N., Bild, D.E., Dishman, R.K., Dubbert, P.M., Marcus, B.H. and Yeager, K.K. (1992). Determinants of physical activity and interventions in adults. *Medicine and Science in Sports and Exercise, 24*(6, Supplement), S221–S236.

Kwak, L., Kremers, S.P.J., van Baak, M.A. and Brug, J. (2007). Formation of implementation intentions promotes stair use. *American Journal of Preventive Medicine, 32*(3), 254–255.

Lawton, R., Conner, M.T. and McEachan, R. (2009). Desire or reason: Predicting health behaviors from affective and cognitive attitudes. *Health Psychology, 28*, 56–65.

Lindsay-Reid, E. and Osborn, R.W. (1980). Readiness for exercise adoption. *Social Science and Medicine, 14*, 139–146.

Liska, A.E. (1984). A critical examination of the causal structure of the Fishbein/Ajzen attitude-behaviour model. *Social Psychology Quarterly, 47*, 61–74.

McAuley, E. and Courneya, K. (1993). Adherence to exercise and physical activity as health promoting behaviors: Attitudinal and self-efficacy influences. *Applied and Preventive Psychology, 2*, 65–77.

McGuire, W.J. (1969). The nature of attitudes and attitude change. In G. Lindzey and E. Aronson (eds), *Handbook of Social Psychology:Vol III* (pp. 136–314). Reading, MA: Addison-Wesley.

Michie, S., van Stralen, M. and West, R. (2011). The behaviour change wheel: A new method for characterising and designing behaviour change interventions. *Implementation Science, 6*(1), 42, http://www.implementationscience.com/content/46/41/42. doi: 10.1186/1748-5908-6-42.

Milne, S., Orbell, S. and Sheeran, P. (2002). Combining motivational and volitional interventions to promote exercise participation: Protection motivation theory and implementation intentions. *British Journal of Health Psychology, 7*, 163–184.

Olson, J.M. and Zanna, M.P. (1993). Attitudes and attitude change. *Annual Review of Psychology, 44*, 117–154.

Orbell, S. (2000). Motivational and volitional components in action initiation: A field study of the role of implementation intentions. *Journal of Applied Social Psychology, 30*, 780–797.

Petty, R.E. and Cacioppo, J.T. (1986). The elaboration-likelihood model of persuasion. In L. Berkowitz (ed.), *Advances in Experimental Social Psychology* (Vol. 19, pp. 123–205). San Diego, CA: Academic Press.

Plotnikoff, R.C., Lubans, D.R., Costigan, S.A., Trinh, L., Spence, J.C., Downs, S. and McCargar, L. (2011). A test of the Theory of Planned Behavior to explain physical activity in a large population sample of adolescents from Alberta, Canada. *Journal of Adolescent Health, 49*, 547–549. doi: 10.1016/j.jadohealth.2011.03.006.

Prentice-Dunn, S. and Rogers, R. (1986). Protection Motivation Theory and preventive health: Beyond the Health Belief Model. *Health Education Research:Theory and Practice, 1*, 153–161.

Prestwich, A., Lawton, R. and Conner, M. (2003). The use of implementation intentions and the decision balance sheet in promoting exercise behaviour. *Psychology and Health, 18*, 707–721.

Rhodes, R.E. and de Bruijn, G-J. (2013). What predicts intention–behaviour discordance? A review of the Action Control framework. *Exercise and Sport Sciences Reviews, 41*(4), 201–207. doi: 0091-6331/4104.

Rhodes, R.E. and Dickau, L. (2013). Moderators of the intention–behaviour relationship in the physical activity domain: A systematic review. *British Journal of Sports Medicine, 47*, 215–225.

Rhodes, R.E., Courneya, K.S. and Jones, L.W. (2002). Personality, the theory of planned behavior, and exercise: A unique role for extroversion's activity facet. *Journal of Applied Social Psychology, 32*, 1721–1736.

Rhodes, R.E., Fiala, B. and Conner, M. (2009). A review and meta-analysis of affective judgments and physical activity in adult populations. *Annals of Behavioral Medicine, 38*, 180–204. doi: 10.1007/s12160-009-9147-y.

Rhodes, S.D., Bowie, D.A. and Hergenrather, K.C. (2003). Collecting behavioural data using the world wide web: Considerations for researchers. *Journal of Epidemiological Community Health, 57*(1), 68–73.

Rogers, R.W. (1983). Cognitive and physiological processes in fear appeals and attitude change: A revised theory of protection motivation. In J.R. Cacioppo and R.E. Petty (eds), *Social Psychology: A sourcebook* (pp. 153–176). New York: Guilford Press.

Rosenstock, I. (1974). Historical origins of the Health Belief Model. *Health Education Monographs, 2*, 328–335.

Sallis, J.F. and Owen, N. (1999). *Physical Activity and Behavioral Medicine*. Thousand Oaks, CA: Sage.

Sandberg, T. and Conner, M. (2008). Anticipated regret as an additional predictor in the theory of planned behaviour: A meta-analysis. *British Journal of Social Psychology, 47*(4), 589–606. doi: 10.1348/014466607X258704.

Schifter, D.E. and Ajzen, I. (1985). Intention, perceived control, and weight loss: An application of the Theory of Planned Behaviour. *Journal of Personality and Social Psychology, 49*, 843–851.

Sechrist, K.R., Walker, S.N. and Pender, N.J. (1987). Development and psychometric evaluation of the exercise benefits/barriers scale. *Research in Nursing and Health, 10*, 357–365.

Sheeran, P. and Abraham, C. (1996). The Health Belief Model. In M. Conner and P. Norman (eds), *Predicting Health Behaviour* (pp. 23–61). Buckingham: Open University Press.

Sniehotta, F.F., Presseau, J. and Araujo-Soares, V. (2014). Editorial: Time to retire the theory of planned behaviour. *Health Psychology Review, 8*(1), 1–7. doi: 10.1080/17437199.2013.869710.

Sonstroem, R.J. (1988). Psychological models. In R.K. Dishman (ed.), *Exercise Adherence: Its impact on public health* (pp. 125–153). Champaign, IL: Human Kinetics.

Stanley, M. and Maddux, J. (1986). Cognitive processes in health enhancement: Investigation of a combined protection motivation and self-efficacy model. *Basic and Applied Social Psychology, 7*, 101–113.

Steinhardt, M.A. and Dishman, R.K. (1989). Reliability and validity of expected outcomes and barriers for habitual physical activity. *Journal of Occupational Medicine, 31*, 536–546.

Stroebe, W. and Stroebe, M.S. (1995). *Social Psychology and Health*. Buckingham: Open University Press.

Sutton, S. (2004). Determinants of health-related behaviours: Theoretical and methodological issues. In S. Sutton, A. Baum and M. Johnston (eds), *The Sage Handbook of Health Psychology* (pp. 94–126). London: Sage.

Symons Downs, D. and Hausenblas, H.A. (2005). The Theories of Reasoned Action and Planned Behavior applied to exercise: A meta-analytic update. *Journal of Physical Activity and Health, 2*, 76–97.

Taylor, A.H. (1999). Adherence in primary health care exercise promotion schemes. In S.J. Bull (ed.), *Adherence Issues in Sport and Exercise* (pp. 47–74). Chichester: Wiley.

Taylor, W.C., Baranowski, T. and Sallis, J.F. (1994). Family determinants of childhood physical activity: A social cognitive model. In R.K. Dishman (ed.), *Advances in Exercise Adherence* (pp. 319–342). Champaign, IL: Human Kinetics.

Terry, D.J. and O'Leary, J.E. (1995). The theory of planned behaviour: The effects of perceived behavioural control and self-efficacy. *British Journal of Social Psychology, 34*, 199–220.

Triandis, H.C. (1977). *Interpersonal Behaviour*. Monterey, CA: Brooks/Cole.

Wallston, B.S. and Wallston, K.A. (1985). Social psychological models of health behaviour: An examination and integration. In A. Baum, S.E. Taylor and J.E. Singer (eds), *Handbook of Psychology and Health: IV. Social psychological aspects of health* (pp. 23–53). Hillsdale, NJ: Erlbaum.

Wankel, L.M. and Mummery, K.W. (1993). Using national survey data incorporating the theory of planned behaviour: Implications for social marketing strategies in physical activity. *Journal of Applied Sport Psychology, 5*, 158–177.

Wurtele, S. and Maddux, J. (1987). Relative contributions of protection motivation theory components in predicting exercise intentions and behaviour. *Health Psychology, 6*, 453–466.

9   Physical activity and motivation

What it is and isn't

There are many common-sense notions about motivation. One, for example, is that we simply need 'to be motivated' in order to be an exerciser or that large amounts of 'willpower' are needed. While the quantity of motivation can be important, the 'quality' of motivation is likely to be more crucial. In other words, motivation is more about 'how' than 'how much'.

The purpose of this chapter is to extend the motivational analysis of physical activity by considering the notion of feelings of perceived control, autonomy and intrinsic motivation, particularly by outlining a popular theory of motivation: Self-Determination Theory. In addition, we will also consider the notion of 'habit' whereby some behaviours may be driven more by unconscious, or less conscious, processes. Of course, many of the chapters in this book are concerned with 'motivation' in a broad sense – attitudes, confidence, stages of change – but in this chapter we also define motivation and consider several perspectives, including a few myths of motivation within the physical activity context. Specifically, in this chapter we aim to:

- define and explore types of motivation;
- consider a framework for the understanding of perceptions of control;
- appreciate the potential of perceptions of control, expectancies and value as determinants of physical activity;
- develop an understanding of intrinsic motivational processes, specifically in terms of Cognitive Evaluation Theory and perceptions of autonomy (Self-Determination Theory);
- consider how rewards and reinforcement might affect intrinsic motivation and behaviour;
- understand the role of beliefs concerning physical activity ability and a 'growth mindset' in motivation;
- define the concept of 'habit' and consider how habits are developed;
- discuss the popular idea of 'nudging' people into healthy behaviours.

Definition and trends in motivation

The study of human motivation has been central to psychology since its earliest days and has developed through many different perspectives. Maehr and Braskamp's (1986) components of motivation will be offered as an operational definition. In particular, we find the following components helpful in addition to the different 'qualities' of motivation expressed through Self-Determination Theory (see later):

- direction and choice
- persistence

- continuing motivation
- intensity.

Direction and choice

The first indicator of motivation is that of direction. This implies that a choice has been made to do something – a decision has been made. In the context of physical activity, for example, there is the basic choice of whether to be active or not, and, if choosing activity, what type of activity is performed. Two important issues arise here. First, to what extent is habitual physical activity consciously chosen? Some may be forced into walking or cycling through a lack of personal resources to travel in any other way. People living in cities will often choose to walk, perhaps coupled with public transport. Different psychological processes may be involved here. Given that exercise is mostly structured and likely to take place in particular locations, such exercise facilities and at certain times choice is important for this type of activity. For more 'active living' behaviours, this may not be the case. Second, one needs to consider the issue of alternative behavioural choices. Someone may not be rejecting exercise in any conscious way, but merely choosing activities that are seen as higher priorities. Some physical activity choices are likely to be made in an effort to reinforce personal perceptions of competence, or behaviours that are coherent with one's sense of self (i.e. they are highly valued).

It is also noteworthy, however, that we are faced with physical activity choices throughout a normal day, and often quite unrelated to self-perceptions of competence. Will I climb the stairs or take the lift? Will I walk or drive? Some choices may be made relatively subconsciously and this in itself provides a challenge to health professionals (see below on 'habit' and 'nudging'). But whatever underlies these disparate physical activity behaviours choices are usually made, and this is the 'direction and choice' component of motivation.

Persistence

Persistence refers to the degree of sustained concentration on one task. Persistence, and hence motivation, may be inferred about someone who walks quite a long way to work alongside a bus route. Lack of persistence is inferred when the walker gives up after five minutes and takes the first available bus. Of course, persistence is also a reflection of choice and decision-making, and is likely to be correlated with how important something is to the individual. In addition, such persistence at a task may be high in order to enhance positive self-presentational aspects: 'I want to be seen walking to work as this confirms my identity (to me and others) that I am an active person.' Persistence is akin to physical activity maintenance.

Continuing motivation

This is when people regularly return to a task after a break. Indeed, Maehr and Braskamp (1986) suggest that 'it is almost as if a certain tension exists when a task is left incomplete; the person simply cannot leave it alone' (p. 4). There is some evidence that a few individuals feel highly committed in this way to structured exercise (Szabo, 2000) – the so-called phenomenon of exercise dependence (see Chapter 2). At a more moderate level, many people report 'feeling good' from physical activity and less good when they have missed their activity for several days.

One aspect of motivation for physical activity that is currently poorly understood involves continuing motivation. Although we have accumulated information on physical activity maintenance over time, we know much less about the processes involved in *resuming* physical activity after a break – the 'relapse' or 'stop-start' syndrome (Sallis and Hovell, 1990). This is the issue of continuing motivation. Seeing that few people adopt physical activity without periods of 'relapse', this would appear to be an important area for study.

Intensity

Behavioural intensity is another indicator of motivation. This is the 'how much' of motivation. It is important in relation to the debate about 'how much physical activity is enough for health gains?', since more moderate forms of activity may require less intense levels of motivation. Certainly we have argued many times before that promoting physical activity on the basis of 'vigorous' exercise only, regardless of any physiological rationale, is often doomed to failure due to the perceived, or actual, motivational effort (intensity) required; i.e. it's too much like hard work!

There is an argument for not only looking at how much motivation is required for some forms of physical activity, and ways to increase that motivation, but to also address the issue of making the physical activity in question more desirable, attractive and easier to do (see http://www.behaviormodel.org/). Sadly we have gone in the opposite direction. One example is where new housing developments are designed with many 'cul-de-sac' (dead-end) configurations requiring car travel to navigate to local facilities such as shops and amenities. Older style layouts were more likely to have had greater connectivity through a grid-like road pattern, encouraging more active forms of transport. Making the activity more difficult, as in the case of newer road designs, means that motivation needs to be even higher if a physically active alternative is to be chosen. In other words, we cannot ignore the interaction between environmental and individual psychological processes when considering motivational intensity.

In addition to the motivational factors just discussed, it may be argued that not all motivation is the same. We express different qualities of motivation, such as being motivated by money, guilt, enjoyment, etc. These qualities will be discussed in more detail when we consider Self-Determination Theory later in the chapter.

> Key point: Motivation involves which behaviours you choose to do, how persistent you are, whether you continue over time, and your intensity of involvement.

Gaining control: recognising the importance of perceptions of control in physical activity motivation

The research and popular literature contains numerous references to the fact that changes in physical activity and other health behaviours are thought to be associated with the need to 'take control' or 'take charge' of personal lifestyles. The information that many of the modern diseases linked with premature mortality are 'lifestyle-related' (Katzmarzyk and Mason, 2009; Powell, 1988) contains the implicit message that we, as individuals, are at least partly responsible for our health and well-being, thus implying the need for personal control and change. Moreover, failure to initiate or maintain physical activity is often attributed to a lack of 'willpower'.

Political ideology towards health is also centred on notions of control. Political parties on the left will legislate more for changes in health behaviours while those on the right believe it is more about personal responsibility. The debate then centres on how much real choice some people have if they are disenfranchised or marginalised in society, or cannot access the necessary places or services supporting health behaviours and care. However, it is recognised that there are potential problems with health messages that consistently encourage personal control as the only way of changing behaviour. This approach is often associated with the 'health fascist' label. Some have argued that a greater emphasis should be placed on social and environmental determinants of health, and others accuse those who over-emphasise the need for personal control of adopting the 'victim blaming approach'. Feelings of guilt can develop when problems arise that are out of one's control (e.g. disease related to environmental pollution), whereas others may blame the victim for a lack of motivation. Similarly, a great deal of good can be achieved by giving control to others, such as doctors, in certain circumstances.

A framework for understanding perceptions of control

Psychological constructs centred on 'control' are numerous, such as self-efficacy, intrinsic motivation and locus of control, all of which have been popular in exercise psychology (Biddle, 1999). In attempting to integrate and make sense of apparently disparate constructs, we draw initially on Skinner's (1995, 1996) agent–means–ends analysis or, to put it simply, a framework linking 'person to behaviour to outcome'. Skinner (1995, 1996) makes the point that one way to conceptualise the vast array of control constructs is to analyse them in relation to their place within the tripartite model of agent (the person), means (the behaviour), and ends (the outcomes). This is illustrated in Figure 9.1.

Person–behaviour (agent–means) connections involve expectations that the individual has the means to produce a response or behaviour (but not necessarily an outcome). This involves *capacity beliefs* – beliefs concerning whether the individual has the ability to produce the appropriate behaviour. For example, if effort is deemed important to be able to cycle to work, then positive capacity beliefs must involve the belief that 'I can put in the effort when cycling to work – I have the capability'. Self-efficacy research has adopted this approach (see Chapter 10). The COM-B approach underpinning the 'behaviour change wheel' (Michie *et al.*, 2011) also highlights the importance of capability (alongside competence and opportunity) as foundations for the adoption of the desired behaviour (see Chapter 12). In this model, capability is seen to be both physical and psychological.

Behaviour–outcomes (means–ends) connections involve beliefs about the link between potential causes and outcomes. This involves *strategy beliefs* – beliefs concerning the necessary availability of behaviours (means) to produce the desired outcomes. For example, 'If I walk to work it will help me lose the weight I want to lose'. There is a belief between the adoption of a behaviour (walking to work) and an expected outcome (losing weight). This does not necessarily predict whether the behaviour will be carried out; there may be barriers preventing the behaviour.

There is also a direct connection between the individual and outcome (agent–ends) (see Figure 9.1). As Skinner (1995) puts it, 'connections between people and outcomes prescribe the prototypical definitions of control' (p. 554); hence this connection involves *control beliefs*.

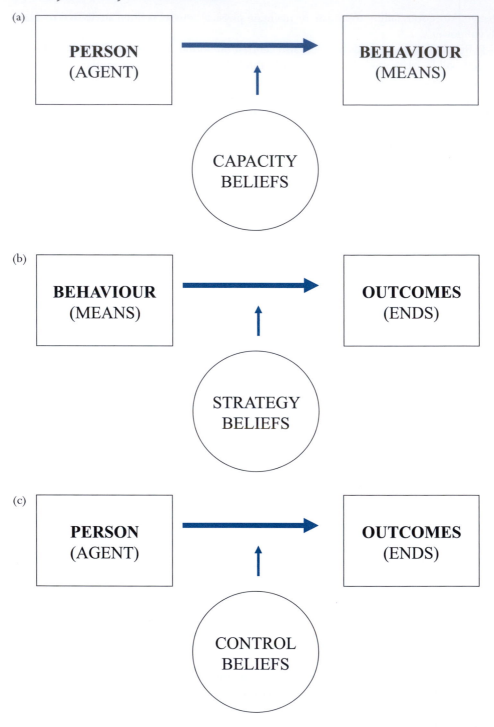

Figure 9.1   (a, b, c) An agent–means–ends (person–behaviour–outcomes) analysis and different types of beliefs mediating such links

Source: Adapted from Skinner (1995, 1996).

These involve the belief by the individual that a desirable outcome is within their capability: 'I do walk to work and, as a result, I am losing weight'. This has to involve both capacity and strategy beliefs.

> Key point: Motivation involves beliefs about capacity ('*Can I* do the behaviour?') as well as strategy ('*How do I* do the behaviour to achieve the desired outcomes?').

I like it! Understanding intrinsic motivation

It is clear from everyday experiences that we prefer, or are more motivated by, situations where some choice, control and 'self-determination' exist. Conversely, we usually prefer not to be controlled and pressured too much. These constructs underpin the link between perceptions of control and motivated behaviour, and are central to intrinsic motivation.

Intrinsic and extrinsic motivation are well-known constructs in psychology and, although often under different names, in everyday situations too. Certainly those involved in promoting physical activity for health believe that intrinsic motivation is key to sustaining involvement. Intrinsic motivation is motivation to do something for its own sake in the absence of external (extrinsic) rewards. Often this involves fun, enjoyment and satisfaction, such as recreational activities and hobbies. The enjoyment is in the activity itself rather than any extrinsic reward such as money, prizes or prestige from others, and participation is free from constraints and pressure. Such intrinsically pursued activities are referred to as 'autotelic' (self-directing) by Csikszentmihalyi (1975), suggesting that intrinsically motivated behaviour is linked to feelings of self-control or self-determination, and 'autonomy' (Deci and Ryan, 2002). Extrinsic motivation, on the other hand, refers to motivation directed by rewards, money, pressure or other external factors. This suggests that if these rewards or external pressures were removed, motivation would decline in the absence of any intrinsic interest. Later, we will introduce motivational constructs that shed extra light on a continuum of motivation, including motivational processes 'between' pure intrinsic and extrinsic motivation.

The development of intrinsic motivation theories

Deci and Ryan (1985, 1991) suggest that four approaches to the study of intrinsic motivation can be identified in the literature. These are free choice, interest, challenge and 'needs'. In the absence of extrinsic rewards, those intrinsically motivated will be those who choose to participate in their own time (free choice). Intrinsically motivated behaviour is also performed out of interest and curiosity, as well as challenge. In addition, Deci and Ryan outline the important role of psychological needs. These have been identified over a long period in psychology through constructs such as 'effectance' (feeling mastery), 'personal causation' (feeling in control), 'competence' (feeling you are capable) and 'self-determination' (feeling you have choice).

It is generally acknowledged that the initiation of the shift towards the study of a cognitive perspective on motivational needs was White's (1959) paper on 'effectance motivation'. White suggested that human beings have a basic need to interact effectively with their environment. He reviewed a wide range of studies and argued convincingly that operant theories (those based on rewards and punishment) could not account for behaviours such as mastery attempts, curiosity, exploration and play. For these types of activities, there seems to be no apparent external reward except for the activity itself, and hence they have been termed 'intrinsically motivating'.

An alternative approach was taken by deCharms (1968). He argued that self-determination is a basic human need and consequently individuals will be optimally and intrinsically motivated when they perceive themselves to be the 'origin' of, or in control of, their own behaviour. DeCharms (1968) used Heider's concept of Perceived Locus of Causality (PLOC) to describe individuals' sense of autonomy or self-determination. PLOC refers to the perception people have about the reasons they engage in a particular behaviour. People with an internal PLOC feel initiators or 'origins' of their behaviour. On the other hand, people feeling that their actions are initiated or strongly influenced by some external force are said to have an external PLOC. External and internal PLOC represent opposite ends of a continuum. According to deCharms, people are more likely to be optimally and intrinsically motivated when they have a more internal PLOC.

Deci and Ryan (1985) propose that three key psychological needs are related to intrinsically motivated behaviour. These are the needs for competence, autonomy and social relatedness (Deci and Ryan, 2000). Competence refers to the need to control outcomes and to experience mastery and effectance. Human beings seek to understand how to produce desired outcomes and are often motivated to 'get better' at tasks. Autonomy is related to self-determination. It is similar to deCharms' notion of being the 'origin' rather than the 'pawn', and to have feelings of perceived control, choice, and to feel that actions emanate from oneself. Finally, social relatedness refers to strivings to relate to, and care for, others; to feel that others can relate to oneself; 'to feel a satisfying and coherent involvement with the social world more generally' (Deci and Ryan, 1991, p. 245).

Deci and Ryan (1991) state that 'these three psychological needs ... help to explain a substantial amount of variance in human behavior and experience' (p. 245). People seek to satisfy these needs, but of more importance from the point of view of enhancing intrinsic motivation is that they predict the circumstances in which intrinsically motivated behaviour can be promoted. We will return to this later. First, let us consider a perspective on intrinsic and extrinsic motivation that has captured some attention in physical activity research.

> Key point: Human beings want to satisfy their need for competence, autonomy and social relatedness. Intrinsic motivation can be enhanced by creating environments that boost these three needs.

Understanding rewards as motivation: Cognitive Evaluation Theory (CET)

The relationship between intrinsic and extrinsic motivation was, at one time, thought to be quite simple – 'more' motivation would result from adding extrinsic motivation to existing intrinsic motivation. This appeared logical given the evidence demonstrating that reinforcements (i.e. extrinsic rewards) will increase the probability of the rewarded behaviour reoccurring. We do it all the time, don't we? We pay people to work, we reward children for good behaviour, we give prizes in sport, etc. However, a number of studies and observations, mainly with children, started to question whether intrinsic motivation could be undermined by the use of extrinsic rewards in some circumstances. This may be explained through 'Cognitive Evaluation Theory' (CET).

CET (Deci, 1975; Deci and Ryan, 1985) suggested that providing individuals with rewards for their participation in an already interesting activity can often lead to a decrease in intrinsic motivation. Deci (1975) theorised that this was due to a shift in PLOC. Thus, individuals who had an internal PLOC for performing an activity shifted their locus of causality to a more external orientation when they received a reward, and consequently their intrinsic motivation decreased. In other words, the focus was on getting the reward rather than the intrinsic interest of the task.

An early seminal study illustrates this (Lepper *et al.*, 1973). These researchers tested the relationship between intrinsic motivation and extrinsic rewards with pre-school children. Baseline data on intrinsic interest were collected. Intrinsic motivation was defined as the amount of time spent playing with brightly coloured highlighting pens during a break in the school day. The children were then assigned randomly to one of three groups:

- *Expected reward condition*: the children agreed to play with the pens and expected a reward for doing so (a certificate with seal and ribbon).
- *Unexpected reward condition*: the children agreed to play with the pens but were not told anything about receiving a reward (although they did receive one afterwards).
- *No reward condition*: these children neither expected nor received a reward for playing with the pens.

The children then participated in the experimental manipulation and were tested individually in a separate room in one of the three conditions. They were later observed, on another occasion, unobtrusively through a one-way mirror. The pens were available in a classroom alongside a variety of other play equipment. The amount of time spent playing with the pens for each of the three groups showed that the expected reward group played for a significantly shorter time than the other two groups.

A similar experiment was conducted by Lepper and Greene (1975) with children of the same age as in the previous study. This time they used two reward conditions: expected reward and unexpected reward. In addition, the researchers had three surveillance conditions. Surveillance is a form of external focus and therefore likely to affect intrinsic interest. Some children were told that while they were playing their performance would be monitored by a video camera most of the time (high surveillance), occasionally (low surveillance) or not at all (no surveillance). Up to three weeks after the experimental manipulation, the children were unobtrusively observed playing. The results showed that intrinsic motivation was lower under surveillance and expected reward conditions.

These two studies supported earlier work by Deci (see Deci and Ryan, 1985), who found that people paid to work on intrinsically motivating tasks spent less time on the tasks when given an opportunity to do so in their free time. Collectively, the results of these studies suggest what has been termed an 'over-justification effect'. By rewarding people for participating in an intrinsically interesting task, subsequent involvement in the task is reduced when the reward is no longer available.

The over-justification effect is based on the premise that the behaviour would have occurred anyway, without the need for extrinsic rewards. However, with the use of expected rewards a shift in perceptions occurs from intrinsic to extrinsic. The task is pursued for reasons of obtaining the reward rather than for intrinsic value. Therefore, the reward 'over-justifies' the behaviour and, in the event of the reward no longer being offered, the individual shows reduced intrinsic motivation.

The studies by Lepper and his co-workers, however, demonstrated that it was not the rewards per se that were the problem, but whether the rewards were expected or not. This suggests, therefore, that rewards need not be detrimental to intrinsic motivation in all situations. This led to the formulation of Cognitive Evaluation Theory which states that rewards are likely to serve two main functions (see Figure 9.2):

- *Information function.* If the reward provides positive information about the individuals' competence then it is likely that intrinsic motivation will be enhanced.
- *Controlling function.* If the rewards are seen to be controlling behaviour (i.e. the goal is to obtain the reward rather than participate for intrinsic reasons), then withdrawal of the reward is likely to lead to subsequent deterioration in intrinsic motivation.

It is important to note that informational events are those events that are perceived to convey feedback about one's competence within the context of autonomy. Events where positive feedback occurs under pressure may be less powerful in influencing intrinsic motivation.

In summarising CET, Deci and Ryan (1985) present three propositions:

- *Proposition 1.* 'External events relevant to the initiation and regulation of behaviour will affect a person's intrinsic motivation to the extent that they influence the perceived locus of causality for that behaviour. Events that promote a more external locus of causality will undermine intrinsic motivation, whereas those that promote a more internal perceived locus of causality will enhance intrinsic motivation' (p. 62).

Deci and Ryan (1985) say that events that lead to an external locus of causality undermine intrinsic motivation because they deny people 'self-determination' – that is, they control people's behaviour. On the other hand, internal locus of causality may enhance intrinsic motivation by facilitating feelings of self-determination, thus creating greater autonomy.

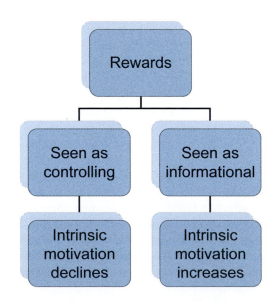

Figure 9.2 Possible links between rewards structures and intrinsic motivation

- *Proposition 2*. 'External events will affect a person's intrinsic motivation for an optimally challenging activity to the extent that they influence the person's perceived competence, within the context of some self-determination. Events that promote greater perceived competence will enhance intrinsic motivation, whereas those that diminish perceived competence will decrease intrinsic motivation' (p.63).

As proposition 2 suggests, intrinsic motivation is not just about feelings of control but also about perceived competence.

- *Proposition 3*. 'Events relevant to the initiation and regulation of behaviour have three potential aspects, each with a functional significance. The informational aspect facilitates an internal perceived locus of causality and perceived competence, thus enhancing intrinsic motivation. The controlling aspect facilitates an external perceived locus of causality, thus undermining intrinsic motivation and promoting extrinsic compliance or defiance. The amotivating aspect facilitates perceived incompetence, thus undermining intrinsic motivation and promoting amotivation (clear lack of motivation). The relative salience of these three aspects to a person determines the functional significance of the event' (Deci and Ryan, 1985, p. 64).

Deci and Ryan (1985) conclude that, generally speaking, choice and positive feedback are perceived as informational, while rewards, deadlines and surveillance tend to be controlling. Negative feedback is seen to undermine motivation and is therefore referred to as 'amotivating'.

Cognitive Evaluation Theory: an appraisal using meta-analysis

Researchers have attempted clarification of the relationships between rewards and intrinsic motivation across various domains and behaviours. The first meta-analysis addressing these issues was reported by Rummel and Feinberg (1988). They included studies that tested the relationship between extrinsic rewards and intrinsic motivation and where the reward was conveyed in such a way as to make it 'controlling'. Only five of the 88 effect sizes contradicted CET and the overall mean effect size was -0.33. It was concluded that rewards do have a moderate detrimental effect on intrinsic motivation and CET was supported.

Cameron and Pierce (1994) conducted a comprehensive meta-analysis of studies investigating the relationships between rewards, reinforcements and intrinsic motivation across various domains of behaviour, including physical activity. Four main measures of intrinsic motivation were analysed: free time on a task, attitude (e.g. self-reported task interest, enjoyment), willingness to volunteer for a task in the future, and performance. They found that intrinsic motivation did not follow the expected trend predicted by CET for any of the measures of intrinsic motivation. However, when they looked at the type of reward being offered, they found that those rewarded with verbal praise or positive feedback had higher intrinsic motivation in comparison with those not rewarded. This trend was reversed for tangible rewards when time on task was the measure of intrinsic motivation, but the effect was small.

Tang and Hall (1995) reported a meta-analysis on the over-justification effect and found support for an undermining effect. Specifically, their results showed that both task-contingent and performance-contingent rewards decreased intrinsic motivation while unexpected rewards showed little or no effect. As a result of the several meta-analyses at the time, and the somewhat inconsistent findings, Deci *et al.* (1999) conducted a comprehensive meta-analysis of their own. This included 128 studies using various measures of intrinsic motivation. They concluded that 'tangible rewards had a significant negative effect on intrinsic motivation for interesting tasks' (p. 653), and this was for when rewards were expected.

From these meta-analyses, therefore, CET is largely supported. The literature in exercise psychology also appears to be supportive, although clearly there are issues still to be developed (Vallerand and Fortier, 1998). One way forward may be to progress beyond the distinction of intrinsic and extrinsic and, instead, to look at a continuum of self-directed behaviour ranging between intrinsic and extrinsic poles and the extent to which people feel self-directed or controlled.

> Key point: Use rewards as recognition of doing well (competence) rather than as a bribe.

Cognitive Evaluation Theory in physical activity: an illustrative study

Since exercise and some forms of physical activity often require persistence, effort, time management and self-regulatory skills, it is relevant to consider the role of intrinsic motivation and self-determination in exercise psychology. An early study by Whitehead and Corbin (1991) tested proposition 2 from CET in the context of fitness testing with children. Studying 12- to 13-year-olds on an agility run test, they sought to test whether changes in perceived competence would vary with changes in intrinsic motivation. They used the Intrinsic Motivation Inventory (IMI) to assess four dimensions of intrinsic motivation: interest/enjoyment, competence, effort/importance, and pressure/tension.

After completing the agility run course, two groups of children were given bogus feedback, stating that they were either in the top or bottom 20 per cent for their age. A third group was given no feedback. Clear support for CET was found, with the low feedback group (low competence) showing less intrinsic motivation than those receiving the more positive feedback. Intrinsic motivation scores were shown to be influenced by perceptions of competence.

Moving towards self-determination

CET involves the processing of information concerning rewards and is part of a wider network of theories within 'Self-Determination Theory' (SDT). Extending this perspective beyond rewards, Deci and Ryan (1985, 1991) have discussed the importance of the psychological needs of competence, autonomy and relatedness. The nature of motivated behaviour, according to Deci and Ryan, is based on striving to satisfy these three basic needs. This, they say, leads to a process of 'internalisation' – internalising behaviours not initially intrinsically motivating. Conversely, intrinsic motivation is less likely when these needs are not met or blocked in some way. Deci and Ryan (1985) have linked the internalisation concept to that of intrinsic and extrinsic motivation. Specifically, they form a continuum of different types of extrinsically and intrinsically regulated behaviour. These are the different qualities of motivation alluded to in the introduction to this chapter.

Types of extrinsic and intrinsic motivation: feel the quality not the weight

While it is common to refer to 'intrinsic' and 'extrinsic' motivation, there are four main types of extrinsic motivation (or external regulation of behaviour): external, introjected, identified and integrated regulation, as well as intrinsic motivation. These are shown in Figure 9.3 and summarised in Table 9.1. These classes of motivational regulations – reasons for engaging in a behaviour – can be meaningfully placed along a continuum of autonomy or self-deter-mination. In addition, there is a state of 'amotivation'. This is where the individual has little or no motivation to attempt the behaviour. Amotivation may be an important construct in physical activity. Many adults report feelings of physical inadequacy that prevent participation in physical activity. They display amotivation.

We have shown how SDT constructs are associated through conducting a meta-analysis (Chatzisarantis *et al.*, 2003) (see Table 9.2). By weighting each subscale, an overall 'Relative Autonomy Index' (RAI) can be computed, with higher scores indicating higher internality or self-determination (see Figure 9.3). Table 9.2 shows that constructs close to each other on the continuum correlate quite highly (0.45 to 0.75 – in bold), while those distal from other constructs are associated more weakly and sometimes in a negative way.

The use of SDT for studying intrinsic motivation in health (Ryan *et al.*, 2008) and physical activity (Chatzisarantis *et al.*, 2003; Hagger and Chatzisarantis, 2005; Standage *et al.*, 2005; Teixeira *et al.*, 2012) now has a large following. In our meta-analysis of the self-determination continuum (Chatzisarantis *et al.*, 2003), we found moderately strong correlations between more self-determined forms of motivation and measures of intention and competence (see Figure 9.4). However, this does not tell us whether the motivational constructs of the theory predict actual behaviour. To this end, Teixeira and colleagues (2012) conducted a systematic review to test various facets of SDT to see if exercise behaviours were associated with SDT constructs.

The review covered all components of SDT, including need satisfaction and motivational regulations, as described in Table 9.1. Specifically, Teixeira *et al.* (2012) tested whether intrinsic, integrated, identified, introjected and external regulations were associated with some measure of exercise involvement. As expected, and as shown in Figure 9.5, the more self-determined forms of regulation were positively associated with exercise involvement, whereas introjection showed mixed findings. External regulation was generally negatively

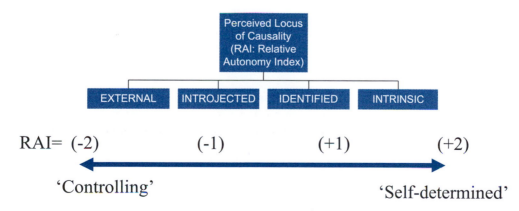

Figure 9.3   A continuum of self-determination in terms of different types of motivation

Table 9.1   Intrinsic and extrinsic forms of motivation (behavioural regulations) according to Self-Determination Theory

Motivation quality	Description	Example in physical activity
External regulation	Where behaviour is controlled by rewards, surveillance or threats	Coercion of patients by medical personnel where physical activity is prescribed for the reduction of health risk factors. 'I'll exercise if I really must.'
Introjected regulation	The individual is acting out of avoidance of negative feelings, such as guilt, or to seek approval from others for their performance or behaviour. The reason for the behaviour has been 'swallowed but not digested'.	It is an 'internally controlling' form of behavioural regulation illustrated by thoughts such as 'I *have* to ...' or 'I *ought* to ...'. This is likely to be quite common in exercise. 'I will go to the gym; otherwise I'll feel guilty.'
Identified regulation	Behaviour acted out of choice where the behaviour is highly valued and important to the individual. Towards the self-determined end of the motivation continuum illustrated by feelings of 'I want to ...' rather than the 'ought' feelings of introjection. The values associated with the behaviour are now 'swallowed *and* digested'.	Action motivated by an appreciation of valued outcomes of physical activity, such as disease prevention or fitness improvement. 'I *want to* exercise to get fit/lose weight.'
Integrated regulation	Behaviour regulated by seeking to achieve important personal goals. The most self-determined extrinsic form of behavioural regulation. The behaviour is volitional 'because of its utility or importance for one's personal goals' (Deci *et al.*, 1994, p. 121). The behaviour is still extrinsically motivated because it may be an instrumental action, done to achieve personal goals rather than for the pure joy of the activity itself.	'I exercise because it is important to me and it symbolises who and what I am.'
Intrinsic motivation	Motivated by the activity itself through feelings of enjoyment.	The individual participates for fun and for involvement in the activity itself. Predicts stronger levels of intention and sustained involvement in physical activity because it involves feelings of personal investment and autonomy. 'I exercise because I enjoy it.'

Table 9.2 Correlation matrix of associations between SDT behavioural regulations (data from Chatzisarantis *et al.*, 2003)

	External	*Introjected*	*Identified*	*Intrinsic*
Amotivation	**.53**	.14	−.15	−.27
External		**.45**	.10	−.12
Introjected			**.55**	.39
Identified				.75

Notes:
1. Correlations are from a meta-analysis of 8 to 18 studies with values adjusted for measurement and sampling error.
2. The measure of intrinsic motivation is for intrinsic motivation 'to experience stimulation'. Other measures of intrinsic motivation were also analysed but are omitted from the table for the sake of clarity.

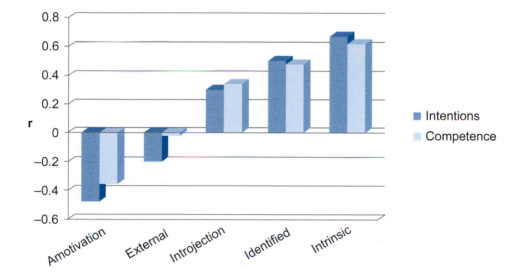

Figure 9.4 Correlations between SDT constructs and intentions and competence calculated from a meta-analysis of studies concerning physical activity

Source: Chatzisarantis *et al.* (2003).

Note: All coefficients are correlations corrected for measurement and sampling error. Intrinsic motivation scores are represented by the subscale of 'intrinsic motivation to experience stimulation'.

associated, or not associated at all, with exercise. Amotivation, predictably, is largely negatively associated with involvement in exercise. Unfortunately, much of the evidence is cross-sectional with rather few or large-scale interventions. This is a development needed for the future.

The second area analysed by Teixeira *et al.* (2012) was that of psychological needs for autonomy, competence and social relatedness. As shown in Figure 9.6, satisfying the need for competence was positively associated with exercise participation, whereas the results for autonomy were surprisingly more mixed. Social relatedness was not strongly associated with exercise, with only 38 per cent of studies showing a positive association. Again, most studies

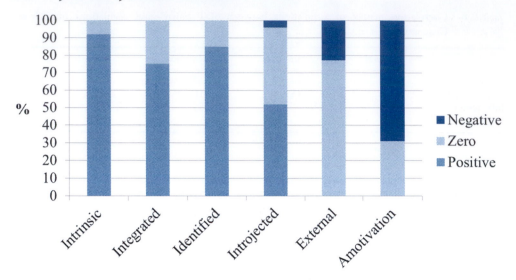

Figure 9.5   Associations between participation in exercise and SDT behavioural regulations

Source: Data from Teixeira *et al*. (2012).

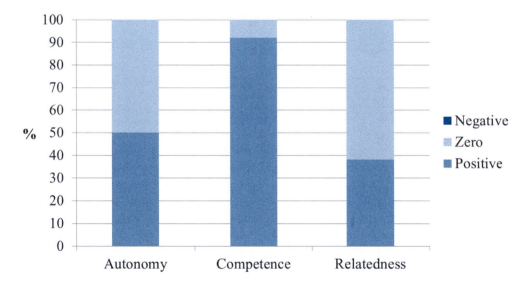

Figure 9.6   Associations between participation in exercise and needs for autonomy, competence and social relatedness

Source: Data from Teixeira *et al*. (2012).

are cross-sectional. In addition, many studies assess exercise or physical activity participation using self-report questionnaires. It is widely known that there is large error in such measures and this can affect the strength of associations. Objective assessment of physical activity is now common and future studies of SDT constructs will include these as routine. These should allow for more valid assessments of the predictive power of SDT variables. Meanwhile, it probably makes sense to support the promotion of both competence and autonomy needs until such a time as more robust evidence tells us otherwise.

> Key point: Always seek to move towards more self-determined forms of motivation through greater feelings of competence and autonomy.

Self-Determination Theory in action: an illustrative study

Silva *et al.* (2010) conducted an intervention designed to enable pre-menopausal overweight and obese women to increase their physical activity and lose weight. The RCT was firmly based on principles of SDT. An intervention group comprised 123 women (n = 115 at one-year follow-up) and 116 in a comparison (control) group (n = 93 at one-year follow-up). Face-to-face meetings took place every one to two weeks with assessments at baseline, four months and 12 months for measures of self-reported physical activity, body composition and psychological variables. For the intervention group, the aim was to create an autonomy-supportive environment allowing participants to feel ownership over their physical activity and weight-loss behaviours. Silva *et al.* outline six key themes designed to achieve this:

1. Build knowledge to support informed choices (this also involved appropriate use of language (e.g. 'could' rather than 'should').
2. Encourage choice and self-initiation.
3. Provide participants with choices (menu of options).
4. Provide clear rationale for choices available.
5. Encourage participants to build a match between their values and goals.
6. Give informational positive feedback.

Five modules were offered to participants with the main themes being increasing knowledge; triggering weight loss/improving diet; adopting and increasing physical activity; addressing barriers, promoting self-regulation, developing autonomy; improving body image; and preparing for weight maintenance.

Results showed that the intervention group reported significantly greater physical activity than controls after 12 months, had more self-determined motivation, and achieved greater weight loss (−7.29% compared to −1.74% in controls). Scores at 12 months for SDT exercise regulations are shown in Figure 9.7. The intervention group showed much greater scores for intrinsic and identified exercise regulation than controls, and also slightly larger scores for introjected regulation. No differences were evident for external regulation.

The authors concluded that the intervention was successful. They said that meaningful changes were achieved for physical activity, and clinically relevant reductions in body composition were evident.

A hierarchical model of intrinsic and extrinsic motivation

Vallerand (1997) organised the constructs of intrinsic and extrinsic motivation into a hierarchical model, as shown in Figure 9.8. Essentially, intrinsic and extrinsic motivation, as well as amotivation, feature at global, contextual and situational levels. At each of these levels, there are antecedents (such as global, contextual or situational factors, and needs for autonomy,

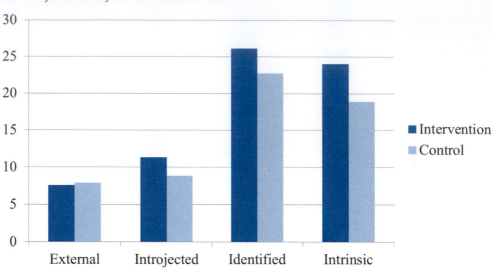

Figure 9.7 Twelve-month SDT behavioural regulation scores following an RCT for overweight and obese women

Source: Data from Silva *et al.* (2010).

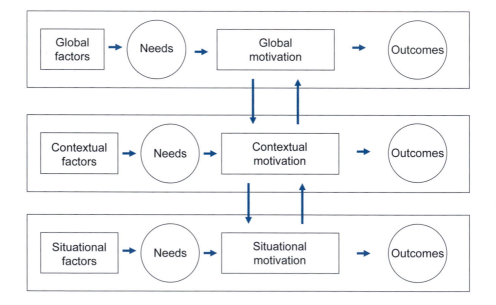

Figure 9.8 A hierarchical model of intrinsic and extrinsic motivation proposed by Vallerand

Source: Vallerand (1997).

competence and relatedness), as well as affective, cognitive and behavioural consequences. The global level refers to a general motivational orientation to which people typically subscribe. The contextual level of the model refers to domains of life, such as education, work, leisure and interpersonal. Finally, the situational level is concerned with situation-specific motivation.

This model is useful for conceptualising the different processes in intrinsic and extrinsic motivation, and should help in the understanding of these constructs in physical activity. For example, patients entering a GP-referral exercise scheme will bring with them their global motivational orientation, yet the personal trainer is in a position to influence situational cues to alter situation-specific motivation. Indeed, Deci and Ryan (1991) suggest that moving individuals to self-determined forms of motivation is more likely by altering situational or contextual factors. These include the following:

1. providing a meaningful rationale for the behaviour;
2. acknowledging the individual's perspective;
3. conveying choice rather than control.

How can we do that? The exercise leader or personal trainer might explain why certain exercises are 'good' and others 'bad' and what effect they may have. Empathy with how exercisers feel concerning incompetence, inadequacy, exertion, etc. will also help. Finally, the leader will allow some choice of activities, pace, difficulty and so on.

Further implications for participation in physical activity

It is generally accepted that intrinsic motivation is a desirable quality for continued involvement in physical activities. However, the complex interrelationship between intrinsic motivation, perceptions of control and autonomy, and extrinsic rewards remains to be fully tested in exercise settings. Early summary evidence on adherence (Dishman *et al.*, 1985) suggested that adults adopt exercise for reasons of health but are more likely to continue participation because of the more intrinsic feelings of well-being and enjoyment. Large population surveys also show that intrinsic reasons, such as 'feeling better', are important to both active and inactive people, although to varying degrees (Canada Fitness Survey, 1983). This suggests that adults may have an intrinsic orientation towards physical activity, whether they are active or not. No doubt the more extrinsic influences of wanting to look 'good' in front of others, or participating to please others, will also be important factors for some people.

Health professionals should be aware, given our previous discussion, of the inter-relationship between rewards and intrinsic motivation. For example, the use of reward systems in health clubs has been a common strategy, though no systematic evaluation of their effectiveness has been reported. While the short-term influence on adherence may be positive, the research reported in this chapter suggests that those wishing to promote greater exercise participation must be cautious in their use of extrinsic rewards, particularly for those already high in intrinsic motivation. Rewarding competence is appropriate, and it may also be better to reward and reinforce good behaviours rather than performance. In other words, encourage the *process* of activity by reinforcing frequency and participation, rather than solely reinforcing the *product* of, say, high fitness scores or the use of comparative reward structures. The rewarding of participation is more likely to lead to feelings of autonomy.

Locus of control (LOC): everything's under control!

An old construct in psychology is that of 'locus of control' (LOC). We could have placed this section at the beginning of the chapter to give things some historical context. However, there is so little new research on LOC per se, including in physical activity, that it seems to fit best here. But we do believe that it is an important construct to understand.

LOC stems from a social learning theory approach to personality (Rotter, 1954) where general beliefs are thought to develop from expectations based on prior outcomes and reinforcements and the value attached to such outcomes. This is a classic expectancy-value approach to motivation. Locus of control of reinforcements refers to the extent people perceive that reinforcements or actions are within their own control, are controlled by others or are due to chance. In Rotter's (1966) seminal monograph on LOC he says, 'it seems likely that, depending on the individual's history of reinforcement, individuals would differ in the degree to which they attributed reinforcements to their own actions' (p. 2). This led Rotter to formalise the construct of LOC and to suggest that a generalised belief existed for internal versus external control of reinforcement. Rotter (1966, p. 1) defined 'internals' and 'externals' as follows:

> If the person perceives that the event (the reinforcement) is contingent upon his/her own behaviour or his/her own relatively permanent characteristics, we have termed this a belief in internal control …
>
> When a reinforcement is perceived … as following some action of his/her own but not being entirely contingent upon his/her action, then … it is typically perceived as the result of luck, chance, fate, as under the control of powerful others, or as unpredictable. … When the event is interpreted in this way … we have labelled this a belief in external control.

In the same monograph Rotter presented psychometric evidence for the measurement of LOC with his internal–external (I–E) scale. This was a measure of 'individual differences in a generalised belief for internal or external control of reinforcement' (Rotter, 1966, pp. 1–2). The 29-item scale yields one score of LOC (high score indicating high externality) thus suggesting that LOC is a uni-dimensional construct. This has been challenged by a number of researchers. It should be noted, however, that Rotter stated that his I–E scale was a measure of *generalised* expectancy and was therefore likely to have a relatively low behavioural prediction but across a wide variety of situations. It was also likely to have greater predictive powers in novel or ambiguous situations, since in specific well-known contexts more specific expectancies will be used (see discussion on self-efficacy in Chapter 10).

Research on physical activity and LOC

Research investigating the link between LOC and participation in physical activity and exercise has taken three routes. First, some researchers have tried to identify links between generalised LOC and exercise, some have used health LOC, and others have used exercise- and fitness-specific measures. Results collectively provide weak support for LOC in predicting fitness and exercise behaviours, although the extent to which this could be a reflection of the inadequacies of the fitness or LOC measures remains to be seen. At best, studies suggest that some group differences may exist between exercisers and non-exercisers at a cross-sectional level on LOC. However, one cannot ascertain whether such differences developed as a result of involvement or whether they were influential in initial decisions to become active. Health LOC does not strongly predict, or relate to, exercise behaviour.

Such an equivocal conclusion has prompted researchers to ask why such is the case. Three main possibilities exist. First, the theory could be wrong or not applicable to exercise; second, the measuring tools are not sensitive or appropriate enough to demonstrate a relationship between LOC and exercise participation, and third, fitness/exercise 'externals' are rare people, thus making it difficult from a research perspective to demonstrate relationships or discriminate among groups. Given the theoretical predictions of LOC research, and the extensive testing of the theoretical constructs involved, one could still propose that a relationship should exist. Most of the studies where no relationship has been found suggest that the LOC measures have not been specific enough to exercise and fitness behaviours, and this includes health LOC. Not all people will perceive exercise as a health-promoting behaviour anyway. Calls for greater specificity in measurement have been met with several studies that have addressed this issue in exercise and physical fitness.

Several researchers have attempted to develop exercise or fitness LOC scales (Noland and Feldman, 1984; Whitehead and Corbin, 1988). However, measures have failed to provide evidence that an LOC measure that is specific to exercise is a better predictor than other LOC measures. Indeed, one could safely argue that they do not predict exercise behaviours at all well. We are not aware of any substantive work being published on this issue in the past decade.

> Key point: The construct of locus of control is well known but has not been a strong predictor of physical activity participation.

Perceptions of the incremental nature of ability

An interesting development in the study of control, goals and motivation has been Dweck's theorising concerning the perceived stability of ability (Dweck, 1999; Dweck and Leggett, 1988; Dweck et al., 1995) or what has popularly become known as the 'growth mindset' (Dweck, 2006). Initially in the domain of intelligence, and then extended to include views of morality and stereotyping, Dweck and colleagues have proposed that two clusters of beliefs underpin people's judgements and behaviours (Dweck and Leggett, 1988). These beliefs centre on the way people view the malleability of attributes, such as intelligence. Those subscribing to the view that a particular attribute (e.g. intelligence) is fixed and relatively stable hold an 'entity' view or 'entity theory'. Conversely, those seeing the attribute as changeable and open to development hold an 'incremental' view or theory – hence reference to the 'growth mindset'.

Research has shown that those holding an entity view are more likely to have negative reactions, such as helplessness, when faced with achievement setbacks (Dweck and Leggett, 1988). Entity theorists are more likely to endorse performance (ego) goals whereas incremental theorists have been shown to endorse learning (task) goals.

There has been little attention given to implicit beliefs in the physical activity domain (Sarrazin et al., 1996). This is despite similar notions in related areas of research, such as ability and effort beliefs in attribution research, or beliefs concerning the causes of success in goal orientations research.

In a small-scale experiment, Kasimatis et al. (1996) told some students that athletic coordination was mostly learned, to create an incremental condition, and told others that coordination was genetically determined (entity condition). After initial success, participants were subjected to a difficult exercise task through video. Results showed that in the face of such difficulty, more positive responses were found for those in the incremental condition. Specifically, such participants reported higher motivation and self-efficacy and less negative affect. However, the implicit beliefs held by the students were not assessed. The nature and extent of entity and incremental beliefs in this sample therefore, as well as the longevity of such effects, are not known.

We developed a scale for young people to assess entity and incremental beliefs in physical activity (Biddle *et al.*, 2003). We reported three studies of over 3,000 young people aged 11 to 19 years and found support for a multidimensional measuring scale that was suitable across age and gender groups. Analyses supported factors of entity and incremental beliefs being underpinned by beliefs that athletic ability is stable and a gift (entity), and open to improvement and being developed through learning (incremental). Incremental (negative) and entity (positive) beliefs predicted self-reported amotivation towards physical education and sport, while a further study provided evidence that enjoyment of physical activity in youth was positively associated with incremental beliefs. Evidence for cross-cultural validity also exists (Wang *et al.*, 2005). The structure of the assessment scale, and modified example items, are shown in Figure 9.9.

The physical activity research reviewed so far suggests that relationships do exist, albeit small at times, between implicit beliefs and goal orientations, as well as other motivational indicators. This could prove to be a useful development because if some individuals feel that exercising 'ability' is fixed and cannot be developed, they are less likely to try. This is supported by the ADNFS data reported in Chapter 7 where over 40 per cent of women said they were 'not the sporty type' and that this presented a significant barrier to physical activity.

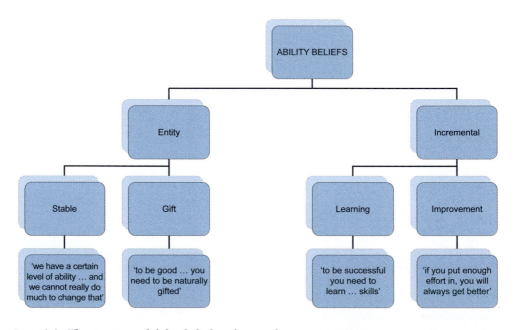

Figure 9.9 The structure of ability beliefs with example assessment items

Source: Adapted from Biddle *et al.* (2003).

Key point: Believing that we can change our capacity to do things, like being physically active, may be important in creating positive motivation – a positive 'mindset'.

Physical activity by stealth: habit and nudging

Health behaviour change may be brought about in two main ways:

- *Deliberative (reflective) processing*: this is where people think about behaviour change such as by weighing up the advantages and disadvantages. This is consistent with many of the psychological constructs discussed in this book, such as theories of attitude and confidence.
- *Automatic processing*: this is where rather little reflection takes place and where the behaviour is driven either by environmental cues (e.g. walking because it's a pedestrian-only zone) or through 'gut feeling' and emotion (e.g. 'I like it').

Automatic processing is associated with notions of 'habit' which involve behavioural patterns learned through context-dependent repetition (see also Chapter 16). This means that when a particular context is encountered, such as sitting down in the lounge at home, it is sufficient to automatically cue the habitual response of, say, switching on the TV. In novel contexts, behaviour is more likely to be regulated by conscious decisions through intentions (reflective processing), but in familiar contexts behaviour will be much more affected by habit (automatic processing). Given the high frequency of many sedentary behaviours, such as sitting at a desk at work or sitting in front of the TV at home, it is easy to see how habitual such behaviours become. Whether this is true for structured exercise is debatable, as it is likely to involve the necessity of more conscious processing. That said, making environments highly conducive to physical activity, or very attractive, will help.

Gardner and colleagues (2011) have reviewed associations between a measure of habit and selected health behaviours. Specifically, they looked at the Self-Report Habit Index which assesses automaticity, frequency and relevance to self-identity. Across a small number of studies, the average strength of correlation between this index and various physical activities was moderate to large, as shown in Figure 9.10.

Recently the popular concept of 'nudging' has been proposed (Marteau *et al.*, 2011). Nudging is when behaviours are encouraged through little or no incentives rather than so-called 'nannying' approaches, such as through government policies and legislation. This is sometimes referred to as the influence of 'choice architecture'. The UK government's 'Behavioural Insights Team' is sometimes referred to as the 'Nudge Unit'.

Examples of nudging would be environmental changes that encourage using stairs by placing attractive-looking staircases in the most accessible positions. That said, the opposite can also happen – we can be nudged into unhealthy behaviours. In fact, the norm in public places, such as hotels, is to find easily accessible and attractive lifts (elevators) and inaccessible stairs, thus nudging us to use the lifts. This has probably happened to people so many times that on encountering the hotel lobby they automatically use the lift with little or no thought about seeking out the stairs. Indeed, as Marteau *et al.* (2011) say, 'nudging certainly works. Shaping environments to cue certain behaviours is extremely effective, *unfortunately often to the detriment of our health*' (p. 263, emphasis added). At the other end of the spectrum is behaviour change through coercion or mandatory rules, such as banning something.

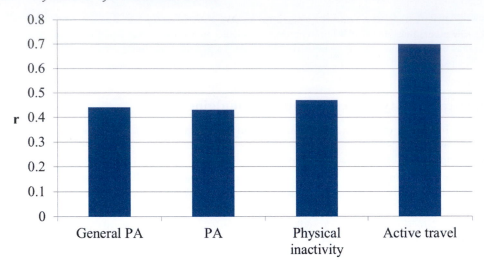

Figure 9.10 Correlations from a meta-analysis of studies assessing the association between a measure of
self-reported habit and different markers of physical activity
Source: Data from Gardner *et al.* (2011).

A report for the UK government's Cabinet Office (Dolan *et al.*, 2010) focuses a great deal on
non-coercive, nudge-type approaches based on behavioural economics. MINDSPACE is their
mnemonic to refer to nine factors which act as a checklist for policy-making:

- Messenger: our behaviours are influenced by the source of communication for
information.
- Incentives: we are influenced by incentives, particularly avoiding losses.
- Norms: we are influenced by what others do.
- Defaults: we 'go with the flow' of pre-set options.
- Salience: novelty and relevance will drive behaviour.
- Priming: we are driven by subconscious cues.
- Affect: our feelings will influence our behaviours (what we like, dislike).
- Commitments: we seek to be consistent with our publicly stated commitments and goals.
- Ego: we act in ways that enhance feeling good about ourselves.

Applications to physical activity might include the source of mass media messaging, use of
incentives, social norms around physical activity or sedentary behaviours, and feeling good
about ourselves through physical activity.

Myths and truths of motivation

In working as consultants on motivation we have come across some misunderstandings of
motivation for physical activity. There are many ways to look at 'motivation'. At its simplest,
motivation is about *direction* (*what* are we motivated about?) and **intensity** (*how much* are
we motivated?). This means that we need to help people to become more focused on both the
what and *how much* of motivation. There seem to be four main myths of motivation:

- **Myth #1: motivation is just about 'how much'.**
- Truth: Motivation is about a focus on something (direction) as well as 'how much'.

In addition, it's not just about 'how much' motivation. It's also about the quality (type) of motivation (Deci and Flaste, 1995) (see previous discussion on intrinsic and extrinsic motivation and the self-determination continuum).

- **Myth #2: motivation is motivation is motivation…**
- Truth: There are different types (forms) of motivation ranging from extrinsic to intrinsic.

We need to move, over time, from being driven by extrinsic motivation to more internal forms of motivation. This will help us stick to our plans and goals. This also tells us that it's not just about 'being motivated' but how we are motivated. People are motivated to achieve their goals in different ways, and exercise is a good example. People can be motivated to exercise through reasons of fitness, health, appearance, social togetherness, etc.

- **Myth #3: we are all motivated to exercise in the same way.**
- Truth: We have different 'motives' for exercise.

Recent evidence, and probably common sense too, tells us, in addition to how and why the individual is motivated, what they actually do (e.g. exercise regularly) which will also be determined by their surroundings and whether the behaviour (exercise) is easy or hard to do (see: http://www.behaviormodel.org/). In addition, we are more likely to come back if we like the experience (Ekkekakis, 2003).

It is often assumed that we need 'willpower' to be a regular exerciser. While some effort is obviously needed, if we make exercise 'easier' to do, it may help us to maintain our involvement.

- **Myth #4: we need high levels of willpower to exercise.**
- Truth: We are more likely to exercise if it's 'easy' or pleasurable to do.

Chapter summary and conclusion

The popular health literature constantly makes reference to the concept of 'control' over lifestyle, fitness and health, about motivation, and about the need for 'willpower'. This suggests that there is a belief that individuals can 'control' their physical activity and, to some extent, their health. While this can be contested, perceptions of control can be important indicators of motivation and mental health. The evidence presented here has been accumulated from one main area – intrinsic motivation – as well as other sources derived from expectancy-value and control theories of motivation, such as locus of control and perceptions of the nature of physical ability.

In summary, therefore, we conclude the following:

- Motivation comprises different elements and qualities.
- Cognitive Evaluation Theory remains a viable theory for the study of motivational processes in physical activity involving rewards.
- Self-Determination Theory is an important perspective for the study of motivation in physical activity and is likely to increase our understanding of motivation, in particular the different types of extrinsic motivation that may exist in physical activity.

- Current research findings are not supportive of locus of control being a strong determinant of physical activity.
- Beliefs concerning the nature of how stable or changeable physical ability can be are important motivational factors in physical activity.
- We should be aware that some behaviours are driven more by unconscious habit than by conscious reflective processes.
- 'Nudging' may act as less conscious motivation for some health behaviours.

References

Biddle, S.J.H. (1999). Motivation and perceptions of control: Tracing its development and plotting its future in exercise and sport psychology. *Journal of Sport and Exercise Psychology, 21*, 1–23.

Biddle, S.J.H., Wang, C.K.J., Chatzisarantis, N.L.D. and Spray, C.M. (2003). Motivation for physical activity in young people: Entity and incremental beliefs about athletic ability. *Journal of Sports Sciences, 21*, 973–989.

Cameron, J. and Pierce, D. (1994). Reinforcement, reward and intrinsic motivation: A meta-analysis. *Review of Educational Research, 64*, 363–423.

Canada Fitness Survey. (1983). *Fitness and Lifestyle in Canada*. Ottawa: Author.

Chatzisarantis, N.L.D., Hagger, M.S., Biddle, S.J.H., Smith, B. and Wang, C.K.J. (2003). A meta-analysis of perceived locus of causality in exercise, sport, and physical education contexts. *Journal of Sport and Exercise Psychology, 25*, 284–306.

Csikszentmihalyi, M. (1975). *Beyond Boredom and Anxiety*. San Francisco, CA: Jossey-Bass.

deCharms, R. (1968). *Personal Causation*. New York: Academic Press.

Deci, E.L. (1975). *Intrinsic Motivation*. New York: Plenum.

Deci, E.L. and Flaste, R. (1995). *Why We Do What We Do: Understanding self-motivation*. New York: Penguin.

Deci, E.L. and Ryan, R.M. (1985). *Intrinsic Motivation and Self-determination in Human Behavior*. New York: Plenum.

———. (1991). A motivational approach to self: Integration in personality. In R.A. Dienstbier (ed.), *Nebraska Symposium on Motivation: Perspectives on motivation (Vol. 38)* (pp. 237–288). Lincoln, NE: University of Nebraska Press.

———. (2000). The 'what' and 'why' of goal pursuits: Human needs and the self-determination of behavior. *Psychological Inquiry, 11*, 227–268.

———. (eds). (2002). *Handbook of Self-determination Research*. Rochester: The University of Rochester Press.

Deci, E. L., Eghrari, H., Patrick, B. C., and Leone, D. R. (1994). Facilitating internalisation: The Self-Determination Theory perspective. *Journal of Personality, 62*, 119–142.

Deci, E.L., Koestner, R. and Ryan, R.M. (1999). A meta-analytic review of experiments examining the effects of extrinsic rewards on intrinsic motivation. *Psychological Bulletin, 125*, 627–668.

Dishman, R.K., Sallis, J.F. and Orenstein, D. (1985). The determinants of physical activity and exercise. *Public Health Reports, 100*, 158–171.

Dolan, P., Hallsworth, M., Halpern, D., King, D. and Vlaev, I. (2010). *MINDSPACE: Influencing behaviour through public policy*. London: Cabinet Office.

Dweck, C. (1999). *Self-theories: Their role in motivation, personality, and development*. Philadelphia, PA: Taylor & Francis.

———. (2006). *Mindset: How you can fulfil your potential*. London: Constable & Robinson.

Dweck, C. and Leggett, E. (1988). A social-cognitive approach to motivation and personality. *Psychological Review, 95*, 256–273.

Dweck, C., Chiu, C.Y. and Hong, Y.Y. (1995). Implicit theories and their role in judgments and reactions: A world from two perspectives. *Psychological Inquiry, 6*, 267–285.

Ekkekakis, P. (2003). Pleasure and displeasure from the body: Perspectives from exercise. *Cognition and Emotion, 17*, 213–239.

Gardner, B., de Bruijn, G.J. and Lally, P. (2011). A systematic review and meta-analysis of applications of the Self-report Habit Index to nutrition and physical activity behaviours. *Annals of Behavioral Medicine, 42*, 174–187.

Hagger, M.S. and Chatzisarantis, N.L.D. (2005). *The Social Psychology of Sport and Exercise*. Milton Keynes: The Open University Press.

Kasimatis, M., Miller, M. and Macussen, L. (1996). The effects of implicit theories on exercise motivation. *Journal of Research in Personality, 30*, 510–516.

Katzmarzyk, P.T. and Mason, C. (2009). The physical activity transition. *Journal of Physical Activity and Health, 6*, 269–280.

Lepper, M.R. and Greene, D. (1975). Turning play into work: Effects of adult surveillance and extrinsic rewards on children's intrinsic motivation. *Journal of Personality and Social Psychology, 31*, 479–486.

Lepper, M.R., Greene, D. and Nisbett, R.E. (1973). Undermining children's intrinsic interest with extrinsic reward: A test of the 'overjustification' hypothesis. *Journal of Personality and Social Psychology, 28*, 129–137.

Maehr, M.L. and Braskamp, L.A. (1986). *The Motivation Factor: A theory of personal investment*. Lexington, MA: Lexington Books.

Mandela, N. (1994). *Long Walk to Freedom*. London: Little, Brown and Company.

Marteau, T.M., Ogilvie, D., Roland, M., Suhrcke, M. and Kelly, M.P. (2011). Judging nudging: Can nudging improve population health? *British Medical Journal, 342*, d228.

Michie, S., van Stralen, M. and West, R. (2011). The behaviour change wheel: A new method for characterising and designing behaviour change interventions. *Implementation Science, 6*(1), 42, http://www.implementationscience.com/content/46/41/42.

Noland, M. and Feldman, R. (1984). Factors related to the leisure exercise behavior of 'returning' women college students. *Health Education, March/April*, 32–36.

Powell, K.E. (1988). Habitual exercise and public health: An epidemiological view. In R.K. Dishman (ed.), *Exercise Adherence: Its impact on public health* (pp. 15–39). Champaign, IL: Human Kinetics.

Rotter, J.B. (1954). *Social Learning and Clinical Psychology*. Englewood Cliffs, NJ: Prentice-Hall.

———. (1966). Generalised expectancies for internal versus external control of reinforcement. *Psychological Monographs, 80, Whole No. 609*, 1–28.

Rummel, A. and Feinberg, R. (1988). Cognitive evaluation theory: A meta-analytic review of the literature. *Social Behavior and Personality, 16*, 147–164.

Ryan, R.M., Patrick, H., Deci, E.L. and Williams, G.C. (2008). Facilitating health behaviour change and its maintenance: Interventions based on self-determination theory. *The European Health Psychologist, 10*, 2–5.

Sallis, J.F. and Hovell, M. (1990). Determinants of exercise behavior. *Exercise and Sport Sciences Reviews, 18*, 307–330.

Sarrazin, P., Biddle, S., Famose, J.P., Cury, F., Fox, K. and Durand, M. (1996). Goal orientations and conceptions of the nature of sport ability in children: A social cognitive approach. *British Journal of Social Psychology, 35*, 399–414.

Silva, M., Vieira, P.N., Coutinho, S.R., Minderico, C.S., Matos, M.G. and Sardinha, L.B. (2010). Using self-determination theory to promote physical activity and weight control: A randomized controlled trial in women. *Journal of Behavioral Medicine, 33*, 110–122.

Skinner, E. (1995). *Perceived Control, Motivation, and Coping*. Thousand Oaks, CA: Sage.

———. (1996). A guide to constructs of control. *Journal of Personality and Social Psychology, 71*, 549–570.

Standage, M., Duda, J.L. and Ntoumanis, N. (2005). A test of self-determination theory in school physical education. *British Journal of Educational Psychology, 75*, 411–433.

Szabo, A. (2000). Physical activity as a source of psychological dysfunction. In S.J.H. Biddle, K.R. Fox and S.H. Boutcher (eds), *Physical Activity and Psychological Well-being* (pp. 130–153). London: Routledge.

Tang, S.H. and Hall, V.C. (1995). The overjustification effect: A meta-analysis. *Applied Cognitive Psychology, 9*, 365–404.

Teixeira, P., Carraca, E., Markland, D., Silva, M. and Ryan, R. (2012). Exercise, physical activity, and self-determination theory: A systematic review. *International Journal of Behavioral Nutrition and Physical Activity, 9*(1), 78.

Vallerand, R.J. (1997). Toward a hierarchical model of intrinsic and extrinsic motivation. In M.P. Zanna (ed.), *Advances in Experimental Social Psychology: Vol 29* (pp. 271–360). New York: Academic Press.

Vallerand, R.J. and Fortier, M.S. (1998). Measures of intrinsic and extrinsic motivation in sport and physical activity: A review and critique. In J.L. Duda (ed.), *Advances in Sport and Exercise Psychology Measurement* (pp. 81–101). Morgantown, WV: Fitness Information Technology.

Wang, C.K.J., Liu, W.C., Biddle, S.J.H. and Spray, C.M. (2005). Cross-cultural validation of the Conceptions of the Nature of Athletic Ability Questionnaire Version 2. *Personality and Individual Differences, 38*(6), 1245–1256.

White, R.W. (1959). Motivation reconsidered: The concept of competence. *Psychological Review, 66*, 297–333.

Whitehead, J.R. and Corbin, C.B. (1988). Multidimensional scales for the measurement of locus of control of reinforcements for physical fitness behaviors. *Research Quarterly for Exercise and Sport, 59*, 108–117.

——. (1991). Youth fitness testing: The effect of percentile-based evaluative feedback on intrinsic motivation. *Research Quarterly for Exercise and Sport, 62*, 225–231.

10 Physical activity and confidence
I think I can, I think I can, I know I can …

Purpose of the chapter

We continue our review of motivational influences on physical activity by reviewing the study of how we perceive our competence and confidence to be physically active. Specifically, in this chapter we aim to:

- outline the basic framework of Social Cognitive Theory (SCT);
- describe and define self-efficacy as a key component of SCT;
- present an overview of research findings concerning self-efficacy in the context of physical activity;
- present some alternative views on confidence relevant to the study of physical activity.

So far, we have discussed a number of issues associated with motivation for physical activity, such as attitude (Chapter 8) and intrinsic motivation (Chapter 9). A dominant perspective on physical activity motivation over the past 20 to 30 years has been 'self-efficacy', and this continues to be a key focus of physical activity research today. Other approaches include theories based on self-presentation, self-perceptions of worth and competence motivation, and perceptions of success and achievement goals.

The need for studying confidence should be self-evident. However, there are a number of issues that need addressing. It is not known whether there are different types of confidence in physical activity, such as the confidence to initiate an exercise programme or the confidence that physical activity will bring about desired results, such as weight loss or gains in fitness. The role of state-versus-trait factors is unclear, although contemporary approaches to the study of self-confidence suggest that situational cues are likely to dominate over and above any trait confidence factors. In addition, the permanence of confidence in particular situations or across different groups (e.g. age, gender, class, ethnicity) is rarely studied. This all suggests that self-confidence, despite a great deal of interest in this area of psychological research, and the intuitive logic and appeal of the topic, requires further study before application can be made in some fields.

The recently published COM-B approach underpinning the 'behaviour change wheel' (Michie *et al.*, 2011a) also highlights the importance of capability (alongside competence and opportunity) as foundations for the adoption of the desired behaviour (see Chapter 12). In this model, capability is seen to be both physical and psychological. Hence capability, a concept close to confidence, is seen as central to behaviour change.

Social Cognitive Theory (SCT) and self-efficacy

The seminal work of Albert Bandura concerning social cognitive influences on behaviour have been most prominent in dealing with feelings of self-efficacy, or confidence, to undertake certain behaviours. However, Bandura's Social Cognitive Theory (SCT) (Bandura, 1986) is more than just self-efficacy (Bandura, 1997).

SCT suggests that we learn and modify our behaviours through an interaction between personal, behavioural and environmental influences. This is the so-called model of 'reciprocal determinism', with all three constructs affecting each other (see Figure 10.1). In other words, we are not merely a function of the environment, nor are we passive in following our psychological characteristics. Moreover, our own and others' behaviour can influence us. Put together, all three factors influence how we think, feel and act.

Key cognitive elements of SCT comprise the ability of human beings to think about the likely consequences of their actions. Bandura refers to this as our 'symbolising capability', or our ability to think about and anticipate future courses of action. Similarly, SCT comprises a self-regulation component in which we regulate our behaviour based on our own goals, behaviours and feelings. For example, people may adopt a certain goal of being physically active that helps motivate action. Attempting to meet that goal regulates our thoughts and behaviour.

We also reflect on our actions, particularly in respect of thinking about the consequences of our behaviours (referred to as 'outcome expectancies') and our own capabilities ('efficacy expectancies'). Thinking about consequences is best illustrated in physical activity by the way we think about the benefits and costs of being more active. I could believe these consequences to be positive, such as improved health, better fitness, good functionality; or negative, such as higher risk of injury, perception of inappropriate use of time or high financial cost.

Motivation and confidence: self-efficacy

Confidence has been identified at the anecdotal and empirical level as an important construct in motivation for physical activity. Statements associated with self-perceptions of confidence are commonplace in studies on exercise and sport. For example, in the Allied Dunbar National

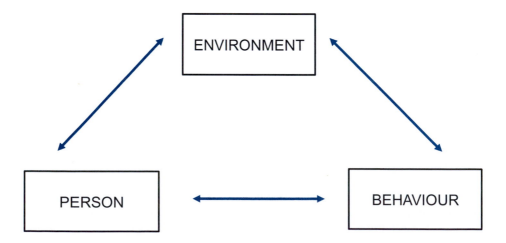

Figure 10.1 Reciprocal determinism underpinning Social Cognitive Theory

Fitness Survey for England (ADNFS) (Sports Council and Health Education Authority, 1992), emotional, motivational and time barriers were identified as factors preventing people from being more physically active. All are likely to be associated, in one way or another, with feelings of confidence to initiate or maintain physical activity.

The self-efficacy construct and framework originated in clinical settings but it has subsequently been tested in a variety of physical activity and health contexts, such as sport (Feltz, 1992), weight loss (Weinberg *et al.*, 1984), exercise (Ewart, 1989; McAuley and Blissmer, 2000), and with other health-related behaviours (Schwarzer, 1992; Strecher *et al.*, 1986). Schwarzer (1992), for example, states that 'self-efficacy has proven to be a very powerful behavioural determinant in many studies, and its inclusion in theories of health behaviour, therefore, is warranted' (p. 223).

Bandura (1986, p. 391) defines perceived self-efficacy as:

> people's judgements of their capabilities to organise and execute courses of action required to attain designated types of performances. It is concerned not with the skills one has but with judgements of what one can do with whatever skills one possesses.

The key phrase here is 'capabilities to organise and execute courses of action', since Bandura has always differentiated between efficacy expectations and outcome expectations. By this it is meant that beliefs related to the ability to carry out a particular behaviour are efficacy expectations, whereas beliefs as to whether the behaviour will produce a particular result are outcome expectations. For example, efficacy expectations might be the belief that one can successfully adhere to a programme of brisk walking five times each week for 30 minutes. However, outcome expectations might refer to whether one believes that such activity will produce the weight loss that was desired at the beginning. This is similar to Skinner's (1995, 1996) control model whereby capacity beliefs are required to produce the behaviour, whereas strategy beliefs are needed to believe that the behaviour will produce the desired outcomes (see Chapter 9).

Although Bandura's self-efficacy framework refers to the two expectancies as being different, they are both part of the self-confidence concept in physical activity. People are likely to be concerned about both types of expectancy and both require study in exercise psychology research. For example, it is important to know whether efficacy expectations are influential in the adoption of exercise programmes, yet it is also likely that outcome expectations will affect the maintenance of such programmes and the reinforcement necessary for continued involvement. Studies apparently testing self-efficacy, however, do not always make it clear whether they are investigating efficacy or outcome judgements.

Key point: Self-efficacy is key to the adoption of many health behaviours.

Sources of efficacy information

Four main sources of information for self-efficacy beliefs have been identified by Bandura (1986, 1997). These are as follows:

- prior success and performance attainment
- imitation and modelling

- verbal and social persuasion
- judgements of physiological states.

PERFORMANCE ATTAINMENT

This is thought to be the most powerful of efficacy sources because it is based on personal experience of success and failure. Bandura (1986) states that 'successes raise efficacy appraisals; repeated failures lower them, especially if the failures occur early in the course of events and do not reflect a lack of effort or adverse external circumstances' (p. 399). Attribution theory predicts that internal and stable causes of failure, such as lack of ability, are more likely to lead to debilitating and demotivating cognitions and negative emotions than factors which appear more changeable, such as lack of effort or poor strategy (Biddle *et al.*, 2001).

IMITATION AND MODELLING

Self-efficacy may also be developed through imitation and modelling. Observing others succeed or fail could affect subsequent efficacy beliefs, particularly if the individual has little or no prior experience to draw on. Bandura (1986) suggests that social comparison information is important in self-efficacy beliefs. For example, confidence may be associated with certain self-presentational processes, such as social physique anxiety (Leary, 1992; Leary *et al.*, 1994), and public exercise behaviours, such as on-street jogging, public swimming or exercise classes, are likely to evoke strong self-presentation influences and could be a major source of motivational variation.

Bandura (1986) suggests that the social comparison element of vicarious experience is important, since in some situations it is not always possible to gauge one's success without some kind of reference point, such as another person's score. 'Because most performances are evaluated in terms of social criteria, social comparative information figures prominently in self-efficacy appraisals' (Bandura, 1986, p. 400).

Another issue concerning vicarious processes in self-efficacy is the use of certain types of individuals in promoting physical activity to inactive people. It is common in the mass media to use elite sport models, or models displaying high levels of fitness or physique development. Bandura contends that vicarious influences, such as modelling, are more likely to have an influence when the individual has some empathy with the model being observed. On the other hand, anecdotal evidence suggests that elite models are 'interesting' and 'motivational'. Indeed, the argument that mega-sports events, such as Olympic and Paralympic Games, create a participation legacy – argued and promoted vigorously for the London 2012 Games – is based on such assumptions. Yet modelling effects according to the self-efficacy framework would suggest that similar role models may be more effective, with elite sport models viewed as being associated with unattainable and unreachable goals. Our own research found that older patients referred into an exercise programme by their family doctor were more confident when exercising with similar individuals. They also reported feeling uncomfortable when around young, 'vigorous' exercisers (Biddle *et al.*, 1994; Fox *et al.*, 1997). More needs to be known about this issue.

VERBAL AND SOCIAL PERSUASION

Depending on the source of such efficacy information, persuasion from others is likely to influence perceptions of self-efficacy. However, it is thought to be a relatively weak source in comparison to the two already mentioned and has not been studied in any systematic way in physical activity. The success of persuasion is also dependent on the realistic nature of the information. Given the potential for regular contact between, say, exerciser and instructor in supervised programmes, or with a personal trainer, verbal persuasion is likely to be a source of self-efficacy worthy of note in some situations. Moreover, medical practitioners can be influential in this regard; hence it is important that they are knowledgeable and encouraging in respect of physical activity. Being a good role model will also help.

JUDGEMENTS OF PHYSIOLOGICAL STATES

The original theorising on self-efficacy was based on experiences in clinical settings, and in particular the modification of reactions to aversive events, such as phobias (Bandura, 1977). In such situations it was found that self-efficacy was related to how one appraised internal physiological states such as heart rate. Bandura (1986) says, 'treatments that eliminate emotional arousal to subjective threats heighten perceived self-efficacy with corresponding improvements in performance' (p. 401). The use of such somatic feedback can be a positive influence on self-efficacy; however, the evidence in sport has been inconsistent (Feltz, 1992) and hardly studied at all, to our knowledge, in exercise, although teaching people how to monitor physiological signs may provide for the possibility of enhancing efficacy perceptions. It seems that studies need to address the links between the concepts of self-efficacy, effort perceptions and the capabilities people have for self-monitoring physical exertion during exercise. This is particularly important for people who may be apprehensive about exertion, such as those in rehabilitation contexts.

> Key point: The enhancement of self-efficacy is based on positive experiences as well as watching others succeed who are similar to you. A non-threatening atmosphere and encouragement will also help.

How do we measure self-efficacy?

Self-efficacy will vary along the dimensions of magnitude, strength and generality (Bandura, 1986):

- *Magnitude* of self-efficacy refers to the ordering of tasks by difficulty, such as feeling that one is capable of sustaining a walking programme but not one for running half marathons.
- *Strength* refers to the assessment of one's capabilities of performing a particular task. For example, people are able to subjectively rate their likelihood of maintaining a programme of walking to work every other day.
- *Generality* of self-efficacy refers to the extent to which efficacy expectations from one situation generalise to other situations, such as efficacy gained through a walking programme generalising to the lifting of weights in an exercise programme. While all studies measure strength of self-efficacy, fewer measure magnitude and generality. The operational measures of self-efficacy in physical activity settings therefore appear to be limited.

Self-efficacy in physical activity: research findings

Self-efficacy is a popular topic of study within the physical activity domain and is often shown to be an important correlate of physical activity (see Chapter 7). Studies on self-efficacy in physical activity settings have investigated non-patient and patient populations.

Early research with patients

Ewart and co-workers conducted a number of the early studies on self-efficacy and exercise, and they shed light on some important issues that are still relevant today (see Ewart, 1989). Ewart *et al.* (1983) studied self-efficacy in the context of treadmill running with post-myocardial infarction (MI) patients. Before and after treadmill exercise, assessment of self-efficacy to take part in walking, running, stair climbing, sexual intercourse, lifting and general exertion (but not all at once!) was made. Results showed that positive changes in self-efficacy took place following treadmill exercise, and that this was greatest for running, suggesting that efficacy effects do generalise but appear to have stronger effects on similar exercise modes – in this case, running.

Ewart *et al.* (1986) investigated the specificity of self-efficacy perceptions of men with coronary heart disease (CHD). Circuit weight training was used and self-efficacy ratings taken prior to a variety of physical fitness tests were shown to correlate more strongly with test results for activities specific to the self-efficacy judgements. For example, efficacy ratings for the performance of lifting activities were significantly correlated with the arm strength test but not with the aerobic endurance treadmill test. Conversely, self-efficacy ratings of jogging were significantly correlated with the aerobic endurance test but not with tests of arm, grip or leg strength.

These two studies have focused on those with known medical symptoms. Given that self-efficacy is a social-cognitive variable open to environmental and perceptual intervention, it may be unwise to generalise from these studies. For example, Ewart (1989) suggests that post-coronary patients are often limited more by fear of exertion than by their actual medical condition. This is quite different from individuals who are free of disease symptoms.

Research with non-patient groups

Many research papers have been published on self-efficacy for exercise and physical activity in non-patient groups. McAuley's work on exercise self-efficacy has been particularly influential (e.g. McAuley *et al.*, 2003a, 2003b). McAuley and Blissmer (2000) summarise evidence on self-efficacy and physical activity in respect of SE being a determinant and an outcome of physical activity, and Figure 10.2 illustrates how self-efficacy has been studied in physical activity.

McAuley and colleagues have studied self-efficacy responses of older adults (although some not that old), a population previously underrepresented in the exercise psychology literature. Several studies by McAuley and co-workers focus on a group of previously inactive 45- to 64-year-olds. These studies have shown that for such adults exercise self-efficacy:

* can be increased through intervention;
* will predict participation, particularly in the early stages of an exercise programme;
* declines after a period of inactivity.

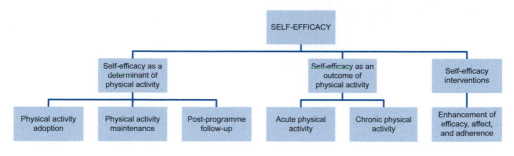

Figure 10.2 A summary of self-efficacy and physical activity

Source: Adapted from McAuley and Blissmer (2000).

McAuley and Blissmer (2000) conclude that while the relationship between self-efficacy and physical activity is well documented, it is also complex. For example, self-efficacy beliefs are likely to be more influential in conditions that are challenging in comparison to circumstances that are more 'habitual' and requiring of less effort. For this reason, the promotion of habitual physical activity through, say, walking to work could involve only minimal amounts of self-efficacy, thus holding much promise for behaviour change. Self-efficacy will be even less important under conditions of behavioural 'nudging' (Marteau *et al.*, 2011) (see Chapter 9).

In summary, the studies investigating self-efficacy in non-patient exercise groups show a consistent relationship between self-efficacy and participation in physical activity.

EVIDENCE FROM SYSTEMATIC REVIEWS

For many years the sources of self-efficacy proposed by Bandura have provided a useful framework for how people might increase their self-efficacy and, ultimately, their physical activity levels. However, it was not until recently that a systematic analysis of such concepts was published. French and colleagues in the UK have analysed what strategies appear to affect self-efficacy and physical activity (Ashford *et al.*, 2010; Williams and French, 2011). First, Ashford and colleagues meta-analysed 27 physical activity intervention studies where self-efficacy was an outcome measure. Research designs included RCTs, non-randomised studies and experiments, quasi-experimental designs and pre-post interventions. Many settings were covered, including the workplace, primary care, media and universities. Lifestyle and recreational physical activities were the focus, thus excluding sport or lab studies. Finally, intervention methods included face-to-face and telephone counselling, email feedback, behaviour change class sessions, discussion groups and watching DVDs.

Table 10.1 shows the frequency of some of the most commonly used strategies in the interventions, with reference made in the table to Bandura's sources of self-efficacy. Overall, there was a small but significant effect for interventions on physical activity self-efficacy, with an effect size (d) of 0.16. Five strategies showed significant effects when included in interventions in comparison with self-efficacy effects for interventions when the strategy was not included. These were graded as mastery experience, vicarious experience, persuasion, feedback (two types) and barriers (with problem-solving), as shown in Figure 10.3. However, not all of these strategies were in the expected direction. To be more precise, Figure 10.3 shows that higher self-efficacy was reported when interventions included vicarious experiences, consistent with Bandura's theorising. Moreover, stronger effects were noted on self-efficacy when feedback was provided both in respect of past behaviour and relative to others. When barriers were identified, self-efficacy was lower. All of these effects are either in line with theory or are logical. However, several findings were counter-intuitive. Graded mastery experience, a key source of self-efficacy according to Bandura (1997), showed lower self-efficacy when included in interventions. In addition, effects for self-efficacy were higher when verbal persuasion was not used. Notwithstanding that the source of the verbal persuasion may be important, as well as the style of delivery, this is a strange finding questioning Bandura's long-standing assumptions, at least for physical activity. Finally, when problem-solving strategies were not used, self-efficacy was higher. Again, this seems counter-intuitive and at odds with other literature, such as the taxonomy of behaviour change techniques (Michie *et al.*, 2011b).

The above review looked only at how self-efficacy might be changed in physical activity interventions. It did not assess whether physical activity itself was associated with certain

Table 10.1 Frequency of intervention strategies grouped by sources of self-efficacy proposed by Bandura and reported in the meta-analysis of physical activity and self-efficacy by Ashford *et al.* (2010)

Sources of self-efficacy proposed by Bandura	Number of intervention groups using the strategy
Mastery experiences	34
Vicarious experiences	9
Persuasion	33
Physiological and fitness feedback	6
Other: goal-setting	27

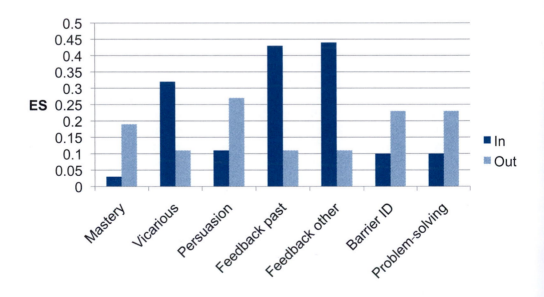

Figure 10.3 Strategies showing significant effects when included in interventions ('in') compared with self-efficacy effects for interventions when the strategy was not included ('out')

Source: Data from Ashford *et al.* (2010).

strategies. This led to a review by Williams and French (2011) of techniques used in physical activity interventions and the degree to which they were associated with changes in self-efficacy and physical activity. This paper reported additional analyses from the review by Ashford *et al.* (2010).

Six strategies were reported to be associated with changes in physical activity, as shown in Figure 10.4. These are as follows:

- provide information on the consequences of the behaviour in general;
- action planning;
- reinforcing effort or progress towards the behaviour;
- provide instruction;
- facilitate social comparison;
- time management.

Unlike the strategies reported by Ashford *et al.* (2010), those found in the review by Williams and French (2011) seem more logical and largely in line with predictions. Essentially, what the review is showing is that the effects of a physical activity intervention are greater when the strategies involve providing information, action planning, reinforcement, instruction and time management. In addition, there was an effect for facilitation of social comparison. However, this is often not recommended and is contrary to much of the motivation literature on self-focused versus other-focused styles of motivation. However, this review did show that changes in self-efficacy were strongly associated with changes in physical activity, although not all strategies changed across self-efficacy and physical activity in the same way or direction.

Finally, Olander *et al.* (2013) conducted a similar systematic review but for physical activity interventions with obese adults. Interventions for physical activity showed a moderate effect

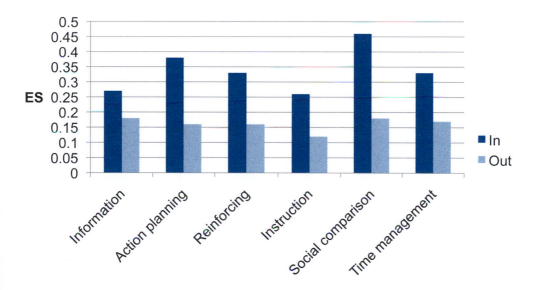

Figure 10.4 Strategies showing significant effects on physical activity when included in interventions ('in') compared with interventions when the strategy was not included ('out')

Source: Data from Williams and French (2011).

size (d = 0.50) with 21 behaviour change techniques being associated with higher levels of physical activity when present. The strategies showing the strongest effects were 'teach to use prompts/cues' and 'prompt rewards contingent on effort or progress towards the behaviour'. However, the association between change in self-efficacy and change in physical activity was small and not significant (rho = -0.18).

Does self-efficacy affect physical activity behaviour in young people?

The discussion thus far has focused on data from studies with adults. Although self-efficacy has been identified as a correlate of physical activity in young people (Biddle *et al.*, 2011), can we say that it is a mediator of physical activity change in this age group? Lubans and colleagues (2008) conducted a review of mediators of physical activity behaviour change in young people. Mediators were categorised as cognitive, behavioural and interpersonal. Self-efficacy was clearly the most studied successful mediator and evidence was strongly in favour of self-efficacy mediating physical activity behaviour change in young people.

Self-efficacy and physical activity: an illustrative study

A study by Luszczynska and Tryburcy (2008) examined whether a self-efficacy intervention would create changes in the frequency of exercise as well as self-efficacy beliefs at six-month follow-up. It was hypothesised that intervention effects will be moderated by having CVD or diabetes and where exercise is used in its prevention and treatment.

Questionnaire measures were completed by 320 adults at baseline. One month later, participants were randomly assigned to experimental (self-efficacy treatment) or control group. Six months after the intervention, further data were collected by email, with a response rate of 58 per cent. In brief, the self-efficacy intervention comprised the following elements:

- information regarding why self-efficacy is important and necessary in pursuing goals for physical activity;
- feedback regarding the participant's self-efficacy;
- discussion of strategies to increase self-efficacy.

Changes in physical activity and self-efficacy are shown in Figure 10.5. Those assigned to the experimental group reported higher levels of both self-efficacy and physical activity after six months from baseline, and the control group also showed increases in self-efficacy, but not in physical activity. Interestingly, greater changes were seen with a diagnosis of CVD or diabetes, suggesting that self-efficacy is particularly important for these individuals. This is consistent with Bandura's theorising insofar that self-efficacy is thought to be more important under conditions of challenge.

Self-efficacy and physical activity: so where are we now?

Linking self-efficacy and physical activity has been ongoing for many years. It is recognised that 'confidence' is important in adopting and maintaining health behaviours, and researchers have enthusiastically embraced the self-efficacy construct. We can now draw on several systematic reviews concerning self-efficacy in physical activity for young people, adults and

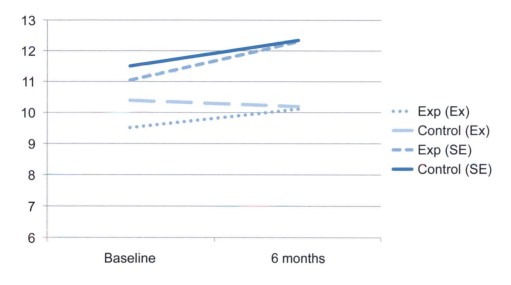

Figure 10.5 Changes at six months between experimental and control groups for exercise (Ex) and self-efficacy (SE)

Source: Luszczynska and Tryburcy (2008).

obese adults. However, the evidence is far from consistent about 'what works'. The following questions and comments address the key issues:

1. Do the sources of self-efficacy proposed by Bandura apply to physical activity? From the reviews summarised, there is mixed evidence for this.
2. Do strategies that increase self-efficacy also increase physical activity? There is support for this.
3. What strategies seem to adversely affect self-efficacy and why? More needs to be known here. The systematic review by Ashford *et al.* (2010) did show some findings that appeared contrary to expectation (see Figure 10.3).

One of the problems in this area is that we are assuming that individual behaviour change techniques (BCTs) act in isolation. So if interventions including the BCT of prompting self-monitoring show no more effectiveness than those without, is this because prompting self-monitoring does not work or that other strategies need to be in place to make it work? Are we fractionating strategies too much in our analyses?

Related to this is that some people are likely to use certain strategies which work while others choose alternative approaches. If people were offered, for example, self-monitoring and goal-setting, not everyone will be equally enthusiastic about both strategies. Yet we have little or no information from qualitative work about such decision-making in physical activity. For the reasons just discussed, it is likely that the development of self-efficacy will require physical activity practitioners to adopt a 'tool box' approach by offering several BCTs and strategies from which people choose what may work for them and what they see as acceptable and palatable.

Key point: Self-efficacy is one of the most consistent correlates of physical activity but more evidence is needed on what strategies work best to increase self-efficacy in physical activity.

Methodological issues in self-efficacy research

It has been argued that self-efficacy needs to be assessed in relation to specific behaviours if better behavioural prediction is to be achieved (Bandura, 1997; McAuley, 1992). Generalised perceptions of confidence are not the same as perceptions of efficacy. Nevertheless, we need more studies on the generalisability of self-efficacy across physical activity settings. Similar to the attitude–behaviour correspondence issue in social psychology (see Chapter 8), the utility of self-efficacy is likely to be greater when measures correspond closely to the behaviour in question, such as cycling three times per week, rather than using a general reference such as 'exercise'. This issue is not always addressed in the measurement of self-efficacy.

The second methodological issue to be considered concerns the behaviours associated with efficacy perceptions. Assessing self-efficacy in any meaningful way requires the behaviour to be associated with effort, potential barriers and behavioural self-regulation. In other words, habitual behaviours, such as tooth brushing, are likely to be unrelated to feelings of efficacy, whereas structured physical exercise may be highly associated with efficacy beliefs, since exercise requires planning, effort and often has some barriers. This is probably why self-efficacy emerges as one of the most consistent predictors of physical activity behaviours, particularly when physical activity includes elements of vigorous exercise. The extent to which less effortful forms of physical activity require self-efficacy remains to be seen. Evidence on 'habit' in physical activity, however, suggests that self-efficacy may be not be so central to undertaking certain behaviours (e.g. active commuting), although no doubt some beliefs of efficacy are required (Gardner *et al.*, 2011; see also Chapter 9).

Other approaches to the study of confidence and physical activity

Although self-efficacy has dominated the literature linking confidence perceptions and physical activity, other perspectives and approaches have been adopted and have potential for further study and application.

Self-presentational processes

Physical appearance, gestures and movement, public self-consciousness, weight, appearance and physique anxiety, and modesty are all constructs listed in the contents page of Leary's (1995) book on 'self-presentation'. Clearly, there is great potential for using such constructs in furthering our understanding of physical activity and perceptions of confidence.

Self-presentational concerns may affect physical activity choice, such as when one perceives the activity to be incompatible with one's image (e.g. dance or strength training), or where anxiety is felt in displaying low levels of physical competence. As Leary (1992) says, 'people are unlikely to devote themselves to activities that convey impressions that are inconsistent with their roles, others' values, or social norms' (p. 342).

Hart and colleagues (1989) have studied the construct of 'social physique anxiety'. Specifically, they propose that people high in such anxiety, in comparison to those who are not anxious, 'are likely to avoid situations in which their physique is under scrutiny of others (e.g. swimming in public) … avoid activities that accentuate their physiques (including aerobic activities that might be beneficial to them) … and attempt to improve their physiques through a variety of means, some of which may be harmful (e.g., fasting)' (p. 96). The ADNFS data showed that concerns about lack of sports competence were major barriers to participation in physical activity (Sports Council and Health Education Authority, 1992). How generalisable such feelings are remains to be seen. For some individuals, feelings of 'not being the sporty type' may generalise across many different physical activities, whereas for others they may only affect one or two specific activities. Indeed, most physical activities, such as sports, occur in public settings and this means that self-presentational issues are hard to ignore. Coupled with this is the widespread social acceptance of and admiration for physical expertise. Social anxiety in physical activity contexts is likely to be common. People are more likely to experience social anxiety when they are motivated to make desirable impressions on others but have low feelings of self-efficacy in being able to do so (Leary, 1995).

Performance estimation

Bandura (1997) clearly differentiates between efficacy and outcome expectations. However, earlier on it was stated that both types of expectancy are likely to be important in physical activity settings. Using a similar construct to outcome expectations, Corbin and his co-workers have investigated the issue of self-confidence in exercise from the viewpoint of performance estimations (see Corbin, 1984). This research programme was based on theorising by Lenney (1977) in the area of women and achievement behaviour. Lenney suggested that while evidence pointed to underachievement by females in some achievement contexts, this was not invariably so and pointed out that female self-confidence was dependent on 'situational vulnerability'. This was determined by three main factors:

- *The sex-typed nature of the task*: confidence is likely to be low in situations where the task is perceived as 'inappropriate'. That is to say, a role conflict may be apparent such as in performing tasks sex-typed as 'masculine'. An example would be women in the context of a weight-training class where some women might lack self-confidence.
- *Social evaluation*: Lenney (1977) has suggested that females will underestimate their ability when they are being evaluated or compared, such as in competition.
- *Feedback*: it has been proposed that females achieve better levels of performance when given objective and accurate feedback.

These factors point to important variables in the physical activity environment and, while originating from the study of women in achievement contexts, could also apply to men in some situations, such as activities sex-typed 'female' or 'feminine' (e.g. some forms of dance). However, given the predominantly masculine stereotyping of many physical activities, particularly sports, the emphasis has been placed on research into female self-confidence (Corbin, 1984). Little research over the past two decades has pursued this topic, but it remains a viable theme related to self-confidence.

Self-perceptions and competence motivation theory

Attempts at explaining human behaviour through an individual's desire to seek situations where he or she can display competence is not new in psychology. A comprehensive interpretation of competence motivation has been made by American developmental psychologist

Susan Harter (Harter, 1978; Harter and Connell, 1984). She conceptualised competence as multidimensional by specifying domains of competence perceptions, such as scholastic and athletic competence. These domains are likely to become more differentiated with age (see Table 6.1). Second, she related self-perceptions of competence to motivational orientations and perceptions of control. Finally, she developed measuring instruments for the assessment of domains of competence and self-perceptions of adequacy.

Harter's theory suggests that individuals are motivated where their competence can be demonstrated, particularly if they also feel intrinsically oriented in that area and see themselves as having a perception of personal control. Clearly, these concepts run in parallel with feelings of confidence. Successful mastery attempts under such conditions are associated with positive emotion and low anxiety.

Differential definitions of competence and success: goal perspectives theory

Early research in sport and exercise psychology followed the theoretical perspectives associated with 'need for achievement' and expectancy-value theories of Murray, Atkinson and McClelland (see Weiner, 1992). However, a major change of direction in the study of achievement motivation and perceptions of ability and competence may be traced to the work of Maehr and Nicholls (1980). They influenced the thinking of many people interested in achievement-related constructs and behaviour, and in particular in education. Such an approach was readily adopted by those in sport psychology, and maintains its relevance to physical activity mainly through the understanding of participation in sport and physical activity by children.

Maehr and Nicholls (1980, p. 228) argued that:

> [S]uccess and failure are not concrete events. They are psychological states consequent on perception of reaching or not reaching goals. ... It follows that, if there is cultural variation in the personal qualities that are seen to be desirable, success and failure will be viewed differently in different cultures.

Maehr and Nicholls (1980) defined three types of achievement motivation: ability-orientated motivation, task-orientated motivation, and social approval-orientated motivation. Ability-orientated motivation is when 'the goal of the behavior is to maximize the subjective probability of attributing high ability to oneself' (Maehr and Nicholls, 1980, p. 237). This has been modified in sport psychology to refer to 'ego' goal orientations where success is defined as the demonstration of superiority over others (Duda, 2001).

According to Maehr and Nicholls (1980), in task-orientated motivation 'the primary goal is to produce an adequate product or to solve a problem for its own sake rather than to demonstrate ability' (p. 239). This is the 'task' goal orientation. The third goal – social approval-orientated motivation – has been investigated less than the other two goals. This dimension of achievement motivation was defined by Maehr and Nicholls (1980) in terms of the demonstration of 'conformity to norms or virtuous intent rather than superior talent' (pp. 241–242).

Nicholls (1989) has argued that the two main orientations here – task and ego – are based on how people construe competence. In a task perspective, cues used to assess competence are effort and task completion, and hence are self-referenced. Ego orientation is where competence is judged relative to others, and ability and effort are differentiated as causes of outcomes. This means that an externally referenced view is adopted.

Key point: People define competence and success in different ways, and this will have implications for their motivation.

A systematic review of the correlates of task and ego goal orientations in physical activity (Biddle *et al.*, 2003) showed associations of varying magnitude between a task orientation and:

- beliefs that effort produces success (positive association: +);
- perceptions of competence (+);
- positive affect (+);
- negative affect (negative association).

Associations of varying magnitude were found between an ego orientation and:

- beliefs that ability produces success (+);
- perceptions of competence (+).

These associations suggest that a task orientation is motivationally positive and may be associated with increased confidence to continue with an activity.

Chapter summary and conclusions

In this chapter, we have attempted to review and synthesise some of the major theoretical approaches in exercise motivation that have focused on self-perceptions of efficacy and competence. In summary, therefore, we conclude the following:

- We have reviewed Social Cognitive Theory, with specific reference to the construct of self-efficacy, and presented a comprehensive overview of research findings, methods and issues.
- We have presented some alternative views on confidence relevant to the study of physical activity, including self-presentational concerns.

From our review, we conclude the following:

- Participation in physical activity is associated with perceptions of competence, in whatever form competence is operationalised.
- Research using self-efficacy with patient groups demonstrates that exercise self-efficacy can be developed.
- Self-efficacy judgements can generalise but will be strongest for activities similar to the activity experienced.
- Research with non-patient groups has shown that exercise self-efficacy can be increased through intervention, will predict participation, particularly in the early stages of an exercise programme, will decline following a period of inactivity, and is associated with positive exercise emotion.
- Self-presentational processes and goal orientations offer additional understanding to physical activity confidence and anxiety.

References

Ashford, S., Edmunds, J. and French, D.P. (2010). What is the best way to change self-efficacy to promote lifestyle and recreational physical activity? A systematic review with meta-analysis. *British Journal of Health Psychology, 15*, 265–288. doi: 10.1348/135910709X461752.

Bandura, A. (1977). Self-efficacy: Toward a unifying theory of behavioral change. *Psychological Review, 84*, 191–215.

———. (1986). *Social Foundations of Thought and Action: A social cognitive theory*. Englewood Cliffs, NJ: Prentice Hall.

———. (1997). *Self-efficacy: The exercise of control*. New York: W.H. Freeman.

Biddle, S.J.H., Fox, K.R. and Edmunds, L. (1994). *Physical Activity Promotion in Primary Health Care in England*. London: Health Education Authority.

Biddle, S.J.H., Hanrahan, S.J. and Sellars, C.N. (2001). Attributions: Past, present, and future. In R.N. Singer, H.A. Hausenblas and C.M. Janelle (eds), *Handbook of Sport Psychology* (pp. 444–471). New York: Wiley.

Biddle, S.J.H., Wang, C.K.J., Kavussanu, M. and Spray, C.M. (2003). Correlates of achievement goal orientations in physical activity: A systematic review of research. *European Journal of Sport Science, 3*(5), http://www.humankinetics.com/ejss.

Biddle, S.J.H., Atkin, A., Cavill, N. and Foster, C. (2011). Correlates of physical activity in youth: A review of quantitative systematic reviews. *International Review of Sport and Exercise Psychology, 4*(1), 25–49.

Corbin, C.B. (1984). Self confidence of females in sports and physical activity. *Clinics in Sports Medicine, 3*, 895–908.

Duda, J.L. (2001). Achievement goal research in sport: Pushing the boundaries and clarifying some misunderstandings. In G.C. Roberts (ed.), *Advances in Motivation in Sport and Exercise* (pp. 129–182). Champaign, IL: Human Kinetics.

Ewart, C.E. (1989). Psychological effects of resistive weight training: Implications for cardiac patients. *Medicine and Science in Sports and Exercise, 21*, 683–688.

Ewart, C.E., Taylor, C.B., Reese, L.B. and DeBusk, R.F. (1983). Effects of early post myocardial infarction exercise testing on self perception and subsequent physical activity. *American Journal of Cardiology, 51*, 1076–1080.

Ewart, C.E., Stewart, K.J., Gillilan, R.E. and Kelemen, M.H. (1986). Self-efficacy mediates strength gains during circuit weight training in men with coronary artery disease. *Medicine and Science in Sports and Exercise, 18*, 531–540.

Feltz, D. (1992). Understanding motivation in sport: A self-efficacy perspective. In G.C. Roberts (ed.), *Motivation in Sport and Exercise* (pp. 93–105). Champaign, IL: Human Kinetics.

Fox, K.R., Biddle, S.J.H., Edmunds, L., Bowler, I. and Killoran, A. (1997). Physical activity promotion through primary health care in England. *British Journal of General Practice, 47*, 367–369.

Gardner, B., de Bruijn, G.J. and Lally, P. (2011). A systematic review and meta-analysis of applications of the Self-report Habit Index to nutrition and physical activity behaviours. *Annals of Behavioral Medicine, 42*, 174–187.

Hart, E.A., Leary, M.R. and Rejeski, W.J. (1989). The measurement of social physique anxiety. *Journal of Sport and Exercise Psychology, 11*, 94–104.

Harter, S. (1978). Effectance motivation reconsidered: Toward a developmental model. *Human Development, 21*, 34–64.

Harter, S. and Connell, J.P. (1984). A model of children's achievement and related self perceptions of competence, control and motivational orientations. In J.G. Nicholls (ed.), *Advances in Motivation and Achievement. III. The development of achievement motivation* (pp. 219–250). Greenwich, CT: JAI Press.

Leary, M.R. (1992). Self presentational processes in exercise and sport. *Journal of Sport and Exercise Psychology, 14*, 339–351.

———. (1995). *Self-presentation: Impression management and interpersonal behavior*. Dubuque, IO: Wm C. Brown.

Leary, M.R., Tchividjian, L.R. and Kraxberger, B.E. (1994). Self-presentation can be hazardous to your health: Impression management and health risk. *Health Psychology, 13*, 461–470.

Lenney, E. (1977). Women's self-confidence in achievement situations. *Psychological Bulletin, 84*, 1–13.

Lubans, D.R., Foster, C. and Biddle, S.J.H. (2008). A review of mediators of behavior in interventions to promote physical activity among children and adolescents. *Preventive Medicine, 47*, 463–470.

Luszczynska, A. and Tryburcy, M. (2008). Effects of a self-efficacy intervention on exercise: The moderating role of diabetes and cardiovascular diseases. *Applied Psychology: An International Review, 57*(4), 644–659. doi: 10.1111/j.1464-0597.2008.00340.x.

Maehr, M.L. and Nicholls, J.G. (1980). Culture and achievement motivation: A second look. In N. Warren (ed.), *Studies in Cross-cultural Psychology – Vol II* (pp. 221–267). New York: Academic Press.

Marteau, T.M., Ogilvie, D., Roland, M., Suhrcke, M. and Kelly, M.P. (2011). Judging nudging: Can nudging improve population health? *British Medical Journal, 342*, d228.

McAuley, E. (1992). Understanding exercise behavior: A self-efficacy perspective. In G.C. Roberts (ed.), *Motivation in Sport and Exercise* (pp. 107–127). Champaign, IL: Human Kinetics.

McAuley, E. and Blissmer, B. (2000). Self-efficacy determinants and consequences of physical activity. *Exercise and Sport Sciences Reviews, 28*, 85–88.

McAuley, E., Jerome, G.J., Elavsky, S., Marquez, D.X. and Ramsey, S.N. (2003a). Predicting long-term maintenance of physical activity in older adults. *Preventive Medicine, 37*(2), 110–118.

McAuley, E., Jerome, G.J., Marquez, D.X., Elavsky, S. and Blissmer, B. (2003b). Exercise self-efficacy in older adults: Social, affective, and behavioral influences. *Annals of Behavioral Medicine, 25*, 1–7.

Michie, S., van Stralen, M. and West, R. (2011a). The behaviour change wheel: A new method for characterising and designing behaviour change interventions. *Implementation Science, 6*(1), 42, http://www.implementationscience.com/content/46/41/42. doi: 10.1186/1748-5908-6-42.

Michie, S., Ashford, S., Sniehotta, F.F., Dombrowski, S.U., Bishop, A. and French, D.P. (2011b). A refined taxonomy of behaviour change techniques to help people change their physical activity and healthy eating behaviours: The CALORE taxonomy. *Psychology and Health, 26*(11), 1479–1498.

Nicholls, J.G. (1989). *The Competitive Ethos and Democratic Education.* Cambridge, MA: Harvard University Press.

Olander, E., Fletcher, H., Williams, S., Atkinson, L., Turner, A. and French, D. (2013). What are the most effective techniques in changing obese individuals' physical activity self-efficacy and behaviour: a systematic review and meta-analysis. *International Journal of Behavioral Nutrition and Physical Activity, 10*(1), 29. doi: 10.1186/1479-5868-10-29.

Schwarzer, R. (1992). Self-efficacy in the adoption and maintenance of health behaviours: Theoretical approaches and a new model. In R. Schwarzer (ed.), *Self-efficacy: Thought control of action* (pp. 217–243). Bristol, PA: Taylor & Francis.

Skinner, E. (1995). *Perceived Control, Motivation, and Coping.* Thousand Oaks, CA: Sage.

———. (1996). A guide to constructs of control. *Journal of Personality and Social Psychology, 71*, 549–570.

Sports Council and Health Education Authority. (1992). *Allied Dunbar National Fitness Survey: Main findings.* London: Author.

Strecher, V.J., DeVellis, B.E., Becker, M.H. and Rosenstock, I.M. (1986). The role of self-efficacy in achieving health behaviour change. *Health Education Quarterly, 13*, 73–92.

Weinberg, R.S., Hughes, H.H., Critelli, J.W., England, R. and Jackson, A. (1984). Effects of pre-existing and manipulated self-efficacy on weight loss in a self-control programme. *Journal of Research in Personality, 18*, 352–358.

Weiner, B. (1992). *Human Motivation.* Newbury Park, CA: Sage.

Williams, S.L. and French, D.P. (2011). What are the most effective intervention techniques for changing physical activity self-efficacy and physical activity behaviour – and are they the same? *Health Education Research, 26*(2), 308–322. doi: 10.1093/her/cyr005.

11 Physical activity and stage-based approaches
Let's do it in stages

Purpose of the chapter

In this chapter we consider models that have been used as potentially better ways of understanding physical activity than more single-theory approaches. In particular, we focus on stage-based approaches and specifically the 'Transtheoretical Model'. Other frameworks are also considered, including the Health Action Process Approach (HAPA). Specifically, in this chapter we aim to:

- outline the 'Transtheoretical Model' approach to physical activity behaviour change;
- consider research findings and the constructs of self-efficacy, pros and cons, and processes of change, including evidence from systematic reviews and interventions;
- outline the 'hybrid' Health Action Process Approach (HAPA) as applied to physical activity;
- discuss the 'natural history' model of exercise proposed by Sallis and Hovell (1990) and suggest which determinants may be important at the different phases of the model;
- consider the relapse prevention model and data from physical activity research.

The theories and approaches discussed so far in this book are what may be termed 'linear' approaches. These include popular theories such as the Theory of Planned Behaviour. Essentially, they operate as continuous and unidirectional models in which specified relationships exist in the prediction of physical activity behaviour. The current chapter deals with models and 'theories' that may best be described as 'stage-based' models of physical activity behaviour. Stage models assume discontinuity between the qualitatively different stages. The best-known such model is the Transtheoretical Model (TTM), sometimes referred to as the 'stages of change' framework.

Several researchers have proposed a stage approach to advance understanding of how people move into or out of participation in physical activity. First, the Transtheoretical Model will be discussed, followed by Sallis and Hovell's (1990) 'natural history of exercise'. This allows for an analysis of possible determinants at different stages of physical activity involvement. A 'hybrid' of continuous and stage models – the Health Action Process Approach (HAPA) (Schwarzer, 1992, 2001) – is also presented briefly.

The Transtheoretical Model (TTM)

Research into the nature of behaviour change in smokers and those presenting themselves for psychotherapy has suggested that recovery from problem behaviours, or successful behaviour change, involves movement through a series of stages (Prochaska and Velicer, 1997; Prochaska *et al.*, 1992, 1994a, 1994b). Literature using the TTM in physical activity is now diverse, including descriptive studies (Marcus *et al.*, 1992b; Mullan and Markland, 1997), interventions (Mutrie *et al.*, 2002), narrative overviews (Prochaska and Marcus, 1994), focused reviews (Nigg, 2005; Rhodes and Nigg, 2011), systematic reviews and a meta-analysis (Hutchison *et al.*, 2009; Marshall and Biddle, 2001; Mastellos *et al.*, 2014; Riemsma *et al.*, 2002; Spencer *et al.*, 2006), and practical guidelines (Marcus and Forsyth, 2003).

Even those attempting self-change, as well as those in therapy, seem to move through 'stages of change'. This approach is popular in psychotherapy and also in other areas of health, including physical activity behaviour change. It features strongly in the ACSM book on behavioural aspects of physical activity (Johnson and Cook, 2014; Symons Downs *et al.*, 2014).

The term 'transtheoretical model' is used to describe the wider framework that encompasses both the 'when' and the 'how' of behaviour change. The 'when' refers to the stages of change and the associated temporal aspects of change, while the 'how' refers to the constructs of self-efficacy, decisional balance (weighing up) of pros and cons, and also the processes of change, the latter being practical strategies used to help people move through the stages. We review the evidence on the TTM and physical activity in this chapter.

Stages of change

Table 11.1 outlines the defining features of the key stages. Typically, studies in physical activity assess pre-contemplation, contemplation, preparation, action and maintenance stages. These stages are outlined below:

- *Pre-contemplation* includes people who are not currently physically active (at the level specified) and have no intention of being so in the near future.
- *Contemplation* includes those who are not currently physically active but have an intention to start in the near future, or at least are considering this.
- *Preparation* includes individuals who are 'currently exercising some, but not regularly' (Marcus and Owen, 1992, p.6), or, as Prochaska and Marcus (1994) suggest, these people are intending to take action in the next month or so.

Table 11.1 Defining stages of the Transtheoretical Model

Stage	Meeting criterion level of physical activity?	Current behaviour	Intention to meet criterion level of physical activity?	Practical label[1]
Pre-contemplation	✗	Little or no physical activity	✗	'I won't' or 'I can't'
Contemplation	✗	Little or no physical activity	✓	'I might'
Preparation	✗	Small changes in physical activity	✓	'I will'
Action	✓	Physically active for less than 6 months	✓	'I am'
Maintenance	✓	Physically active for more than 6 months	✓	'I have'

Note:
1. Provided by Symons Down *et al.* (2014).

- *Action* is a stage represented by people who are currently active, but have only recently started. As such, Prochaska and Marcus (1994) suggest that it is an unstable stage during which individuals are at high risk of relapse.
- *Maintenance* is a stage that includes those who are currently physically active and have been so for some time, usually for at least six months.

Other 'stages' sometimes considered include 'termination' and 'relapse'. Termination has not been used in physical activity research but does feature in other TTM research, such as on smoking and alcohol abuse. Prochaska and Marcus (1994) define this stage as the point at which people have 'no temptation to engage in the old behaviour and 100% self-efficacy in all previously tempting situations' (p. 163). Relapse has not been tested much in physical activity research but is consistent with Sallis and Hovell's (1990) model, discussed below. While data are available from smoking and alcohol research on the risk of relapse from the maintenance phase, little data are available on physical activity. However, Marcus and Simkin (1994) suggest that perhaps 15 per cent fall into the category of being 'relapsers' (i.e. regressive movement back to either contemplation or pre-contemplation).

Attempts to estimate the prevalence within each stage are fraught with difficulties because such efforts will be reliant on how the criterion level of behaviour is defined. For example, one would expect more people to be in the maintenance group if the criterion measure of physical activity is moderate activity for 30 minutes on three days each week in comparison to the internationally accepted target of at least five days (150 minutes) per week. However, estimates from our meta-analysis (Marshall and Biddle, 2001) shown in Figure 11.1 suggest that even this is inconsistent, leading to the conclusion that sampling in TTM studies may be biased. This is supported by data showing that for studies that actively recruited participants, far more were in the pre-contemplation stage (25%) than when passive methods were used (8%). We estimated the stage distributions for our total sample of 68,580 derived from 68 samples, as well as for four countries. These are shown in Figure 11.2.

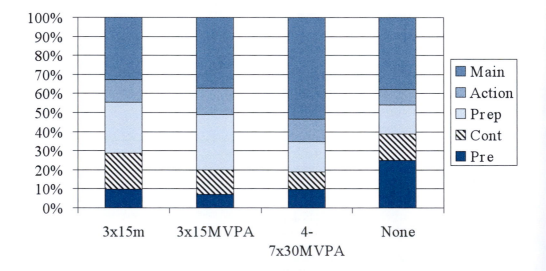

Figure 11.1 Prevalence estimates for stages of change by different levels of physical activity and exercise
Source: Data from Marshall and Biddle (2001).

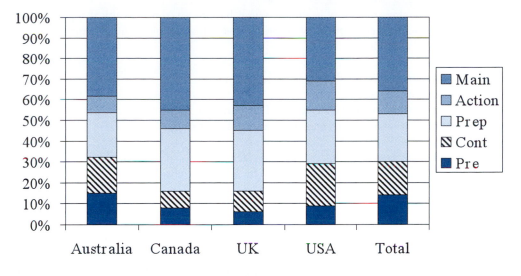

Figure 11.2 Prevalence estimates for stages of change across four countries

Source: Data from Marshall and Biddle (2001).

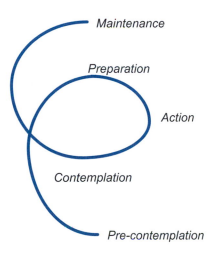

Figure 11.3 Cyclical stages of behaviour change

The stages outlined above suggest a steady linear progression from one stage to the next. However, certainly in addictive behaviours, where the TTM approach has been investigated extensively, a linear pattern has given way to the belief that change is cyclical, as suggested in Figure 11.3. In the context of physical activity, Marcus and Simkin (1994) suggest that several attempts at change are likely before maintenance is reached. Indeed, Prochaska *et al.* (1992) say that for many the process of 'cycling' back and forth through the stages may help strengthen behaviour change in the long run as people learn from their mistakes and relapses. However, 'much more research is needed to better distinguish those who benefit from recycling from those who end up spinning their wheels' (Prochaska *et al.*, 1992, p. 1105).

More recently, stage models of health behaviour have received more critical appraisal. For example, Weinstein and colleagues (1998) present what they see as defining features of stage theories. These are as follows:

- a classification system for defining stages;
- an ordering of stages;
- common barriers to change facing people in the same stage;
- different barriers to change facing people in different stages.

They suggest that cross-sectional comparisons across stages have limited value in testing whether a true stage process is followed in health behaviour change.

Processes of change

The stages of change discussed thus far refer to the temporal patterning of behaviour change. By also identifying processes of change we are able to better understand why and how this temporal shift might take place. Processes of change, therefore, are important for interventions – for moving people between stages. We outline the proposed processes of change and report on summary meta-analytic data.

Processes of change are defined by Marcus *et al.* (1992c) as 'the cognitive, affective, and behavioral strategies and techniques people use as they progress through the different stages of change over time' (p. 425). Table 11.2 describes 10 processes of change. Five of these processes are described as cognitive or 'thinking' strategies and the other five as behavioural or 'doing' strategies. The results of our meta-analysis showed that individuals use all 10 processes of change when trying to modify their physical activity behaviour. Cognitive processes tended to peak during the action stage and behavioural processes in the maintenance stage. However, the pattern of change for behavioural processes differed from that described in narrative reviews (Prochaska and Marcus, 1994; Reed, 1999). Behavioural processes have been hypothesised to increase in a linear fashion up to the stage of action and then level off during maintenance. However, the meta-analytic evidence showed that pre-contemplation to contemplation and preparation to action are characterised by sharper increases in behavioural process use compared to other transitions.

Nine of the 10 processes followed similar patterns of change across the stages and this is important because it argues against the presence of a stage-by-process interaction, whereby some processes are thought to be more important or likely at certain stages (Johnson and Cook, 2014). The distinction between the higher order cognitive and behavioural processes, therefore, may not apply in the physical activity domain. We said that in our 2001 paper but little seems to have been done to test this further.

Few studies are available that make process-specific predictions at each stage of change. It has been suggested that increasing knowledge is particularly important when moving from pre-contemplation to contemplation, and our meta-analysis supported this.

Decisional balance

One strategy that can assist people to make successful behaviour change is to weigh up the advantages of change ('pros') against the disadvantages or costs of change ('cons'). This 'decisional balance' exercise is one that has been at the core of the TTM. Examples of items in a decisional balance questionnaire for exercise are shown in Table 11.3. Research has shown

Table 11.2 Processes of change applied to physical activity (Marcus and Forsyth, 2003)

Process	Description
COGNITIVE / THINKING PROCESSES	
Increasing knowledge	Increasing information about oneself and physical activity.
Being aware of risks	Understanding the risks of inactivity and sedentary living.
Caring about consequences to others	Recognising how inactivity might affect others, such as family and co-workers.
Increasing healthy alternatives	Increasing awareness of alternatives for being physically active.
Understanding the benefits	Increasing awareness of the benefits of physical activity.
BEHAVIOURAL/ DOING STRATEGIES	
Substituting alternatives	Seeking ways of being physically active when encountering barriers of time, etc.
Enlisting social support	Seeking support from others for your physical activity efforts.
Rewarding yourself	Praising and rewarding yourself, in a healthy way, for making successful efforts in physical activity.
Committing yourself	Making plans and commitments for physical activity.
Reminding yourself	Establishing reminders and prompts for physical activity, such as diary time slots and making equipment easily available.

Table 11.3 Example items assessing decisional balance ('pros' and 'cons') for exercise (Marcus and Owen, 1992). A 5-point Likert scale is used to score responses (not at all important = 1 to extremely important = 5)

1	I would be healthier if I exercised regularly
2	I would feel better about myself if I exercised regularly
3	Other people would respect me more if I exercised regularly
4	My family and friends would get to spend less time with me if I exercised regularly
5	I would feel that I was wasting my time if I exercised regularly
6	I would probably be sore and uncomfortable if I exercised regularly

that at the early stages of behaviour change cons outweigh pros. Those in preparation may have more equality between the pros and cons, whereas those who are in maintenance will perceive more pros than cons. This suggests that influencing perceptions of pros and cons may assist in behaviour change and that reaching the stage of action may be dependent on having pros outweigh cons. This is illustrated by the 'cross-over' point shown in Figure 11.4 where the change from one stage to another is shown. Essentially, this is where people say it's worth changing and feel that they can change.

Self-efficacy

Evidence has shown consistently that increasing self-efficacy is associated with greater readiness for physical activity – that is, a more 'advanced' stage (Marcus and Owen, 1992; Marshall and Biddle, 2001; Prochaska and Marcus, 1994). Results from our meta-analysis showed that self-efficacy increased with each stage of change, as proposed by the TTM.

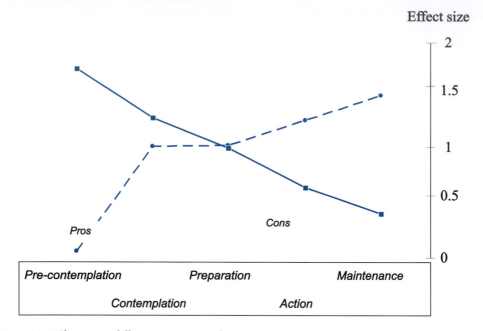

Figure 11.4 Changes or differences in pros and cons across stages
Source: Data from Marshall and Biddle (2001).

However, although the pattern of increase appears to be linear in Figure 11.5, the pattern of effects was as follows and is suggestive of some non-linearity, contrary to predictions:

- moderate change from pre-contemplation to contemplation;
- small to moderate change from contemplation to preparation;
- moderate change from preparation to action;
- moderate to large change from action to maintenance (see Figure 11.5).

Key point: The Transtheoretical Model involves both the 'when' and 'how' of behaviour change.

Conclusions from systematic reviews of the TTM in physical activity

There are several reviews of the TTM in physical activity contexts (Hutchison *et al.*, 2009; Marshall and Biddle, 2001; Mastellos *et al.*, 2014; Riemsma *et al.*, 2002; Spencer *et al.*, 2006). The only meta-analysis was reported by Marshall and Biddle (2001).

The first meta-analysis reported in 2001

The objective of Marshall and Biddle's (2001) meta-analysis – the first on the TTM and physical activity – was to identify the strength of difference between stages in the core constructs of the TTM so that it is possible 'to identify and describe more accurately factors that may facilitate transitions between stages' (p. 230). They had available for analysis 91

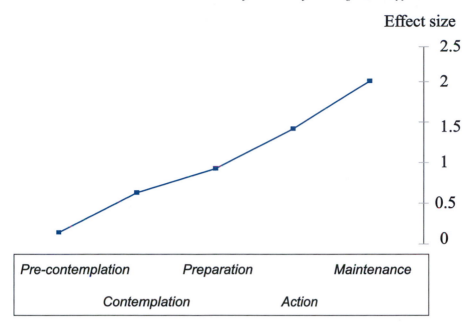

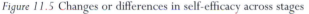

Figure 11.5 Changes or differences in self-efficacy across stages
Source: Data from Marshall and Biddle (2001).

independent samples from 71 published reports. Most of these were cross-sectional designs (n = 54), with six being longitudinal, 10 quasi-experimental and one RCT.

Some results have already been reported in this chapter but may best be summarised as follows:

- *Physical activity*: As expected, physical activity increased by stage. The largest different (d = 0.85) was from preparation to action.
- *Self-efficacy*: This increased by stage, although with some non-linear trends (see earlier). The largest change was from action to maintenance.
- *Decisional balance*: The 'pros' of change increased by stage, with the largest effect from pre-contemplation to contemplation. The 'cons' of change diminished across stages with small to moderate strength.
- *Processes of change*: The largest effects were from pre-contemplation to contemplation. Results suggest that the 10 main processes are used across all stages.

Three conclusions were stated from this meta-analysis. First, there is no need for additional cross-sectional studies which merely confirm that stage membership is associated with differences in the core constructs, such as self-efficacy. More diverse designs are needed, including experimental trials and studies to test moderators and mediators of stage transitions. Second, there is a need to standardise and improve the measurement of constructs in the TTM, including having one response format for stage assessment. Finally, it was concluded that the role of processes of change in physical activity research remains unclear. Further work is still required to ascertain how relevant the 10 processes are to physical activity.

A systematic review of the TTM in the context of interventions reported in 2002 and 2005

A review by Riemsma and colleagues (2002) sought to judge the effectiveness of health behaviour interventions that were based on the TTM. In addition to physical activity, they reviewed RCTs on smoking cessation, diet, multiple lifestyle change, screening mammography, treatment adherence, and smoking and alcohol use. There were seven studies meeting their inclusion criteria for physical activity. Five were from the USA, and one each from Australia and the UK. The same seven papers also appear to have been reviewed in Bridle *et al.* (2005).

All seven of the trials reported on physical activity comparing a stage-based intervention arm with either a control arm receiving information only or one that had no intervention. Two trials compared a stage-based intervention with one that was not stage based. One of these showed no difference and for the other the outcome was unclear. Three trials showed no effects; three showed some effects but only in the short term. This led the authors to conclude that 'there is little evidence for the effectiveness of stage-based interventions to promote physical activity' (p. 22).

When looking at the effectiveness of TTM-based interventions across all health behaviours, Riemsma and colleagues reported that 17 of 37 trials showed no significant differences between stage-based and other comparison conditions, suggesting that it is not physical activity studies that seem to have trouble supporting the TTM in interventions. One of the problems, as stated by Marshall and Biddle (2001), is that methodological quality and consistency is low, including measurement of key variables.

A systematic review of the TTM in exercise reported in 2006

Spencer *et al.* (2006) published a review of TTM studies in physical activity focusing on interventions, population-based studies, and studies aimed at measurement validation. Unfortunately, the searches finished in August 2003, even though the paper was published three years later. Of the 150 included studies, 38 were interventions, 70 were population-based studies, and 42 were validation studies. The authors concluded quite positively about intervention effectiveness, with 17 studies showing positive effects for stage matching, with a further eight showing just short-term effects. It was not clear how successful the 17 studies were long term. Five studies were inconclusive and three did not support the TTM. Overall, it was concluded that the TTM was moderately successful for physical activity behaviour change. However, the review was scant in its reporting of the methods used to conduct the review.

An updated systematic review of the TTM in the context of interventions reported in 2009

Hutchison *et al.* (2009) also reviewed physical activity interventions that used the TTM. Their argument was that many of the studies failed to incorporate all features of the TTM; thus it may be erroneous to conclude that interventions using the TTM are unsuccessful. Their review showed the following:

- Eighteen of 24 studies (75%) showed significant short-term effects for TTM-based interventions.
- Eight of 24 interventions (33%) showed significant long-term effects for TTM-based interventions.

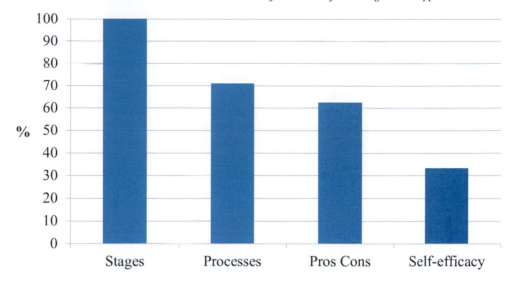

Figure 11.6 Percentage of studies using the four dimensions of the TTM in intervention development
Source: Data from Hutchinson *et al.* (2009).

Figure 11.6 shows the percentage of studies using the four dimensions of the TTM in intervention development. It is clear that only stage of change has been included in all interventions, thus showing that interventions are incomplete tests of the model. Hutchinson and colleagues found that only seven interventions used all four dimensions of the TTM, and six showed significant intervention effects in the short term.

A Cochrane review of the TTM in the context of physical activity and diet interventions for overweight and obese adults

A Cochrane review is also available, appraising the TTM in the context of weight-management interventions with adults. Both dietary and physical activity behaviours were included for trials that assessed the sustainability of behaviour change (i.e. one year or longer). Only three trials met inclusion criteria. Although there were trends for increases in physical activity, the authors concluded that the methodological quality of the studies was too low to allow for firm conclusions. Key shortcomings included inadequate reporting of outcomes and over-reliance on self-reported outcome measures.

The TTM and physical activity: an illustrative study

The TTM was becoming a popular framework in exercise psychology and physical activity research in the 1990s, stimulated by several key papers and chapters from Beth Marcus (e.g. Marcus *et al.*, 1992a, 1992b, 1994; Prochaska and Marcus, 1994). One of the first interventions designed to increase physical activity using the TTM was also reported by Marcus and colleagues (1998).

Men and women, with an average age of 44 years and not meeting national guidelines for physical activity, were recruited, and 150 completed all assessments at baseline, one month, three months and six months. Participants were randomly assigned to one of the following two groups:

- *Individually tailored intervention*: These individuals received materials for behaviour change matched to their 'stage' according to the TTM. They received feedback on their scores for their stage of readiness, self-efficacy, ratings of pros and cons, and their use of processes of change for physical activity adoption.
- *Standard intervention*: These individuals received a standard self-help manual in the form of four booklets developed by the American Heart Association.

Results showed that the individually tailored stage-matched intervention group was more likely to reach the physical activity guidelines of 30 minutes on five days per week at the end of the intervention, and to reach the action stage by one month. These trends are shown in Figure 11.7. Both groups increased their physical activity across the six-month period of the intervention. Interestingly, both groups showed increases in self-efficacy, the pros of physical activity, and both cognitive and behavioural processes of change, thus it was not possible to attribute intervention effects to any of these potential TTM-based mechanisms.

Based on this design, it should be noted that the stage-matched arm of the trial was not compared to a control condition but, rather, to an alternative intervention. Based on these findings, the stage-matched strategy was successful but not because it changed any of the underlying constructs of the TTM. Moreover, it was not possible to conclude how well individuals would have fared when in comparison with a stage-mismatched condition. The latter would have been a truer test of the model.

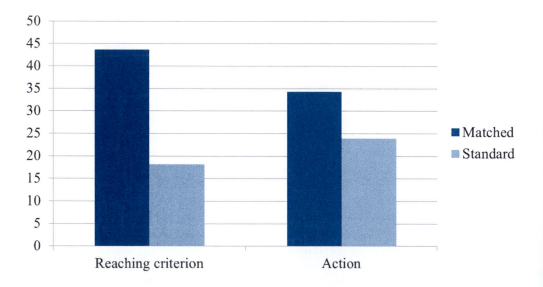

Figure 11.7 Results showing that the individually tailored stage-matched intervention group was more likely to reach the physical activity guidelines of 30 minutes on five days per week at the end of the intervention, and to reach the action stage by one month

Source: Data from Marcus *et al.* (1998).

Conclusions and critique of the Transtheoretical Model

There is no doubt that a dynamic approach to understanding physical activity that includes different stages of 'readiness' is an appropriate framework to understand behaviour and behaviour change. The success of the TTM in other health settings initially led to confidence in its application to physical activity. Similarly, Marcus and co-workers, as well as other researchers, have shown the utility of the TTM in physical activity across several countries and in adults of differing ages. With processes of change also proposed, the likelihood of TTM being applied successfully in intervention trials seems logical. Indeed, many interventions have used the TTM as its theoretical framework for interventions (Cox *et al.*, 2003; Dunn *et al.*, 1999).

The majority of studies investigating the TTM in physical activity (Marshall and Biddle, 2001) and other health behaviour contexts (Sutton, 2000) are cross-sectional. This presents difficulties in establishing causal relationships between constructs and stages. Moreover, many studies using such a design provide support for what Weinstein and colleagues (1998) have called 'pseudo-stage' models where there is a linear pattern of 'change', or 'difference' in a cross-sectional design, between variables, rather than having an a priori assumption of discontinuity whereby a variable is predicted to act differently at different stages (Sutton, 2000). Data from our meta-analysis are more supportive of a pseudo-stage model. For example, physical activity differences between stages followed an essentially linear pattern, with only a hint of discontinuity. In Figure 11.5, self-efficacy has a hint of discontinuity – and statistically this is true – but some might describe the pattern as essentially linear. Future studies on the TTM and physical activity need to test for the discontinuity of variables across stages and establish whether the variable is an antecedent or consequence of stage transition (Sutton, 2000).

Non-linear patterns and support for stage assumptions have also been found. Lippke and Plotnikoff (2006), for example, reported the strongest support for discontinuity patterns for perceptions of vulnerability (subjective chances of contracting a disease if one is not physically active). Individuals in the pre-contemplation stage felt least vulnerable, those in contemplation and action reported the highest vulnerability, and individuals in preparation and maintenance had reduced vulnerability. The higher level of vulnerability in the contemplation stage, in comparison to pre-contemplation, is in accordance with the stage definition. Individuals in pre-contemplation are either unaware of the risk behaviour (such as being not physically active enough) or subjectively reduce their vulnerability due to an incorrect optimistic mindset. In contemplation, individuals become aware of their risk. However, if they plan to start performing the behaviour in question in the near future, or if they are already performing a certain behaviour, their vulnerability estimation now becomes relevant and they may express feelings of vulnerability. Individuals in action are likely to be more realistic and those in maintenance are actually reducing their vulnerability because of their behaviour.

A study by Gorely and Bruce (2000) has also located differences within a stage. This may suggest that future research needs to address not only the distinction between stages, but the possible existence of subgroups within stages. Specifically, Gorely and Bruce found that three subgroups of contemplators existed: early and mid-contemplators, and those in 'pre-preparation'. Self-efficacy was progressively higher as the sub-stage became more 'advanced', and there were subgroup differences in pros (lowest in pre-preparation) and cons (lowest in early contemplation). Although these subgroup differences may appear to confirm predictions, analysis of the whole sample using cluster analysis did confirm three distinct clusters, as labelled above.

Based on the findings from our meta-analytic study (Marshall and Biddle, 2001), three general conclusions were offered. First, the majority of study designs are cross-sectional, limiting their utility. Cross-sectional studies provide the weakest evidence of true stage theories. More conclusive evidence would come from experimental studies of stage-matched and mismatched interventions (see illustrative study above). Studies that simply stage participants or examine cross-sectional differences between core constructs of the TTM are now of limited use because, it may be argued, we now have sufficient data to confirm that stage membership is associated with different levels of physical activity, self-efficacy, pros and cons, and processes of change. Future studies should examine the moderators and mediators of stage transition.

Second, the growing number of studies that incorporate TTM concepts means that there is an increasing need to standardise and improve the reliability of measurement. Researchers may wish to consider using a consistent response format for staging participants.

Third, the role of processes of change for physical activity behaviour remains unclear. The presence of higher order constructs is not apparent in applications of the model to physical activity, and stage-by-process interactions are not evident. Because the 10 processes emerged from change systems used in psychotherapy to treat addictions, their relevance or importance in the physical activity domain remains uncertain, and little progress has been made on this since our 2008 edition of this book. If processes of change are used in interventions, it would be prudent to select on the basis of logic and pilot testing, particularly given that it is likely to be impractical to use all processes at all stages.

In conclusion, there is still some debate about the use of the TTM. The model makes good sense to some researchers, and certainly to health professionals, and offers many logical applications for behaviour change. But, equally, doubts have been expressed about some of its assumptions, few studies have tested all elements together, and most show only short-term changes. It is prudent to continue to test this model in physical activity with these issues in mind.

Hybrid model: the Health Action Process Approach (HAPA)

The Health Action Process Approach (HAPA) (Schwarzer, 1992, 2001) explicitly integrates linear and stage assumptions, and is thereby a 'hybrid model' (see summary at http://userpage.fu-berlin.de/health/hapa.htm). The HAPA model also integrates motivational and behaviour-enabling models. The former include predictions of intention while the latter include post-decisional facets such as implementation intentions (see Chapter 8).

The HAPA makes a distinction between a motivation phase and a volition/post-decision phase of health behaviour change (see Figure 11.8). The basic idea is that individuals experience a shift in mindset when moving from the first phase (motivational) to the second (volitional). The moment when people commit themselves to an intention to exercise, they enter the volitional phase. Here, a division into two sub-phases appears to be meaningful where people can be labelled as either intenders or actors. First, they intend to act but they remain inactive (akin to contemplators in the TTM). Second, they have initiated the intended action. Thus three phases or stages may be distinguished, as shown in Figure 11.8. In the non-intentional stage, a behavioural intention is being developed which is similar to the contemplation stage in the TTM. Afterwards, individuals enter the intentional stage, where the person has already formed an intention but still remains inactive (or at least not active at the recommended level), while the exercise behaviour is being planned and prepared. If these plans are translated into action, individuals reside in the action stage. They are then physically active at the recommended or criterion level.

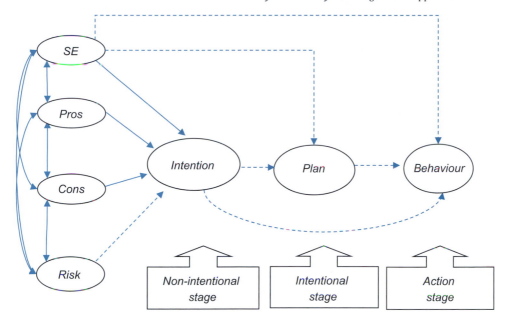

Figure 11.8 The Health Action Process Approach

In the non-intentional stage, an intention has to be developed. Risk perception may enable the undecided person to form an intention. Furthermore, it is a prerequisite for a contemplation process and further elaboration of thoughts about consequences and capacities. Risk perception operates at a stage-specific level and therefore its effect on intention is represented by a dashed line in Figure 11.8; in the intentional stage, risk perception has no effect (Lippke *et al.*, 2005). The belief in one's capabilities to perform a desired action (self-efficacy) is necessary. That is, perceived self-efficacy promotes intention formation and behaviour implementation in all stage groups (Lippke *et al.*, 2005) and the arrow is therefore drawn as a solid line, not dashed, in Figure 11.8.

After a decision has been made, the intentional stage is entered. The individual has a high intention but is not performing the behaviour – this is the intention–behaviour gap we discussed in Chapter 8. The intention has to be transformed into plans on how to perform the behaviour. These state when, where and how the goal behaviour will be initiated (Lippke *et al.*, 2004); thereby cognitive links between concrete opportunities and the intended behaviour will be built. Risk perception has no further influence while outcome-expectancies remain important. Self-efficacy is also important in the planning and initiation process, especially if barriers occur. Self-efficacy keeps intentions high and the plans flexible to compensate for setbacks and to stay on track.

If exercise has been started, the individual enters the action stage. To enhance maintenance, self-regulatory skills are important. Effort has to be invested, situations for implementation of the new behaviour identified, and distractions resisted. The behaviour will mainly be directed by self-efficacy (Schwarzer, 2001) because it regulates effort and persistence in the face of barriers and setbacks. Behaviour has to be maintained, and relapses have to be managed by different strategies.

Due to individuals having to first set a goal which may then be translated into plans and behaviour, this process is stage-specific; only persons in intentional and action stages are more likely to make plans and subsequently perform the goal behaviour (dashed lines in Figure 11.8) (Lippke *et al.*, 2005). In addition, the influence of self-efficacy on post-decisional processes, such as planning and behaviour, depends on whether one has decided to change (here it is crucial to believe in one's own competences) or not (here only intention formation can be supported by self-efficacy).

The HAPA model combines several psychological constructs appearing elsewhere in this book, including stages (this chapter), self-efficacy (Chapter 10), the intention–behaviour gap, and implementation intentions (Chapter 8). It therefore appears to be a useful model for further testing in physical activity.

A natural history model of exercise

Early studies investigating differences between 'adherers' and 'dropouts' gave the mistaken impression that physical activity participation was an 'all-or-none' phenomenon (Sonstroem, 1988) rather than a process open to considerable change over time. As suggested by stage and hybrid models, such as the TTM and HAPA, people move between stages of contemplation, decision-making and behavioural involvement, and even then maybe not in any linear fashion.

In reviewing the determinants of exercise, Sallis and Hovell (1990) produced a 'natural history' model that has considerable utility in understanding the process of involvement in physical activity. Their model is shown in Figure 11.9 and depicts the three important transition phases:

- from physical inactivity to physical activity adoption;
- from physical activity adoption to maintenance or dropout;
- from dropout to resumption.

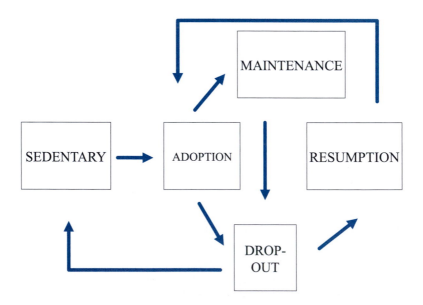

Figure 11.9 Sallis and Hovell's natural history model of exercise

Source: Sallis and Hovell (1990).

We still know relatively little about the physical activity adoption process, and hardly anything about resumption. We stated this in all previous editions of this book! The following additional factors should be taken into account when considering the natural history model:

- There are degrees of being physically active, or 'exercising'. When is someone 'inactive', for example? For the sake of clarity, the natural history model assumes that exercise, for example, is a dichotomous rather than a continuous variable. The notion of sporadic activity, and its determinants, is a challenge for research.
- The model is simply a useful device for focusing on the dynamic process of physical activity and exercise. There are many other factors to be considered to obtain a full picture of determinants across the life span. For example, we need to consider developmental/life span stages, socio-demographic characteristics and actual activity differences. All are likely to operate slightly differently across the phases described here. There are potentially hundreds of permutations of determinants on the basis of catego- rising determinants into major categories (e.g. social and environment, attitude, etc.), developmental periods and stages of the natural history model.

Determinants may differ across phases of physical activity

'Those who study determinants of exercise behavior must carefully define which transition they are studying, because the determinants are likely to be different at each transition point' (Sallis and Hovell, 1990, p. 310). Given the extensive discussion on possible determinants that has already taken place in the preceding chapters (e.g. see Chapter 7), this section will consider the factors that could be most influential at each of the phases, or transitions, in the natural history model. For the sake of clarity, we shall describe the model in terms of phases as follows and as shown in Figure 11.9:

- *Phase 1*: Moving from being inactive to adopting physical activity.
- *Phase 2*: Maintaining involvement in physical activity.
- *Phases 3 and 4*: Ceasing involvement in physical activity.
- *Phase 5*: Resuming physical activity after previously ceasing participation.

Starting physical activity

Sallis and Hovell (1990) were pessimistic about this phase of their model. They concluded that 'we understand almost nothing about why some people start exercising' (p. 313). Sallis' own work (Sallis *et al.*, 1986) is one of the few population-based studies of exercise adoption, but by his own admission the study of determinants lacked a theoretical focus. Their work did show, however, that self-efficacy, knowledge and attitudes were generally associated with the adoption of vigorous and moderate exercise. Logic also dictates that much of the material reviewed in the previous chapters on attitudes (Chapter 8) and self-efficacy (Chapter 10) appears to be appropriate for understanding the adoption process. Similarly, research on the TTM in physical activity has shown that self-efficacy levels of contemplators are usually lower than for those in the action or maintenance stages, and that those not yet exercising hold more negative beliefs about exercise. The natural history model deals with exercise and it is not known how appropriate such a model is for lifestyle physical activity, such as walking or stair climbing.

Maintaining physical activity

We are on much firmer ground when proposing determinants of the maintenance phase. In addition to the factors identified for adoption, two important issues need to be considered as far as psychological determinants are concerned. First is the issue of psychological reinforcement from physical activity or exercise, and second is the issue of self-regulation.

The reinforcement associated with exercise has also been raised by Sallis and Hovell (1990). They proposed a closer look at learning theories and the role of reinforcement and punishment in exercise. Studies have shown that many people do not find the higher effort of physical activity pleasant (Ekkekakis *et al.*, 2010) (see Chapter 2).

What appears to be emerging, therefore, is the important role of psychological outcomes from physical activity. Typically, the so-called 'mental health' benefits have largely been studied from the point of view of outcomes (see Chapters 2 to 6). From the view of determinants of physical activity maintenance, however, we should also consider the mental health outcomes as *re-enforcers* of subsequent behaviour (Ekkekakis, 2003, 2009). Although Sallis and Hovell (1990) suggest that 'the punishment of vigorous exercise remains immediate and salient, while the reinforcers of improved health or weight loss are greatly delayed and silent' (p. 320), it is possible to suggest that the mood-enhancing and 'feel-better' effects of physical activity or exercise may also be perceived in the short term. The key is to structure activity experiences such that the probability of perceiving physical activity as rewarding is increased. We suggest that the message for more vigorous exercise has not served us well, despite obvious physiological benefits. Such benefits will never accrue if the experience is so unpleasant.

The maintenance of involvement in exercise or physical activity is also likely to be enhanced through the operation of self-regulatory strategies and skills. Evidence from the TTM suggests that those in the action and maintenance phases are more likely to have arrived at a positive 'balance' of physical activity 'pros' (benefits) and 'cons' (costs), and this process of decisional balance is itself a conscious exercise in self-regulation.

Ceasing physical activity

The study of physical activity and exercise 'dropout' has been controversial, mainly because early studies were not able to identify if those ceasing participation in a structured programme had quit altogether or had merely gone elsewhere to exercise. The word 'dropout', therefore, was difficult to define. The cessation of activity may also be dependent on a variety of life cycle influences, such as work, family or illness.

Resuming physical activity

In discussing the determinants of resumption of physical activity or exercise after dropout, Sallis and Hovell (1990, p. 315) are quite clear:

> [T]his phase of the natural history of exercise has been completely neglected by both theoreticians and empirical investigators. The extent to which drop-outs resume exercise later has never been studied, to our knowledge. Thus, there are no studies on the determinants of resumption of exercise. Research on these issues is desperately needed with both participants in specialised programs and with the general population.

Sallis and Hovell's comment has sparked interest in the resumption process but few data have emerged and we are left to speculate about possibilities, one of which is the process of relapse studied in other health fields. This repeats the statement we made in the previous edition of this book, so little progress appears to have been made.

Marlatt (1985) has proposed a 'relapse prevention' model for the explanation of poor adherence to abstaining from various addictions and negative health behaviours, such as excessive alcohol and nicotine consumption. Marlatt (1985) defines relapse as 'a breakdown or setback in a person's attempt to change or modify any target behavior' (p. 3).

Although this definition, as well as the relapse prevention model, provides a starting point for the analysis of exercise resumption, it may not be wholly suitable. Knapp (1988), for example, notes that the behaviours addressed in addiction relapse are high-frequency, undesired behaviours, yet exercise is low frequency and desired. Nevertheless, it provides us with a workable model in which to identify possible determinants of exercise resumption. Marlatt's model, modified for possible application to exercise, is illustrated in Figure 11.10.

The starting point is identified in Figure 11.10 as the high-risk situation of ceasing exercise. This risk situation is the threat to self-control that could produce 'relapse' back to physical inactivity. For those with addiction problems, Marlatt (1985) has identified inter-personal conflict, negative emotional states and social pressure as the three primary high-risk situations. Certainly the latter two have been identified as predictors of (in)activity. Whether these situations lead to relapse will be dependent on the adequacy of the individual's coping skills and responses. A high-risk situation for lack of exercise may be extra work pressures,

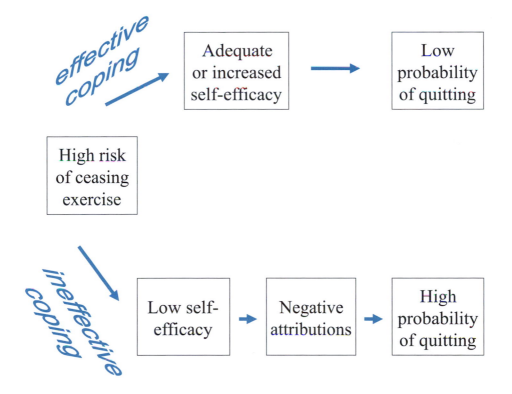

Figure 11.10 Relapse prevention model applied to exercise

thus producing a perception of reduced time for exercise. The probability of relapse from this is associated with the adequacy of coping response, such as time management skills, as well as self-efficacy towards exercise. A lack of coping response may lead to decreased efficacy and an expectation of less exercise taking place. The 'abstinence violation effect' could lead on from this and is where the individual displays feelings of guilt and self-blame, depending on the attributions made for the relapse. For example, attributions reflecting negative personal characteristics and feelings of helplessness and lack of control will increase the probability of a sustained relapse.

Relapse prevention has been successfully applied in physical activity research. King and Frederiksen (1984) demonstrated its success, alongside social support, for a small group of previously inactive college women attempting increases and maintenance in the frequency of jogging. Belisle and colleagues (1987) tested Marlatt's relapse prevention model in an experimental design with adult exercisers. In comparison to a standard control group receiving a regular exercise programme, those in the experimental condition also received health education through elements of the relapse prevention model. These included information on overcoming critical situations, awareness of the abstinence violation effect and principles of habit maintenance. Small but consistent effects in favour of the experimental group were noted across three studies. Similarly, positive coping responses were found by Stetson *et al.* (2005) to reduce the likelihood of an exercise 'slip' in high-risk situations. They concluded that 'exposure to high-risk situations per se does not precipitate slips and relapse; rather, it is the manner in which individuals cope with the situations that impacts outcome' (p. 33).

The relapse model is consistent with other physical activity determinants research in playing a central role for self-efficacy. In addition, attributions for relapse or dropout may be important factors in determining the strength of the motivational deficit associated with relapse and the ability that people feel they can cope in high-risk situations.

> Key point: Determinants will differ across different phases or stages of involvement in physical activity.

Chapter summary and conclusions

The research and theorising on the psychological determinants of physical activity is becoming increasingly complex. Theories have been borrowed, adapted and developed from other branches of the psychological and behavioural sciences, and, as such, there is a need to not only review the contribution of these theories to the understanding of physical activity behaviour, as we have done elsewhere in this book, but also to consider more dynamic, process-oriented, stage-based approaches to behaviour.

In this chapter, we have:

- reviewed and critiqued the Transtheoretical Model of behaviour change applied to physical activity; specifically, we reviewed evidence concerning the role of self-efficacy, pros and cons (decisional balance), and processes of change;
- considered the HAPA 'hybrid' model applied to physical activity;
- outlined a 'natural history' model of physical activity and exercise, and discussed determinants appropriate for different phases of the model, including relapse.

In summary, therefore, we conclude the following:

- The TTM provides an important advance on static linear models of exercise and physical activity determinants by hypothesising both the 'how' and 'when' of behaviour change. Measures of stages and processes of change are now available and require validation across more diverse samples.
- TTM research needs to advance beyond description of predictable cross-sectional differences between stages.
- Review-level evidence broadly supports elements and structure of the model, although the classification of processes of change into two higher order categories is questioned.
- Review-level evidence is less clear about how effective interventions are when based on the TTM.
- The hybrid HAPA model allows for the distinction between non-intentional, intentional and action stages of behaviour.
- A natural history model of exercise is a useful framework for identifying key phases in physical activity behaviour.
- Relapse prevention may depend on the ability to operate appropriate coping strategies.

References

Belisle, M., Roskies, E. and Levesque, J-M. (1987). Improving adherence to physical activity. *Health Psychology, 6*, 159–172.

Bridle, C., Riemsma, R.P., Pattenden, J., Sowden, A.J., Mather, L., Watt, I.S. and Walker, A. (2005). Systematic review of the effectiveness of health behavior interventions based on the transtheoretical model. *Psychology and Health, 20*(3), 283–301. doi: 10.1080/08870440512331333997.

Cox, K.L., Gorely, T.J., Puddey, I.B., Burke, V. and Beilin, L.J. (2003). Exercise behaviour change in 40–65 year old women: The SWEAT study (Sedentary Women Exercise Adherence Trial). *British Journal of Health Psychology, 8*, 477–495.

Dunn, A.L., Marcus, B.H., Kampert, J.B., Garcia, M.E., Kohl, H.W. and Blair, S.N. (1999). Comparison of lifestyle and structured interventions to increase physical activity and cardiorespiratory fitness: A randomized trial. *Journal of the American Medical Association, 281*, 327–334.

Ekkekakis, P. (2003). Pleasure and displeasure from the body: Perspectives from exercise. *Cognition and Emotion, 17*, 213–239.

———. (2009). The Dual-Mode Theory of affective responses to exercise in metatheoretical context: I. Initial impetus, basic postulates, and philosophical framework. *International Review of Sport and Exercise Psychology, 2*(1), 73–94.

Ekkekakis, P., Lind, E. and Vazou, S. (2010). Affective responses to increasing levels of exercise intensity in normal-weight, overweight, and obese middle-aged women. *Obesity, 18*(1), 79–85. doi: 10.1038/oby.2009.204.

Gorely, T. and Bruce, D. (2000). A 6-month investigation of exercise adoption from the contemplation stage of the transtheoretical model. *Psychology of Sport and Exercise, 1*, 89–101.

Hutchison, A.J., Breckon, J.D. and Johnston, L.H. (2009). Physical activity behavior change interventions based on the Transtheoretical Model: A systematic review. *Health Education and Behavior, 36*, 829–845.

Johnson, S.S. and Cook, B. (2014). Building motivation: How ready are you? In C.R. Nigg (ed.), *ACSM's Behavioral Aspects of Physical Activity and Exercise* (pp. 103–128). Philadelphia, PA: Lippincott Williams & Wilkins.

King, A.C. and Frederiksen, L.W. (1984). Low-cost strategies for increasing exercise behaviour: Relapse prevention training and social support. *Behavior Modification, 8*, 3–21.

Knapp, D.N. (1988). Behavioral management techniques and exercise promotion. In R.K. Dishman (ed.), *Exercise Adherence: Its impact on public health* (pp. 203–235). Champaign, IL: Human Kinetics.

Lippke, S. and Plotnikoff, R.C. (2006). Stages of change in physical exercise: A test of stage discrimination and non-linearity. *American Journal of Health Behavior, 30*(3), 290–301.

Lippke, S., Ziegelmann, J.P. and Schwarzer, R. (2004). Initiation and maintenance of physical exercise: Stage-specific effects of a planning intervention. *Research in Sports Medicine, 12,* 221–240.

———. (2005). Stage-specific adoption and maintenance of physical activity: Testing a three-stage model. *Psychology of Sport and Exercise, 6,* 585–603.

Marcus, B.H. and Forsyth, L.H. (2003). *Motivating People To Be Physically Active.* Champaign, IL: Human Kinetics.

Marcus, B.H. and Owen, N. (1992). Motivational readiness, self-efficacy and decision making for exercise. *Journal of Applied Social Psychology, 22,* 3–16.

Marcus, B.H. and Simkin, L.R. (1994). The transtheoretical model: Applications to exercise behavior. *Medicine and Science in Sports and Exercise, 26,* 1400–1404.

Marcus, B.H., Selby, V.C., Niaura, R.S. and Rossi, J.S. (1992a). Self-efficacy and stages of exercise behavior change. *Research Quarterly for Exercise and Sport, 63,* 60–66.

Marcus, B.H., Rossi, J.S., Selby, V.C., Niaura, R.S. and Abrams, D.B. (1992b). The stages and processes of exercise adoption and maintenance in a worksite sample. *Health Psychology, 11,* 386–395.

Marcus, B.H., Banspach, S.W., Lefebvre, R.C., Rossi, J.S., Carleton, R.A. and Abrams, D.B. (1992c). Using the stages of change model to increase the adoption of physical activity among community participants. *American Journal of Health Promotion, 6,* 424–429.

Marcus, B.H., Eaton, C.A., Rossi, J.S. and Harlow, L.L. (1994). Self-efficacy, decision-making and stages of change: An integrative model of physical exercise. *Journal of Applied Social Psychology, 24,* 489–508.

Marcus, B.H., Bock, B.C., Pinto, B.M., Forsyth, L.H., Roberts, M.B. and Traficante, R.M. (1998). Efficacy of an individualized, motivationally-tailored physical activity intervention. *Annals of Behavioral Medicine, 20*(3), 174–180.

Marlatt, G.A. (1985). Relapse prevention: Theoretial rationale and overview of the model. In G.A. Marlatt and J.R. Gordon (eds), *Relapse Prevention: Maintenance strategies in the treatment of addictive behaviours* (pp. 3–70). New York: Guilford Press.

Marshall, S.J. and Biddle, S.J.H. (2001). The Transtheoretical Model of behavior change: A meta-analysis of applications to physical activity and exercise. *Annals of Behavioral Medicine, 23,* 229–246.

Mastellos, N., Gunn, L.H., Felix, L.M., Car, J. and Majeed, A. (2014). Transtheoretical model stages of change for dietary and physical exercise modification in weight loss management for overweight and obese adults. *Cochrane Database of Systematic Reviews, Issue 2,* Art. No. CD008066. doi: 10.1002/14651858.CD008066.pub3.

Mullan, E. and Markland, D. (1997). Variations in self-determination across the stages of change for exercise in adults. *Motivation and Emotion, 21,* 349–362.

Mutrie, N., Carney, C., Blamey, A., Crawford, F., Aitchison, T. and Whitelaw, A. (2002). 'Walk in to work out': A randomised controlled trial of self help intervention to promote active commuting. *Journal of Epidemiology and Community Health, 56,* 407–412.

Nigg, C.R. (2005). There is more to stages of exercise than just exercise. *Exercise and Sport Sciences Reviews, 33*(1), 32–35. doi: 0091-6331/3301/32-35.

Prochaska, J.O. and Marcus, B.H. (1994). The transtheoretical model: Application to exercise. In R.K. Dishman (ed.), *Advances in Exercise Adherence* (pp. 161–180). Champaign, IL: Human Kinetics.

Prochaska, J.O. and Velicer, W. (1997). The transtheoretical model of health behavior change. *American Journal of Health Promotion, 12,* 38–48.

Prochaska, J.O., DiClemente, C.C. and Norcross, J.C. (1992). In search of how people change: Applications to addictive behaviors. *American Psychologist, 47,* 1102–1114.

Prochaska, J.O., Norcross, J.C. and DiClemente, C.C. (1994a). *Changing for Good.* New York: Avon.

Prochaska, J.O., Velicer, W.F., Rossi, J.S., Goldstein, M.G., Marcus, B.H., Rakowski, W. and Rossi,

S.R. (1994b). Stages of change and decision balance for 12 problem behaviors. *Health Psychology*, *13*, 39–46.

Reed, G.R. (1999). Adherence to exercise and the transtheoretical model of behaviour change. In S.J. Bull (ed.), *Adherence Issues in Sport and Exercise* (pp. 19–46). Chichester: Wiley.

Rhodes, R.E. and Nigg, C.R. (2011). Advancing physical activity theory: A review and future directions. *Exercise and Sport Sciences Reviews, 39*(3), 113–119. doi: 0091-6331/3903/113-119.

Riemsma, R.P., Pattenden, J., Bridle, C., Sowden, A., Mather, L., Watt, I. and Walker, A. (2002). A systematic review of the effectiveness of interventions based on a stages-of-change approach to promote individual behaviour change. *Health Technology Assessment, 6*(24).

Sallis, J.F. and Hovell, M. (1990). Determinants of exercise behavior. *Exercise and Sport Sciences Reviews, 18*, 307–330.

Sallis, J.F., Haskell, W., Fortmann, S., Vranizan, K., Taylor, C.B. and Solomon, D. (1986). Predictors of adoption and maintenance of physical activity in a community sample. *Preventive Medicine, 15*, 331–341.

Schwarzer, R. (1992). Self-efficacy in the adoption and maintenance of health behaviours: Theoretical approaches and a new model. In R. Schwarzer (ed.), *Self-efficacy: Thought control of action* (pp. 217–243). Bristol, PA: Taylor & Francis.

——. (2001). Social-cognitive factors in changing health-related behaviors. *Current Directions in Psychological Science, 10*(2), 47–51.

Sonstroem, R.J. (1988). Psychological models. In R.K. Dishman (ed.), *Exercise Adherence: Its impact on public health* (pp. 125–153). Champaign, IL: Human Kinetics.

Spencer, L., Adams, T.B., Malone, S., Roy, L. and Yost, E. (2006). Applying the Transtheoretical Model to exercise: A systematic and comprehensive review of the literature. *Health Promotion Practice, 7*(4), 428–443. doi: 10.1177/1524839905278900.

Stetson, B.A., Beacham, A.O., Frommelt, S.J., Boutelle, K.N., Cole, J.D., Ziegler, C.H. and Looney, S.W. (2005). Exercise slips in high-risk situations and activity patterns in long-term exercisers: An application of the relapse prevention model. *Annals of Behavioral Medicine, 30*, 25–35.

Sutton, S. (2000). Interpreting cross-sectional data on stages of change. *Psychology and Health, 15*, 163–171.

Symons Downs, D., Nigg, C.R., Hausenblas, H.A. and Rauff, E.L. (2014). Why do people change physical activity behavior? In C.R. Nigg (ed.), *ACSM's Behavioral Aspects of Physical Activity and Exercise* (pp. 1–38). Philadelphia, PA: Lippincott Williams & Wilkins.

Weinstein, N.D., Rothman, A.J. and Sutton, S.R. (1998). Stage theories of health behavior: Conceptual and methodological issues. *Health Psychology, 17*, 290–299.

Part IV

Physical activity behaviour change

12 Physical activity interventions
Planning and design

The Toronto Charter and its companion document, the seven investments that work (see Chapter 1), have provided strong evidence that changing people's physical activity and sedentary behaviour could have a major impact on their physical and mental well-being. In particular, the seven investments show very clearly the areas in which we would be best to invest our efforts in trying to change physical activity (see Table 12.1). However, physical activity behaviours in any of these seven areas have shown themselves to be difficult to change, particularly in the long term.

Many studies have used cross-sectional designs to highlight potential influences on behaviour (see Chapter 7), but these cannot establish causal links and are only a small step in building evidence for actual behaviour change. Intervention research that attempts to manipulate correlates to facilitate behaviour change offers much stronger evidence and is critical to the continued development of the field. The purpose of this chapter, therefore, is to highlight key issues in the design and evaluation of physical activity behaviour change interventions, including the following:

- frameworks for intervention design and evaluation;
- the importance of theory;
- behaviour change techniques;
- mediation analysis;
- the importance of process evaluation.

Frameworks for intervention design and evaluation

The development of a behaviour change intervention takes time, and careful consideration of a number of factors is required. Interventionists must understand the target behaviour, give consideration to the context in which they wish to change the behaviour and/or deliver the intervention, be aware of what is already known and what knowledge gaps exist, choose a theory or theories to underpin the intervention, develop the intervention strategies and resources, and finally implement and evaluate the intervention. Several frameworks have been developed to guide this process and encourage a systematic approach to intervention development. These frameworks will be outlined in the following sections.

MRC framework for the development of complex interventions

One of the most influential guides has been provided by the Medical Research Council (MRC) in the United Kingdom (Campbell et al., 2000; Craig et al., 2008). The original MRC

Table 12.1   Seven best investments for physical activity (Global Advocacy Council for Physical Activity International Society for Physical Activity and Health, 2011)

Approach	Requirements
'Whole-of-school' programmes	This approach involves encouraging schoolchildren to be active on the journey to and from school, during school break times, and after school and via quality physical education programmes at all ages. It includes the provision of suitable environments and resources to support this.
Transport policies and systems that prioritise walking, cycling and public transport	This approach would involve the development and implementation of policies on land use, access to footpaths, cycle paths and public transport, plus promotional programmes to encourage and support walking, cycling and public transport.
Urban design regulations and infrastructure that provide for equitable and safe access for recreational physical activity, and recreational and transport-related walking and cycling across the life course	This approach means that urban planning and design regulations would require mixed-use zoning (i.e. placing homes, shops, services and jobs near each other), access to public open space and recreation facilities, plus complete networks of footpaths, cycle paths and public transport.
Physical activity and non-communicable disease prevention integrated into primary health care systems	This approach requires health care systems to include physical activity within regular behavioural risk factor screening, patient education and referral. The focus should be on practical brief advice and links to community-based supports for behaviour change. May require additional training of health professionals.
Public education, including mass media to raise awareness and change social norms on physical activity	This approach suggests the use of media (e.g. print, audio, electronic, point of decision prompts) to raise awareness, increase knowledge, shift norms and values, and motivate the population. Community-based events.
Community-wide programmes involving multiple settings and sectors and that mobilise and integrate community engagement and resources	This approach supports the development of whole-of-community approaches across the life span. Such approaches would integrate policies, programmes and education aimed at encouraging physical activity.
Sports systems and programmes that promote 'sport for all' and encourage participation across the life span	This approach builds on the universal appeal of sport and requires the development of a comprehensive sport system that includes adaption of sports to match the interests of diverse groups within the population as well as coaching and training opportunities. It would involve policies and programmes that reduce social and financial barriers to access and participation.

framework (Campbell *et al.*, 2000) suggested that several stages of design and development are required for complex interventions (i.e. an intervention with many parts to it, such as one aimed at increasing physical activity in a community through a variety of means). Initial stages involve exploration of the literature, perhaps in the form of a systematic review, to ensure that the best theoretical base and intervention is chosen. Systematic reviews have become the preferred approach to synthesising evidence because they follow a systematic and explicit process to (1) identify as much relevant research as possible, (2) critically appraise this research, and (3) analyse and synthesise the data from the included studies. Statistical methods such as meta-analysis or meta-regression may or may not be used to synthesise the results (Higgins and Green, 2011).

Following on from the literature review, the next steps involve identifying intervention strategies and demonstrating how they might influence the target behaviour. The strategies chosen will be determined from the literature review, the theoretical perspective(s) chosen, and from engagement with potential participants as to what might be acceptable or unacceptable. Within the guidance it is considered critical that there is a good theoretical understanding of how the intervention causes, or might cause, behaviour change, and the importance of theory is discussed later in this chapter. Engaging with potential participants and other stakeholders (sometimes referred to as 'Patient and Public involvement' or 'PPI'; see http://www.publications.parliament.uk/pa/cm200607/cmselect/cmhealth/278/278i. pdf and http://www.nice.org.uk/getinvolved/patientandpublicinvolvement), conducting feasibility studies and pilot work of both the intervention and outcome measures are all important elements during this step. This preparatory work is important so that the intervention itself is not undermined by problems of acceptability to participants which may result in non-compliance by either intervention deliverers or the participants. In addition, this early work can highlight potential recruitment and retention problems that may impact upon the intervention process and outcomes. A mixture of qualitative and quantitative methods is likely to be needed at this stage (e.g. to understand barriers to participation or to estimate recruitment rates).

> Key point: It is important to engage with potential participants and stakeholders when developing an intervention.

Once an intervention has been developed, including feasibility and pilot trials, the next major step is to conduct a definitive trial to determine the effect of the intervention. This trial will usually involve randomisation and a control group. The final stage of this framework involves the implementation of the findings in more ecologically valid settings to determine whether the intervention has the same effects in less controlled conditions. This stage is similar to the final stage of the behavioural epidemiology framework (see Chapter 1).

In response to criticism that the original MRC framework was too rigid, a revised version was developed (Craig *et al.*, 2008). This new version continues to emphasise the importance of undertaking a series of development steps but highlights that these steps may not occur in the linear fashion suggested by the original guidance. In addition, there is recognition that designs other than randomised control trials (such as non-randomised control studies, or case control studies) are potentially suitable for behaviour change interventions. Greater emphasis is also placed on process evaluation in order to understand why an intervention was or was not successful (see later in this chapter for more detail on process evaluation). Finally, the authors of the revised guidance stressed the importance of researchers reporting their interventions with enough detail to make replication possible.

National Institute for Health and Clinical Excellence guidance on effective behaviour change interventions

The National Institute for Health and Clinical Excellence (NICE) in the UK (now the National Institute for Health and Care Excellence) has also published guidance on the principles for effective behaviour change interventions (National Institute for Health and Clinical Excellence, 2007, 2014). This guidance provides a systematic, coherent and evidence-based approach for health behaviour change interventions. Similar to the MRC framework, the NICE guidance highlights the need for careful planning of interventions that clearly specifies the behaviour(s) to be targeted, and takes into account the context in which the intervention will take place and the needs and resources of the target population. The guidance also emphasises the importance of the theoretical underpinning that links intervention content to behavioural outcomes and the clear definition of behaviour change techniques so that each component may be replicated. In addition, the guidance stresses the importance of outcome and process evaluation and also recommends that data for cost-effectiveness analysis be collected. It is also recommended that interventions should help individuals maintain their behaviour change in the long term (i.e. longer than one year after the intervention) by providing feedback and monitoring at regular intervals.

The NICE guidance (2014) also recommends that before an intervention is implemented the researchers should develop a manual that provides a detailed and comprehensive overview of the intervention. The manual should include: the objectives, evidence base, and an explanation of how the intervention is hypothesised to work; detail of the resources, setting and context for the intervention; expected outcomes; a clear definition of the behaviour change techniques employed, preferably described using a taxonomy such as the CALO-RE taxonomy discussed in a following section; details of how to tailor the intervention to individual needs; plans for long-term maintenance of behaviour change; and implementation details such as who will deliver what, to whom, when and how. It is recommended that these manuals are made publicly available (e.g. through a website; published as protocol papers) to aid replication, evidence synthesis and knowledge transfer.

The Behaviour Change Wheel

Michie and colleagues (2011a) suggest that the process of designing behaviour change interventions involves understanding the nature of the behaviour to be changed, determination of the broad approach or type of intervention to be adopted, and then working on the specifics of intervention design/components. They acknowledge that behaviour change may need to take place at multiple levels: individual, practitioner/professional (service delivery) and/or organisational level (guidelines, policy). This thinking is reflected in the Behaviour Change Wheel (BCW) (see Figure 12.1).

To understand the behaviour to be changed, intervention developers need to be able to answer the question: Who needs to do what differently, when, where and how? To answer this question fully the target behaviour must be understood within the context in which it occurs. Consideration should also be given to why the behaviours are as they are and what needs to change for the desired behaviours to occur. Answering these questions is helped by the COM-B model, which underpins the Behaviour Change Wheel. This model suggests that behaviour occurs as an interaction among three necessary 'COM' conditions – capability, opportunity, motivation – leading to the behaviour (B):

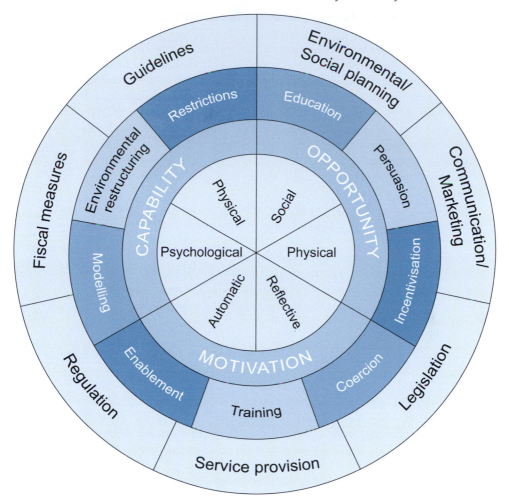

Figure 12.1 The Behaviour Change Wheel

Source: Michie *et al.* (2011a).

- Capability (psychological or physical ability to perform the behaviour, including having the necessary knowledge and skills);
- Opportunity (physical and social environment that enables the behaviour);
- Motivation (includes reflective and automatic mechanisms that facilitate or inhibit the behaviour).

The COM-B model forms the centre of the Behaviour Change Wheel. An intervention might target one or more of these conditions. The COM-B model does not prioritise the individual over the group or the environment; rather all components are given equal status in controlling behaviour. An initial step in intervention design would be to talk to members of the target group with questions framed around the COM-B characteristics; the questions at this stage would not be about how to change, but would focus on identifying what needs to change.

The inner ring of the wheel incorporates nine intervention functions, or more specifically the activities that are designed to change behaviours. This level identifies the broad approach for the intervention. Michie and colleagues (2011a) propose that each of these functions is associated with one or more specific behaviour change technique. Examples include the following:

- education would be associated with strategies to increase knowledge or understanding;
- restriction would include using rules to increase or reduce the opportunity to engage in the target behaviour;
- environmental restructuring would involve strategies to change the physical or social context;
- modelling involves strategies to provide a model for people to aspire to or imitate;
- enablement includes strategies to reduce barriers to increase participants' capability or opportunity;
- training involves strategies to increase skills;
- coercion uses strategies to create an expectation of punishment or cost, while conversely incentivisation would use strategies to create an expectation of reward;
- persuasion would use communication strategies to induce positive or negative feelings, or stimulate action.

These functions may be mapped to the needs identified from the COM-B analysis. For example, if psychological capability needed to be targeted, then education, training and enablement would be appropriate functions to include in an intervention. As another example, if physical opportunities needed to be addressed, then restriction, environmental restructuring and enablement would be appropriate. If automatic motivation (involving less conscious processing) were a target of the intervention, then coercion, environmental restructuring, modelling and enablement might be appropriate functions.

The outside ring of the wheel comprises seven policy categories in which authorities make decisions that could enable or support the interventions to occur. The policy categories are as follows:

- communication/marketing (including using print, electronic, telephone or broadcast media), guidelines (documents that recommend or mandate practice or levels of a behaviour);
- fiscal (using the tax system to increase or decrease cost);
- regulation (establishing rules or principles of behaviour or practice);
- legislation (making or changing laws);
- environmental/social planning (designing and/or controlling the physical or social environment);
- service provision (delivering a service).

The intervention functions identified at the inner ring suggest which of the policy categories are likely to be appropriate. For example, if education or persuasion were identified as important functions to target, then the following policy categories would be appropriate: communication/marketing, guidelines, regulation, legislation, and service provision. However, if modelling was identified as a function, then the policy categories would be communication/marketing and service provision.

Michie and colleagues (2011a) suggest that using the BCW has several advantages. First, it encourages consideration of all potential intervention functions and policy categories, and therefore could prevent intervention developers from neglecting important options. Second, it provides the basis for systematic analysis of how to choose what to do – by selecting the intervention function(s) most likely to be effective for a given behaviour, these may be linked to specific behaviour change techniques (BCTs). Third, the BCW emphasises context through the opportunity spoke of the wheel, and therefore places context as a starting point in intervention design. Finally, the BCW looks beyond conscious processing models to include automatic processing, such as habit.

Intervention mapping

Bartholomew *et al.* (2001) outline an intervention mapping protocol to assist in the planning, design and evaluation of theoretically based health promotion interventions. A central tenet of intervention mapping is that theories and empirical evidence should form the basis for decisions made during intervention planning, development and evaluation (Kok *et al.*, 2004). Intervention mapping is a very detailed process and the six broad steps are outlined in Table 12.2. Although presented as a series of steps, intervention mapping is seen as iterative rather than linear, with planners moving back and forth between the steps as they develop an 'intervention map' that guides the design, implementation and evaluation of an intervention. Core to the intervention mapping process is an understanding of existing evidence about the specific problem to identify what is already known about factors that influence it (e.g. correlates/determinants), previous intervention attempts, and identification of theories that can help in the development of a comprehensive explanation. If gaps are identified in the evidence base, it may be necessary to collect new data before the intervention is developed.

The RE-AIM framework

It is important to consider the public health impact of all interventions, taking into account the extent and ease with which they can be rolled out and delivered to large numbers of people. However, much intervention research focuses on demonstrating efficacy – that is, demonstrating that an intervention works and facilitates behaviour change. Such efficacy trials are typically well-controlled studies, with good internal validity, but limited external validity, as they are delivered to carefully selected populations under ideal conditions. This makes it difficult to generalise or translate the results of research interventions into more

Table 12.2 Intervention mapping steps (adapted from Bartholomew *et al.*, 2001)

(1) Needs assessment
(2) Specification of the objectives of the intervention
(3) Selection of theory(s) that are relevant to the target behaviours
(4) Development of practical strategies based on the theory(s) chosen to achieve the objectives
(5) Specification of adoption and implementation plans
(6) Generating an evaluation plan.

ecologically valid settings. Estabrooks and Gyurcsik (2003) argue that less attention has been given to the 'translatability' and public health impact of interventions in comparison to the assessment of the efficacy of an intervention. The RE-AIM framework (Glasgow *et al.*, 1998; see also http://www.re-aim.org), developed to evaluate the dimensions most important for implementation, provides a wider view for judging intervention effectiveness (King *et al.*, 2010). It was designed to enhance the quality, speed and public health impact of efforts to translate research into practice. The goal of RE-AIM is to encourage all those involved in intervention design and evaluation to pay more attention to essential programme elements that can improve the sustainable adoption and implementation of effective, generalisable, evidence-based interventions (http://www.re-aim.org).

RE-AIM is an abbreviation for the five factors of Reach, Effectiveness, Adoption, Implementation and Maintenance (see Table 12.3). These dimensions occur at multiple levels (e.g. individual, organisation, community) and interact to determine the public health or population-based impact of an intervention programme.

The RE-AIM model is intended to guide planning and evaluation of health behaviour interventions. All of the dimensions should be considered during the intervention design phase. For example, in the planning phase, intervention developers can ask themselves the following questions:

- How will we optimise reach?
- How do we reach the target population with the intervention?
- How will we demonstrate effectiveness?
- How do we develop organisational support for the intervention?
- How do we optimise the number of people who are willing to deliver the intervention?
- How do we ensure that the intervention is delivered properly?
- How can we observe implementation differences?
- What do we need to do to generate sustainability?

Table 12.3 Elements of the RE-AIM framework

RE-AIM elements	Descriptions
R: Reach	Concerned with the numbers of people taking part in the intervention as well as their participation rate and how representative they are of the population.
E: Effectiveness	Concerned about the impact of the intervention on important outcomes, including potential negative effects and economic outcomes.
A: Adoption	Refers to the reach of the intervention at the level of the setting or organisation, such as the number of worksites adopting the intervention and characteristics of the worksites which adopt the intervention.
I: Implementation	Refers to whether the intervention was delivered as intended, including consistency of delivery across intervention sites, and time and cost of the intervention.
M: Maintenance	Concerned with the extent to which behaviour change is maintained or whether relapse effects are noted. Maintenance may be considered both at the individual level and at the level of the organisation, such as the number of organisations continuing to support the intervention in the long term.

Then, during the evaluation, the questions become:

- Who did participate?
- Were there changes in the important outcomes?
- Did the outcomes vary by setting?
- What were the differences?
- Were the intervention effects maintained?
- Did the organisations involved continue with intervention activities?

Key point: The RE-AIM principles offer a public health perspective on how to evaluate interventions.

Exemplar of intervention planning and design using walking

We have followed the MRC's framework for developing and evaluating complex inter-ventions in our work related to walking. Our early work suggested that it was feasible to encourage short-term changes in walking in a workplace setting when workers were encouraged by behavioural strategies to consider more active ways to travel to work (Mutrie *et al.*, 2002). We then undertook a systematic review to determine the current evidence for walking promotion and to identify gaps in the evidence. We established from that systematic review that it is feasible to increase walking by 30 to 60 minutes per week with promotional efforts (Ogilvie *et al.*, 2007). We concluded that people can be encouraged to walk more by interventions that are tailored to their needs; that are targeted to the most inactive or to those most motivated to change. The evidence came from interventions delivered at the level of the individual, households or group-based approaches. In that review we also noted that pedometers were promising tools for promoting walking but that more research was needed on their use. For example, none of the studies that used pedometers found more than short-term change.

Our next step was to design and pilot an intervention using pedometers. That led us to refine the intervention and we then conducted a randomised controlled trial which showed that, by using a pedometer and providing a graduated programme of step count targets over 12 weeks, individuals can be encouraged to increase their activity levels and maintain them for 12 months (Baker *et al.*, 2008; Fitzsimons *et al.*, 2012). In terms of implementation, we have shown that this approach is successful with adults (Baker *et al.*, 2008), older adults (Mutrie *et al.*, 2012) and overweight men (Hunt *et al.*, 2014). 'Paths for All' have used our evidenced-based approach in their latest advice about increasing walking with pedometers (http://www.pathsforall.org.uk/pfa/community-pedometer-pack/pedometers.html). We have also shown that such increases in walking are associated with improved positive mood and perceived quality of life, and are cost-effective (Shaw *et al.*, 2011).

The importance of theory

Theory is strongly emphasised in all the frameworks and guidance for the development of interventions (Bartholomew *et al.*, 2001; Campbell *et al.*, 2000; Craig *et al.*, 2008; Michie *et al.*, 2011a; National Institute for Health and Clinical Excellence, 2007, 2014), and this is further emphasised by systematic reviews of interventions which show that interventions based on theory are generally more effective than those that are not (e.g. Greaves *et al.*, 2011; Ogilvie *et al.*, 2007). According to Michie and Prestwich (2010), the explicit use of theory has several benefits: (1) theory identifies constructs that are hypothesised to lead to behaviour change and are therefore targets within interventions; (2) examining behaviour change within a theoretical framework aids the synthesis of evidence across contexts, population and behaviours; and (3) the use of theory provides a mechanism for understanding why an intervention was effective or not, and as a result leads to the refinement of theory. Despite the many potential benefits of theory to intervention design, few authors give more than a passing reference to the theoretical underpinnings of their interventions and fewer still explain how the theory was actually linked to their behaviour change strategies (Michie and Prestwich, 2010). To help improve the use and reporting of theory within interventions, Michie and Prestwich (2010) have developed a method for assessing the extent to which theory has been employed in the development and evaluation of behaviour change interventions. The Theory Coding Scheme considers the extent to which theoretical constructs are targeted, how theory is used, or not used, to select participants or to tailor the intervention, the measurement of theoretical constructs and whether the theory is tested and/or refined. Referring to this scheme provides a systematic way for interventionists to use and report theory within interventions. In addition, the scheme could be used in systematic reviews and meta-analyses to provide a more rigorous examination of theory use and to more effectively examine the impact of different theories on behaviour change.

One of the challenges facing interventionists is to choose between the myriad theoretical perspectives (e.g. Social Cognitive Theory, Theory of Planned Behaviour, Health Belief Model – see chapters in Part III) that could be employed in an attempt to change physical activity behaviour. Although the frameworks outlined earlier all emphasise the importance of theory, they do not specify how to select a theory (Michie *et al.*, 2011a). Choosing one theoretical perspective may make the design of an intervention easier but runs the risk of limiting effectiveness as key constructs from other theories are ignored (Michie *et al.*, 2011a). Indeed, the frameworks outlined earlier tend to lead the interventionist to draw on multiple theories in order to develop the most comprehensive intervention strategies. The use of multiple theories makes it even more important that links between theory and behaviour change techniques are clearly articulated. Furthermore, the frameworks for intervention design suggest that for an intervention to be truly theory based, rather than simply theory informed, it is essential that explicit links are made, and reported, between the theoretical constructs (e.g. social norms, attitudes) and the techniques employed to change them. Unfortunately many existing physical activity interventions do not provide this detail, and it is not always clear how the behaviour change techniques used within interventions actually influence the theoretical constructs hypothesised to lead to behaviour change (Brug *et al.*, 2005).

> Key point: Use of theory helps to identify constructs that are hypothesised to lead to behaviour change and provides a mechanism for understanding why an intervention was effective or not.

Behaviour change techniques (BCTs)

BCTs are the 'active ingredients' within an intervention and are designed to change the target behaviour. Just as there are a variety of factors (e.g. barriers, self-efficacy, social support) that may influence physical activity participation, there are a number of BCTs that have been used to try to facilitate behaviour change. This has created a lack of clarity in the literature, particularly as a lack of consistency in terminology across interventions has led to the same label being used for different techniques (e.g. behavioural counselling being used as a label for 'education of participant' and for 'feedback on self-monitoring') or a different label being used for the same technique (Michie *et al.*, 2011b). Furthermore, reports of interventions often do not adequately describe the behaviour change techniques employed, making replication of studies difficult and limiting what can be learned from research syntheses. There is a need for a common language and definition of behaviour change techniques to aid both researchers and practitioners in the identification of effective techniques.

Michie *et al.* (2011b) have developed a taxonomy of behaviour change techniques that have been used in interventions to help people change their physical activity and healthy eating behaviours. Using the original behaviour change taxonomy (Abraham and Michie, 2008) as a starting point, Michie *et al.* (2011b) conducted systematic reviews to see which behaviour change techniques could be used to identify core components of physical activity and healthy eating behaviour change interventions. The resulting CALO-RE taxonomy contains 40 behaviour change techniques and provides a definition of each technique and the construct it is hypothesised to change (see Table 12.4). The BCTs are defined in such a way as to remove overlap. The CALO-RE taxonomy does not suggest which techniques to use or which are most effective. However, according to Michie *et al.* (2011b), they offer several advantages. First, the use of standardised BCTs facilitates identification of the BCTs that actually contribute to intervention effectiveness. Second, the taxonomy provides authors with a common language to accurately describe their intervention, thereby facilitating the ability for intervention evidence to be replicated and synthesised. Third, standardisation improves the mapping of BCTs to constructs identified in behavioural theory and through this is likely to aid the development and refinement of behaviour change theory. Finally, having standardised BCT definitions helps in the effective implementation of interventions, thereby maximising the chance that BCTs are delivered as intended across different contexts.

In a study focused on interventions to increase physical activity and/or healthy eating, Michie *at al.* (2009) sought to examine the effectiveness of different BCTs within interventions. Pooling data across 122 studies, they reported an overall small positive effect size of 0.31, indicating that those receiving the interventions achieved significantly better outcomes than those in control groups. The analysis also showed that the most effective interventions included self-monitoring of behaviour and at least one of the following techniques: feedback on performance, prompt intention formation, prompt specific goal setting, and prompt review of behavioural goals.

Key point: Behaviour change techniques are the 'active ingredients' in an intervention.

Mediation analysis

Health behaviour interventions are designed to target change in correlates of a behaviour which are hypothesised to lead to changes in the actual behaviour (MacKinnon and Fairchild, 2009). These correlates are often derived from theoretical models. For example, within Social Cognitive Theory (SCT), it is hypothesised that self-efficacy influences physical activity participation (i.e. a person with higher self-efficacy for physical activity will be more likely to participate in physical activity). Interventions based on SCT would, therefore, seek to employ

Table 12.4 Summary of CALO-RE behaviour change techniques with definitions (Michie *et al.*, 2011b)

Behaviour change technique	Definition
1. Provide information on consequences of behaviour in *general*	Information about the relationship between the behaviour and its possible or likely consequences in the general case, usually based on epidemiological data, and not personalised for the individual.
2. Provide information on consequences of behaviour *to the individual*	Information about the *benefits and costs* of action or inaction to the individual or tailored to a relevant group based on that individual's characteristics (i.e. demographics, clinical, behavioural or psychological information). This may include any costs/benefits and not necessarily those related to health (e.g. feelings).
3. Provide information about others' approval	Involves information about what other people think about the target person's behaviour. It clarifies whether others will like, or approve or disapprove of what the person is doing or will do.
4. Provide normative information about others' behaviour	Involves providing information about what other people are *doing*, i.e. indicates that a particular behaviour or sequence of behaviours is common or uncommon among the population or among a specified group – presentation of case studies of a few others is not normative information.
5. Goal-setting (behaviour)	The person is encouraged to make a behavioural resolution (e.g. take more exercise next week). This is directed towards encouraging people to decide to change or maintain change.
6. Goal-setting (outcome)	The person is encouraged to set a general goal that may be achieved by behavioural means but is not defined in terms of behaviour (e.g. to reduce blood pressure or lose/maintain weight), as opposed to a goal based on changing behaviour as such. The goal may be an expected consequence of one or more behaviours, but is not a behaviour per se (see also techniques 5 and 7). This technique may co-occur with technique 5 if goals for both behaviour and other outcomes are set.
7. Action planning	Involves detailed planning of what the person will do including, as a minimum, when, in which situation and/or where to act. 'When' may describe frequency (such as how many times a day/week) or duration (e.g. for how long). The exact content of action plans may or may not be described, in this case code as this technique if it is stated that the behaviour is planned contingent to a specific situation or set of situations, even if exact details are not present.
8. Barrier identification/ problem-solving	This presumes having formed an initial plan to change behaviour. The person is prompted to think about potential barriers *and* identify ways of overcoming them. Barriers may include competing goals in specified situations. This may be described as 'problem-solving'. If it is problem-solving in relation to the performance of a behaviour, then it counts as an instance of this technique. Examples of barriers may include behavioural, cognitive, emotional, environmental, social and/or physical barriers.
9. Set graded tasks	Breaking down the target behaviour into smaller easier-to-achieve tasks and enabling the person to build on small successes to achieve target behaviour. This may include increments towards a target behaviour, or incremental increases from baseline behaviour.
10. Prompt review of behavioural goals	Involves a review or analysis of the extent to which previously set *behavioural* goals (e.g. take more exercise next week) were achieved. In most cases this will follow previous goal-setting (see technique 5) and an attempt to act on those goals, followed by a revision or readjustment of goals, and/or means to attain them.

Behaviour change technique	Definition
11. Prompt review of outcome goals	Involves a review or analysis of the extent to which previously set *outcome* goals (e.g. to reduce blood pressure or lose/maintain weight) were achieved. In most cases this will follow previous goal-setting (see technique 6) and an attempt to act on those goals, followed by a revision of goals, and/or means to attain them.
12. Prompt rewards contingent on effort or progress towards behaviour	Involves the person using praise or rewards for attempts at achieving a behavioural goal. This may include efforts made towards achieving the behaviour, or progress taken in preparatory steps towards the behaviour, but not merely participation in intervention. This may include self-reward.
13. Provide rewards contingent on successful behaviour	Reinforcing successful performance of the specific target behaviour. This may include praise and encouragement as well as material rewards but the reward/incentive must be explicitly linked to the achievement of the specific target behaviour; i.e. the person receives the reward if they perform the specified behaviour but not if they do not perform the behaviour. This may include self-reward. Provisions of rewards for completing intervention components or materials are not instances of this technique. References to provision of incentives for being more physically active are not instances of this technique unless information about contingency to the performance of the target behaviour is provided.
14. Shaping	Contingent rewards are first provided for any approximation to the target behaviour (e.g. for any increase in physical activity). Then, later, only a more demanding performance (e.g. brisk walking for 10 minutes on three days a week) would be rewarded. Thus, this is graded use of contingent rewards over time.
15. Prompting generalisation of a target behaviour	Once a behaviour is performed in a particular situation, the person is encouraged or helped to try it in another situation. The idea is to ensure that the behaviour is not tied to one situation but becomes a more integrated part of the person's life that can be performed at a variety of different times and in a variety of contexts.
16. Prompt self-monitoring of behaviour	The person is asked to keep a record of specified behaviour/s as a method for changing behaviour. This should be an explicitly stated intervention component, as opposed to occurring as part of completing measures for research purposes. This could take the form of a diary or completing a questionnaire about their behaviour, in terms of type, frequency, duration and/or intensity.
17. Prompt self-monitoring of behavioural outcome	The person is asked to keep a record of specified measures expected to be influenced by the behaviour change (e.g. blood pressure, blood glucose, weight loss, physical fitness).
18. Prompting focus on past success	Involves instructing the person to think about or list previous successes in performing the behaviour (or parts of it).
19. Provide feedback on performance	This involves providing the participant with data about their own recorded behaviour (e.g. following technique 16) or commenting on a person's behavioural performance (e.g. identifying a discrepancy between behavioural performance and a set goal – see techniques 5 and 7) or a discrepancy between one's own performance in relation to others' – note: this could also involve technique 28.
20. Provide information on *where and when* to perform the behaviour	Involves telling the person about when and where they might be able to perform the behaviour (e.g. tips on places and times participants can access local exercise classes). This may be in either verbal or written form.

Behaviour change technique	Definition
21. Provide instruction on how to perform the behaviour	Involves *telling* the person *how* to perform a behaviour or preparatory behaviours, either verbally or in written form. Examples of instructions include how to use gym equipment (without getting on and showing the participant), instruction on suitable clothing, and tips on how to take action. *Showing* a person how to perform a behaviour without verbal instruction would be an instance of technique 22 only.
22. Model/Demonstrate the behaviour	Involves *showing* the person how to perform a behaviour (e.g. through physical or visual demonstrations of behavioural performance) in person or remotely.
23. Teach to use prompts/ cues	The person is taught to identify environmental prompts which may be used to remind them to perform the behaviour (or to perform an alternative, incompatible behaviour in the case of behaviours to be reduced). Cues could include times of day, particular contexts or technologies such as mobile phone alerts which prompt them to perform the target behaviour.
24. Environmental restructuring	The person is prompted to alter the environment in ways so that it is more supportive of the target behaviour (e.g. altering cues or reinforcers). For instance, they might be asked to lock up or throw away their high-calorie snacks, or take their running shoes to work. Interventions in which the interveners directly modify environmental variables (e.g. the way food is displayed in shops, provision of sports facilities) are not covered by this taxonomy and should be coded independently.
25. Agree behavioural contract	Must involve written agreement on the performance of an explicitly specified behaviour so that there is a written record of the person's resolution witnessed by another.
26. Prompt practice	Prompt the person to rehearse and repeat the behaviour or preparatory behaviours numerous times. Note that this will also include parts of the behaviour (e.g. refusal skills in relation to unhealthy snacks). This could be described as 'building habits or routines' but is still practice so long as the person is prompted to try the behaviour (or parts of it) during the intervention or practice between intervention sessions (e.g. as 'homework').
27. Use of follow-up prompts	Intervention components are gradually reduced in intensity, duration and frequency over time (e.g. letters or telephone calls instead of face to face) and/or provided at longer time intervals.
28. Facilitate social comparison	Involves explicitly drawing attention to others' performance to elicit comparisons.
29. Plan social support/social change	Involves prompting the person to plan how to elicit social support from other people to help him or her achieve their target behaviour/ outcome. This will include support during interventions (e.g. setting up a 'buddy' system) or other forms of support and following the intervention including support provided by the individuals delivering the intervention: partner, friends, family.
30. Prompt identification as role model/position advocate	Involves focusing on how the person may be an example to others and affect their behaviour (e.g. being a good example to children). Also includes providing opportunities for participants to persuade others of the importance of adopting/changing the behaviour; for example, giving a talk or running a peer-led session.

Behaviour change technique	Definition
31. Prompt anticipated regret	Involves inducing expectations of future regret about the performance or non-performance of a behaviour. This includes focusing on how the person will *feel* in the future and specifically whether they will feel regret or feel sorry that they did or did not take a different course of action.
32. Fear arousal	Involves presentation of risk and/or mortality information relevant to the behaviour as emotive images designed to evoke a fearful response (e.g. 'smoking kills!' or images of the grim reaper).
33. Prompt self-talk	Encourage the person to use talk to themselves (aloud or silently) before and during planned behaviours to encourage, support and maintain action.
34. Prompt use of imagery	Teach the person to imagine successfully performing the behaviour or to imagine finding it easy to perform the behaviour, including component or easy versions of the behaviour. Distinct from recalling instances of previous success without imagery (technique 18).
35. Relapse prevention/ coping planning	This relates to planning how to maintain behaviour that has been changed. The person is prompted to identify in advance situations in which the changed behaviour may not be maintained and develop strategies to avoid or manage those situations. Contrast with techniques 7 and 8 which are about initiating behaviour change.
36. Stress management/ emotional control training	This is a set of specific techniques (e.g. progressive relaxation) which do not target the behaviour directly but seek to reduce anxiety and stress to facilitate the performance of the behaviour. It may also include techniques designed to reduce negative emotions or control mood or feelings that may interfere with performance of the behaviour, and/or to increase positive emotions that might help with the performance of the behaviour.
37. Motivational interviewing	This is a clinical method including a specific set of techniques involving prompting the person to engage in change talk in order to minimise resistance and resolve ambivalence to change (includes motivational counselling).
38. Time management	This includes any technique designed to teach a person how to manage their time in order to make time for the behaviour. These techniques are not directed towards performance of target behaviour but rather seek to facilitate it by freeing up times when it could be performed.
39. General communication skills training	This includes any technique directed at general communication skills but not directed towards a particular behaviour change. Often this may include role play and group work focusing on listening skills or assertive skills.
40. Stimulate anticipation of future rewards	Create anticipation of future rewards without necessarily reinforcing behaviour throughout the active period of the intervention. Code this technique when participants are told at the onset that they will be rewarded based on behavioural achievement.

strategies to increase self-efficacy for physical activity which should then lead to increases in physical activity. A correlate, therefore – in this case self-efficacy – acts as a mediator of physical activity behaviour change (see Chapter 7).

A mediator may be defined as 'an intervening variable that is necessary to complete a cause–effect link between intervention program and physical activity' (Bauman *et al.*, 2002, p. 8). The mediation pathway is illustrated in Figure 7.1. While many interventions are based on psychological theories, many studies do not systematically measure the mediating variables or assess the mediation pathways in the analysis (Baranowski *et al.*, 1998; Lubans *et al.*, 2008). This is a significant limitation in the literature for several reasons. Mediation analysis helps to identify critical components of interventions (MacKinnon *et al.*, 2000) providing evidence of 'what works' for changing behaviour (Lubans *et al.*, 2008). This allows more effective interventions to be developed as factors identified as mediators can become the focus of future interventions, and other factors shown not to mediate the behaviour change may be ignored (Bauman *et al.*, 2002; MacKinnon and Fairchild, 2009). In addition, mediation analysis may be used to refine and develop better theories of behaviour change. For example, if an intervention results in behaviour change, but this change is not explained by the hypothesised mediating variables within the underlying theoretical models, then this indicates that the theory is incomplete and needs further development (Baranowski *et al.*, 1998).

There are several approaches to mediation analysis (Baron and Kenny, 1986; MacKinnon, 2008) but it is beyond the scope of this book to outline them here. However, mediation analysis should become a fundamental component of intervention evaluation so that key mechanisms of behaviour change are identified (see Cerin, 2010). This will enable the development of increasingly effective interventions and enhance our understanding of how to facilitate health behaviour change (Lubans *et al.*, 2008).

The importance of process evaluation

The various frameworks for intervention design all suggest that process evaluation of interventions should be considered as an integral part of intervention design and ideally be considered at the planning stage prior to intervention delivery. Many interventions focus on the evaluation of primary and secondary outcomes and measures to demonstrate that the intervention did or did not result in the targeted behaviour change. However, outcome results cannot tell the full story, as they do not provide information on why an intervention was or was not successful. This means that alongside an outcome evaluation researchers should also conduct a process evaluation. Process evaluation helps interventionists understand why a programme was or was not successful. It is used to monitor the implementation of the intervention and helps in understanding the relationship between programme elements and programme outcomes (Baranowski and Jago, 2005; Saunders *et al.*, 2005).

Process evaluation focuses on how an intervention operates. It is designed to answer questions of what was actually done, when, by whom and to whom. An effective process evaluation will address the question of whether the intervention operated as intended and is critical to understanding the outcomes achieved. A process evaluation can help distinguish between interventions that fail because they are inherently faulty and those that fail because they were poorly implemented or failed to reach sufficient numbers of the target audience (Oakley *et al.*, 2006; Saunders *et al.*, 2005). It will also provide information that may be used to refine and enhance the intervention in the future, and will identify unexpected challenges and barriers encountered during the programme.

A process evaluation is an ongoing process and does not just occur at the end of the intervention. It occurs during recruitment, intervention implementation and follow-up (Hughes *et al.*, 2008). It includes a focus on participants' perceptions and reactions to the intervention. The actual questions asked vary but should address the following issues (Hughes *et al.*, 2008; Saunders *et al.*, 2005):

1. *Exposure*: The extent to which the target group is engaged and aware of the intervention, resource or message being implemented. It includes both initial and continued awareness and use.
2. *Reach*: Addresses the question 'Are all parts of the intervention reaching all parts of the target group?' It examines the proportion of the target group who participate in the intervention, and numbers and characteristics of those who drop out at different stages. It may also address recruitment procedures.
3. *Satisfaction*: Assesses whether participants were happy with and liked the intervention. Covers interpersonal issues (e.g. Is the participant comfortable in the intervention? Is the facilitator or intervention leader approachable?), service issues (e.g. Is it at a convenient time or location?), and content issues (e.g. Is the intervention material relevant and interesting and at an appropriate level?).
4. *Fidelity or quality of implementation*: Assesses whether all parts of the intervention were delivered as planned. It includes quality assurance and assessment of consistency both between sessions and across different intervention deliverers and sites.
5. *Dose*: Assesses how much of the programme was delivered. It also examines to what extent participants received and used materials or other resources.
6. *Context*: Explores aspects of the environment (physical and social) that may have influenced either implementation of the intervention or outcomes (e.g. other initiatives, staff turnover). This is particularly important when the intervention is delivered across multiple sites and settings.

Both qualitative and quantitative methods are used in process evaluation. Quantitative methods will usually be used to assess reach, delivery and exposure components, and qualitative methods may be employed to assess elements of satisfaction, fidelity and context. Typical process evaluation data sources include attendance records, logs of activities conducted, log books of difficulties or barriers encountered during implementation, interviews with participants and intervention deliverers, and observations. By better understanding how an intervention works, programmes can evolve and become increasingly effective.

> Key point: Process evaluation can help in understanding why an intervention was successful or not in achieving behaviour change.

Process evaluation example: lessons from active winners

Pate and colleagues reported on the 'Active Winners' intervention, designed to increase physical activity in 10- to 11-year-old children in the USA (Pate *et al.*, 2003). The intervention targeted school students with home, school and community components over 18 months. Social Cognitive Theory was chosen to underpin the intervention. There were no differences after the intervention between the intervention and control communities in physical activity, nor on most psychosocial variables.

Pate *et al.* (2003) reported on a comprehensive process evaluation to ascertain why the intervention failed to achieve the intended behaviour change. The process evaluation focused on issues of intervention planning, development and implementation. Three key questions were asked:

1.   Was the programme implemented as planned?
2.   To what extent were the participants actually exposed to the intervention?
3.   Did the programme adhere to the theoretical model and philosophy as intended? The plan was for activities to be fun, inclusive and confidence building.

Both qualitative and quantitative methods were used in the process evaluation. These included participant attendance records, surveys of participants and staff, individual and focus group interviews, a review of records, and heart rate monitoring in activity sessions.

Of the 255 students in the target group, 82 per cent had at least one exposure to the intervention elements, but only 5 per cent attended at least half of the sessions offered. Moreover, not all staff and peer leaders appeared to understand the philosophy of the programme.

Implementation of the programme includes an appraisal of fidelity (was the programme implemented as intended?) and completeness (proportion of activities and other elements delivered). Process evaluation indicated that the summer programme and after-school elements were delivered as intended. However, this was not the case for the home, school and community elements.

As a result of the process evaluation, Pate *et al.* (2003) provided 10 recommendations for school and community physical activity interventions with similar target groups. These addressed resources, planning issues, staff training, issues around consistency, and organisational structures and responsibilities. Even though the intervention itself did not achieve the intended increase in physical activity, valuable lessons were learned through the process evaluation for future interventions.

Chapter summary

The design of interventions is not simple, and takes time and careful consideration of a number of factors. Several frameworks have been proposed to guide the process of intervention development, and while they differ from each other some common themes emerge. These include a systematic review of what is already known, the importance of theory, and the choosing of behaviour change strategies that are linked to the chosen theory(s). Understanding the target group, the target behaviour and the intervention context is also fundamental to effective interventions. Potential participants and key stakeholders should be involved at all stages of intervention design, development and evaluation. The importance of pilot work and refinement is stressed. Finally, there is a need to look beyond outcome measures and to use process evaluation to understand the intervention experience from the participant's perspective.

References

Abraham, C. and Michie, S. (2008). A taxonomy of behavior change techniques used in interventions. *Health Psychology, 27*(3), 379–387.

Baker, G., Gray, S., Wright, A., Fitzsimons, C., Nimmo, M., Lowry, R. and the Scottish Physical Activity Research Collaboration. (2008). The effect of a pedometer-based community walking intervention 'Walking for Wellbeing in the West' on physical activity levels and health outcomes: A 12-week randomized controlled trial. *International Journal of Behavioral Nutrition and Physical Activity, 5*(1), 44–49.

Baranowski, T. and Jago, R. (2005). Understanding mechanisms of change in children's physical activity programs. *Exercise and Sport Science Reviews, 33*(4), 163–168.

Baranowski, T., Anderson, C. and Carmack, C. (1998). Mediating variable framework in physical activity interventions. How are we doing? How might we do better? *American Journal of Preventive Medicine, 15*, 266–297.

Baron, R. and Kenny, D. (1986). The moderator–mediator variable distinction in social psychology research: Conceptual strategies and statistical concerns. *Journal of Personality and Social Psychology, 51*, 1173–1182.

Bartholomew, K., Parcel, G., Kok, G. and Gottleib, N. (2001). *Intervention Mapping: Designing theory- and evidence-based health promotion programs.* California: Mayfield.

Bauman, A., Sallis, J., Dzewaltowski, D. and Owen, N. (2002). Toward a better understanding of the influences on physical activity: The role of determinants, correlates, causal variables, mediators, moderators, and confounders. *American Journal of Preventive Medicine, 23*(2S), 5–14.

Brug, J., Oenema, A. and Ferreira, I. (2005). Theory, evidence and intervention mapping to improve behavior nutrition and physical activity interventions. *International Journal of Behavioral Nutrition and Physical Activity, 2*(2). doi: 10.1186/1479-5868-2-2.

Campbell, M., Fitzpatrick, R., Haines, A., Kinmouth, A., Sandercock, P., Spiegelhalter, D. and Tyrer, P. (2000). Framework for the design and evaluation of complex interventions to improve health. *British Medical Journal, 321*, 694–696.

Cerin, E. (2010). Ways of unraveling how and why physical activity influences mental health through statistical mediation analyses. *Mental Health and Physical Activity, 3*, 51–60.

Craig, P., Dieppe, P., Macintyre, S., Michie, S., Nazareth, I. and Petticrew, M. (2008). Developing and evaluating complex interventions: The new Medical Research Council guidance. *British Medical Journal, 337*, 979–983.

Estabrooks, P. and Gyurcsik, N. (2003). Evaluating the impact of behavioral interventions that target physical activity: Issues of generalizability and public health. *Psychology of Sport and Exercise, 4*, 41–55.

Fitzsimons, C., Baker, G., Gray, S., Nimmo, M., Mutrie, N. and The Scottish Physical Activity Research Collaboration. (2012). Does physical activity counselling enhance the effects of a pedometer-based intervention over the long-term: 12-month findings from the Walking for Wellbeing in the West study. *BMC Public Health, 12*(1), 206.

Glasgow, R., Vogt, T. and Boles, S. (1998). Evaluating the public health impact of health promotion interventions: The RE-AIM framework. *American Journal of Public Health, 89*(9), 1322–1327.

Global Advocacy Council for Physical Activity International Society for Physical Activity and Health. (2011). Investments that work for physical activity.

Greaves, C., Sheppard, K., Abraham, C., Hardeman, W., Roden, M., Evans, P. and the Image Study Group. (2011). Systematic review of reviews of intervention components associated with increased effectiveness in dietary and physical activity interventions. *British Medical Council Public Health, 11*, 119.

Higgins, J. and Green, S. (2011). *Cochrane Handbook for Systematic Reviews of Interventions Version 5.1.0* [updated March 2011].

Hughes, R., Black, C. and Kennedy, N. (2008). *Public Health Nutrition Intervention Management: Process evaluation.* JobNut Project, Trinity College Dublin.

Hunt, K., Wyke, S., Gray, C.M., Anderson, A.S., Brady, A., Bunn, C. and Treweek, S. (2014). A gender-sensitised weight loss and healthy living programme for overweight and obese men delivered by Scottish Premier League football clubs (FFIT): A pragmatic randomised controlled trial. *Lancet*. doi: 10.1016/S0140-6736(13)62420-4.

King, D., Glasgow, R. and Leeman-Castillo, B. (2010). Reaiming RE-AIM: Using the model to plan, implement, and evaluate the effects of environmental change approaches to enhancing population health. *American Journal of Public Health, 100*, 2076–2084.

Kok, G., Schaalma, H., Ruiter, R., Van Empelen, P. and Brug, J. (2004). Intervention mapping: A protocol for applying health psychology theory to prevention programmes. *Journal of Health Psychology, 9*, 85–97.

Lubans, D., Foster, C. and Biddle, S. (2008). A review of the mediators of behavior in interventions to promote physical activity among children and adolescents. *Preventive Medicine, 47*, 463–470.

MacKinnon, D. (2008). *Introduction to Statistical Mediation Analysis*. Mahwah, NJ: Erlbaum.

MacKinnon, D. and Fairchild, A. (2009). Current directions in mediation analysis. *Current Directions in Psychological Science, 18*, 16–20.

MacKinnon, D., Krull, J. and Lockwood, C. (2000). Equivalence of the mediation, confounding and suppression effect. *Prevention Science, 1*, 173–181.

Michie, S. and Prestwich, A. (2010). Are interventions theory-based? Development of a theory coding scheme. *Health Psychology, 29*, 1–8.

Michie, S., Abraham, C., Whittington, C., McAteer, C. and Gupta, S. (2009). Effective techniques in healthy eating and physical activity interventions: A meta-regression. *Health Psychology, 28*(6), 690–701.

Michie, S., van Stralen, M. and West, R. (2011a). The behaviour Change Wheel: A new method for characterising and designing behaviour change interventions. *Implementation Science, 6*, 42.

Michie, S., Ashford, S., Sniehotta, F., Dombrowski, S., Bishop, A. and French, D. (2011b). A refined taxonomy of behaviour change techniques to help people change their physical activity and healthy eating behaviours: The CALO-RE taxonomy. *Psychology and Health, 26*(11), 1479–1498.

Mutrie, N., Carney, C., Blamey, A., Crawford, F., Aitchison, T. and Whitelaw, A. (2002). 'Walk in to work out': A randomised controlled trial of a self help intervention to promote active commuting. *Journal of Epidemiology and Community Health, 56*(6), 407–412.

Mutrie, N., Doolin, O., Fitzsimons, C., Grant, P.M., Granat, M., Grealy, M. and Skelton, D. (2012). Increasing older adults' walking through primary care: Results of a pilot randomized controlled trial. *Family Practice, 29*(6), 633–642. doi: 10.1093/fampra/cms038.

National Institute for Health and Clinical Excellence. (2007). *Behaviour Change: The principles for effective interventions NICE public health guidance 6*. Retrieved from http://www.nice.org.uk.

———. (2014). *Behaviour Change: Individual approaches, NICE public health guidance 49*. Retrieved from http://www.nice.org.uk.

Oakley, A., Strange, V., Bonell, C., Allen, E., Stephenson, J. and RIPPLE Study Team. (2006). Process evaluation in randomised controlled trials of complex interventions. *British Medical Journal, 332*, 413–416.

Ogilvie, D., Foster, C., Rothnie, H., Cavill, N., Hamilton, V., Fitzsimons, C. and SPARColl. (2007). Interventions to promote walking: Systematic review. *British Medical Journal, Online First*, 10.

Pate, R., Saunders, R., Ward, D., Felton, G., Trost, S. and Dowda, M. (2003). Evaluation of a community-based intervention to promote physical activity in youth: Lessons from Active Winners. *American Journal of Health Promotion, 17*(3), 171–182.

Saunders, R., Evans, M. and Joshi, P. (2005). Developing a process-evaluation plan for assessing health promotion program implementation: A how-to guide. *Health Promotion Practice, 6*(2), 134–147.

Shaw, R., Fenwick, E., Baker, G., McAdam, C., Fitzsimons, C. and Mutrie, N. (2011). 'Pedometers cost buttons': The feasibility of implementing a pedometer based walking programme within the community. *BMC Public Health, 11*(1), 200.

13 Physical activity interventions for young people
Get 'em young!

Purpose of the chapter

There has been great academic and media attention concerning physical activity of children and adolescents. While activity levels are sometimes low, and often lower than we would recommend for health, this age group is also the most active in society. Physical activity among children is often reported to be quite high, especially if it is assessed using self-report methods. However, objective assessment using movement sensors (accelerometers) suggest quite low values. For example, physical activity statistics from the British Heart Foundation (Townsend *et al.*, 2012), as illustrated in Figure 13.1, show that young people meeting national recommendations, when assessed objectively, fall to only 7 per cent of boys and no girls at the age of 11 to 15 years. Such data support the need to increase physical activity levels of young people.

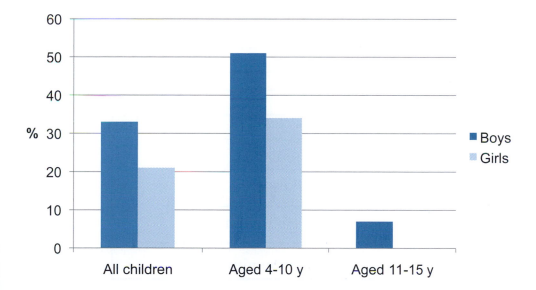

Figure 13.1 Percentage of young people in the UK meeting national physical activity recommendations, when assessed by objective monitor

Source: Data from Townsend *et al.* (2012).

Interventions to change physical activity may be categorised in different ways, including populations and settings. Interventions can target the following in the context of young people and are nested within each other, as shown in Figure 13.2:

- individuals, such as one-to-one counselling or advice by, for example, a medical practitioner;
- groups, such as educational or physical activity classes;
- organisations and communities, such as in schools or local open spaces;
- populations (society), such as through government policies.

Interventions may target certain populations, such as young girls, or adolescents, and may target change through psychological, social or environmental manipulation. Finally, it is common to attempt behaviour change in certain settings. For young people, many interventions target the school setting (Stratton *et al.*, 2008). In this chapter, we will address the evidence for how effective interventions have been in increasing physical activity for young people. In addition to looking at overall trends and mediators of behaviour change, we will summarise evidence on girls, school-based interventions, those taking place in the after-school period, active travel, the use of pedometers, community and family interventions, and those using mass media. Specifically, in this chapter we aim to:

- summarise the evidence concerning the effectiveness of physical activity interventions for children and adolescents;
- focus on interventions that have involved girls;
- appraise intervention effectiveness in different settings, including schools, after school, active travel, and communities and families;
- evaluate whether interventions using pedometers and mass media are effective for young people.

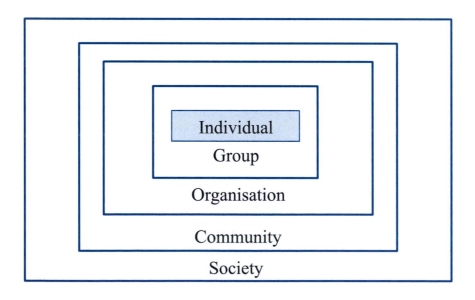

Figure 13.2 Different levels of interventions for young people

Overview of intervention effectiveness: do interventions work?

Van Sluijs and colleagues (2007) reviewed evidence on the effectiveness of interventions designed to increase physical activity in children and adolescents. Only controlled trials were analysed and were classified as educational interventions (children n = 19; adolescents n = 17), environmental or policy interventions (children n = 4; adolescents n = 1) and multi-component interventions (children n = 10; adolescents n = 6). The latter category included at least two of the former three categories. A positive intervention effect was shown in 67 per cent of trials, but only in 47 per cent of cases overall was this significant. Effectiveness was greater for adolescents (54%) than for children (42%). Results concerning the types of interventions are summarised in Table 13.1.

There were five key settings analysed: school, school plus community or family, family, community, and primary care. Results for these are summarised in Table 13.2. Again, little or no evidence for effectiveness was shown for children, and only one setting was effective for adolescents. There was 'strong' evidence for effectiveness for the school plus community or family setting. This conclusion came from two of three high-quality trials showing statistically significant positive results for the intervention.

Overall, therefore, the evidence from controlled trials for successful behaviour change interventions with children and adolescents is rather pessimistic. This could be for several reasons, including poor design of trials (only a few were rated as high quality by van Sluijs *et al.*, 2007), weak delivery (fidelity) of the intervention, inadequate statistical power to detect differences, use of self-report outcome measures, and the difficulty in combating competing behavioural demands outside of the intervention setting. The strongest evidence appears to be for adolescents using multi-component interventions or in the school setting where family components were also included.

> Key point: There is little evidence for increases in physical activity from trials with children and adolescents. The best evidence is with adolescents for multi-component interventions.

Mediators of change: what works?

From large reviews it can be difficult to conclude what may have brought about successful behaviour change (see Chapter 12). In individual trials, one way to do this is to conduct mediation analysis or to conduct a process evaluation. These allow conclusions to be drawn about what 'active ingredients' seemed to be associated with behaviour change.

Table 13.1 A summary of the main findings for types of physical activity interventions for young people (based on van Sluijs *et al.*, 2007)

Type of intervention	Children	Adolescents
Educational	No overall effect; only two rated as high quality	No overall effect; four rated as large and high quality
School environment	Limited evidence of effectiveness	Inconclusive evidence; only one trial
Multi-component	Inconclusive evidence	Strong evidence of effectiveness; includes three large high-quality trials

Table 13.2 A summary of the main findings for settings of physical activity interventions for young people (based on van Sluijs *et al.*, 2007)

Type of intervention	Children	Adolescents
School interventions	Inconclusive evidence	Inconclusive evidence
School plus family or community environment	Inconclusive evidence	Strong evidence of effectiveness; includes two large high-quality trials
Family interventions	No evidence	Inconclusive evidence
Community interventions	No evidence	Inconclusive evidence
Primary care interventions	No studies	Inconclusive evidence

Lubans and colleagues (2008) conducted a systematic review of the mediators of physical activity behaviour change in children and adolescents. Three categories of mediators were analysed: cognitive, behavioural (behaviour change strategies) and interpersonal (e.g. social support). Only seven papers were included. Self-efficacy was the main cognitive mediator of physical activity behaviour change. All studies had self-efficacy included and five showed evidence of some form of mediation (see Chapter 10). Outcome expectancies and perceived benefits of physical activity also showed some evidence of mediation. Changes in enjoyment only showed partial mediation effects, and changes in barriers did not support mediation.

Such analyses by Lubans *et al.* (2008) enable the identification of the factors that seem most likely to actually change behaviour. Too often in interventions, variables are identified as potential mediators but without being tested as such. In addition, it is often assumed in psychology that some variables are associated with behaviour change. Two such variables in the analysis by Lubans and colleagues are enjoyment and barriers. Neither supported the claim that they are mediators of physical activity behaviour change in young people. That said, the number of papers available for inclusion in the systematic review was very small. It is clear that much more work is needed to identify mediating variables, even though Baranowski *et al.* (1998) advocated this a long time ago.

> Key point: Self-efficacy is a key factor for increasing physical activity in young people.

Interventions by population groups: the case of girls

Girls are nearly always shown to have lower levels of physical activity than boys and have thus been identified as an important population group to work with (see Figure 13.1). One of the first reviews of the effects of physical activity interventions in young people was reported by Stone *et al.* (1998), who recommended that future research involve studies which investigate the success of interventions that attempt to prevent the decline in physical activity in females and adolescents. The most comprehensive review to date is that by van Sluijs and colleagues (2007), as reported earlier in this chapter. Interventions conducted with adolescents generally showed no or inconclusive effectiveness; only two categories ('school plus community plus family' and 'multi-component') showed 'strong' evidence for effectiveness. However, only eight of the included studies were exclusively on girls, and no distinction was made in the results for studies including both boys and girls where there were results for girls separately. This suggests that we need to know more about how interventions may be effective when targeting girls, either alone or in settings with boys.

Camacho-Miñano and co-workers (2011) reviewed the evidence for the effectiveness of physical activity interventions when aimed only at girls. Studies where boys and girls were together were excluded, leaving 21 interventions in their review. Results showed that 10 of the 21 interventions were successful, with seven being rated as high in methodological quality, and five of these targeted adolescent girls. Of six interventions aimed at young girls, only two were effective.

Most studies were from the USA and took place in schools. Although 14 interventions used a behavioural theory as the framework for the intervention, the review was not able to identify whether theory-based interventions were more effective or which theories might be more successful. One of the problems is that many interventions were poor in explaining how the theory was applied.

Overall, while showing some evidence for intervention effectiveness, the review by Camacho-Miñano *et al.* (2011) also showed mixed findings. The authors did conclude that they believed their results suggested that the most effective interventions were likely to be for girls in a school setting with enjoyable physical education being one intervention component, but also addressing multiple levels of influence. The latter point is consistent with the findings of van Sluijs *et al.* (2007).

We have recently conducted two meta-analyses to quantify the effect of physical activity interventions for both pre-adolescent and adolescent girls by including all intervention studies that provided results for girls separately. This was from girls-only studies as well as boys and girls in the same study but where data on girls were reported separately (Biddle *et al.*, 2014; Pearson *et al.*, 2014). This adds extra information to the reviews by van Sluijs *et al.* (2007) and Camacho-Miñano *et al.* (2011) because neither review reported all intervention studies where data for girls were available. Van Sluijs *et al.* reported findings without splitting results by gender, while Camacho-Miñano *et al.* reviewed studies on girls only but did not include studies where both girls and boys were together but where data on girls were also available.

In our two meta-analyses, the overall effect sizes for both pre-adolescent and adolescent girls were small but significant, as shown in Figure 13.3. This may suggest that changing physical activity in girls is possible, but also challenging. Current environments are not conducive to being physically active as routine and there are many competing demands on young girls' time, including wide-scale availability of sedentary pursuits.

When investigating moderators of this overall effect, it was shown that studies using multi-component interventions were more successful than those using educational or environmental approaches alone, as shown in Figure 13.3. This was true for both age groups and the larger effect sizes are clear to see. It appears, therefore, that interventions need to use various approaches together, such as combining educational and environmental approaches, as proposed when using a socio-ecological framework (Stokols, 1992). This may also be indicative of not just using psychological approaches but also embedding such methods within social and environmental changes. Seeing the 'bigger picture' – beyond just psychology – is important.

Another consistent finding across both pre-adolescent and adolescent girls was that interventions targeting just girls seemed to work better than when girls were included in interventions alongside boys. As shown in Figure 13.4, intervention effects were larger for girls-only studies, especially for pre-adolescents, although even for adolescents the effect size was almost double that for the girls-only studies in contrast to the studies with boys and girls. However, the larger effect for pre-adolescent girls was based on only six studies, so caution is needed. Nevertheless, there appears to be a clear trend in favour of girls-only interventions.

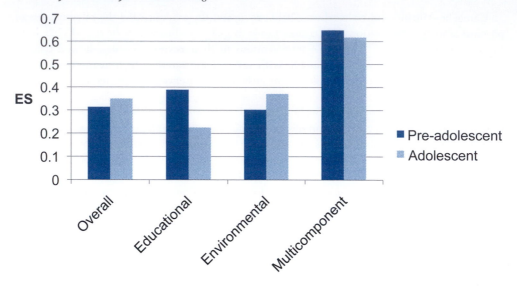

Figure 13.3 Effect sizes for three intervention types from meta-analyses of physical activity interventions for both pre-adolescent and adolescent girls
Source: Data from Biddle *et al.*, (2014); Pearson, *et al.* (2014).

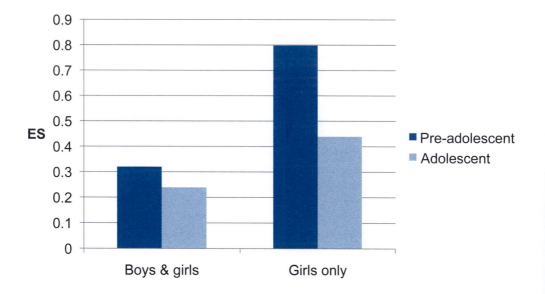

Figure 13.4 Effect sizes for studies with girls only and boys and girls combined (but data for girls' physical activity) from meta-analyses of physical activity interventions for both pre-adolescent and adolescent girls
Source: Data from Biddle *et al.* (2014); Pearson *et al.* (2014).

This may be due to girls feeling more comfortable in such environments, where comparisons with boys are eliminated, body image and self-presentational concerns reduced, and possibly greater gains in self-efficacy are evident.

Key point: Evidence suggests that physical activity for girls can be increased by having girls-only initiatives and multi-component interventions.

Interventions by settings: schools

In the reviews discussed thus far, the school setting is usually the most common location for interventions. This is not surprising, as there are a number of advantages in using schools for physical activity behaviour change studies. These include ease of recruitment and data collection and a ready-made infrastructure, including facilities and staffing.

Dobbins and colleagues have reported two Cochrane reviews on school-based physical activity interventions (Dobbins *et al.*, 2009). The latter review is a modification and update of the review reported in 2009. For the more recent review, Dobbins *et al.* include only RCTs with a minimum duration of 12 weeks and reviewed 44 studies. In addition to secondary outcomes that were mainly physiological, including blood pressure and BMI, two primary physical activity outcomes were assessed:

1. physical activity rates: percentage of the sample engaged in MVPA;
2. physical activity duration: time spent in MVPA.

Nine studies investigated physical activity rates and results were largely mixed. All studies attempted to increase MVPA in school hours, and more successful interventions involved physical education rather than other 'classroom' teachers. The quality of evidence, however, was rated as 'low', and this was interpreted as 'further research is very likely to have an important impact on our confidence in the estimate of effect and is likely to change the estimate' (Dobbins *et al.*, 2013, p. 4).

For interventions assessing the duration of MVPA, 23 studies were reviewed. While changes in the expected direction were noted, these were described as modest and the quality of evidence was again rated as 'low'. Studies that did report an effect tended to have a longer duration of intervention, and included changes to the school curriculum, often using printed educational resources.

The updated systematic review by Dobbins *et al.* (2013) led to the conclusion that there is only limited evidence that school-based interventions are successful in increasing rates and duration of MVPA, but that effects are more obvious in younger children. Studies of longer duration tended to be more successful. It was recommended to include changes to the school curriculum and to have printed educational materials. The latter supports the earlier findings that multi-component strategies may be more effective than those using single strategies (Biddle *et al.*, 2014; De Meester *et al.*, 2009; Pearson *et al.*, 2014; van Sluijs *et al.*, 2007).

A more focused review was published by De Meester *et al.* (2009) whereby they reviewed studies only for teenagers from European countries, 20 of which were school-based interventions. From these they concluded that interventions in schools do increase levels of physical activity but only in the short term. Effectiveness was also confined to school-based physical activity rather than physical activity outside of school. This is an important conclusion, as one possible outcome may be to increase school physical activity which then leads to decreases outside of school due to some kind of compensation effect. While this is plausible, more evidence is needed. Ideally, we want to see increases in and out of school time.

De Meester *et al.* (2009) drew their conclusions from whether interventions produced statistically significant differences between intervention and control groups. Crutzen (2010) conducted further analysis of the studies included in De Meester *et al.*'s review by calculating effect sizes. Crutzen confirmed that there is an increase in levels of physical activity from school-based interventions, but only in the short term. However, he also found that effect sizes showed very large variability.

A review of reviews was reported by Kriemler and colleagues (2011). In addition, they updated their review with additional primary studies. Kriemler *et al.* concur with what we have reported here, namely that interventions in schools can be effective, at least in the short term, and that such changes tend to take place in schools rather than outside. In addition, physical activity interventions tended to be more effective when only physical activity was targeted rather than being included alongside other health behaviours. Of note is that the 20 additional intervention studies reviewed by Kriemler *et al.* showed more optimistic findings and higher quality than had been the case previously.

> Key point: Interventions in schools are common but success has been patchy. Short-term changes are possible involving physical education curricula and printed support materials.

Illustrative study: use of school playground markings to increase physical activity

A long-standing context in which young people are physically active is the school break (recess) time, using the school playground (yard). Extensive research on playground modifications, such as painting playground markings, has generally been positive for physical activity, with much of this research being led by Gareth Stratton and colleagues (Stratton, 2000; Stratton *et al.*, 2008; Stratton and Leonard, 2002).

Ridgers *et al.* (2007) evaluated the effect of playgrounds being redesigned in 15 schools in areas of deprivation in England. Specifically, playgrounds were divided into three different zones and painted, as follows:

- Red: sports zone.
- Blue: multi-activity zone.
- Yellow: quiet zone.

Children were assessed prior to the markings being in place (baseline) and again at six weeks and six months. Assessments of physical activity were made using both heart rate monitors and accelerometers. Schools were allocated to intervention (n = 15) and control (n = 11) conditions. Intervention schools received extra equipment and some fencing for the active areas. Equipment was available at control schools.

As shown in Figure 13.5, there was a significant intervention effect for the playground markings. Intervention schools showed an increase in the percentage of time during break (recess) spent in MVPA. The effects show an increase from baseline to six weeks with levels largely maintained at six months. Control schools showed no changes. Boys were also more active than girls, although the effect of the intervention was effective for both sexes.

These findings suggest that simple strategies, such as zoning and painting school playgrounds, may be highly effective for increasing levels of physical activity. However,

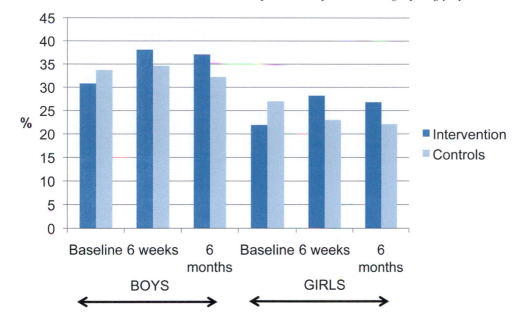

Figure 13.5 Percentage of time children spend in MVPA during break (recess) time for schools exposed to playground markings (intervention) and no markings (controls) determined by accelerometer measures

Source: Data from Ridgers *et al.* (2007).

this is likely to be most appealing to children and may decrease in its effectiveness in some adolescent age groups.

Interventions by settings: the after-school period

The interventions discussed thus far concern studies that target young people in the school setting, and usually in curriculum time. There are also studies that have focused solely on the after-school period; three systematic reviews exist and all were published around the same time (Atkin *et al.*, 2011; Beets *et al.* 2009; Pate and O'Neill, 2009).

A brief review reported by Pate and O'Neill (2009) gave very little information on their method of selecting papers, but they included 12 after-school intervention studies between 2003 and 2008. Three of five RCTs which used objective physical activity assessment showed successful behaviour change whereas the results were more mixed for three studies using self-reported measures. Although Pate and O'Neill recognised that there are some advantages to after-school programmes, including the provision of a safe environment with role models to hand, the overall results were rather mixed.

Atkin *et al.* (2011) also reported on a systematic review of after-school intervention studies published between 2002 and 2008. They reviewed nine studies and found only three which reported positive intervention effects. There was a trend for single behaviour interventions, focusing just on physical activity, to be more effective. But design and measurement issues probably account for the mixed findings.

Beets and colleagues (2009) reported a meta-analysis of 11 after-school intervention studies. As shown in Figure 13.6, there was a moderate effect on physical activity from six studies, but a small effect for physical fitness, also from six studies, and a very small effect on body composition (10 studies). However, all three effect sizes were significantly different from zero. These authors concluded that after-school programmes hold promise for increasing physical activity in youth. Interestingly, Jago and Baranowski (2004), when reviewing a range of non-curricular approaches for youth physical activity, said that the uptake of after-school programmes is typically low, yet few studies seemed to have addressed this. One issue may be that such programmes may be appealing to those who are already active, such as those playing sport. It is much less common to hear about after-school or extra-curricular physical activity initiatives specifically aimed at the less active.

> Key point: After-school programmes have had mixed success in increasing physical activity. Uptake may be low or be appealing only to those who are already active.

Interventions by settings: families and communities

The majority of interventions have focused on the school setting, including the after-school period in some cases, for understandable reasons. However, potentially key non-school settings may involve the family and wider community (Dzewaltowski, 2008; Saelens and Kerr, 2008). As stated earlier in this chapter through the findings of the comprehensive review by van Sluijs *et al.* (2007), and shown in Table 13.2, evidence for effectiveness of physical activity interventions on family and community settings alone has not been seen

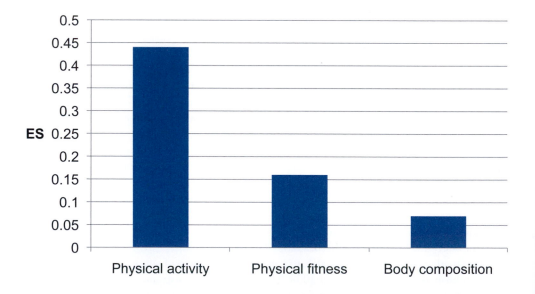

Figure 13.6 Effect sizes reported for after-school interventions on the outcomes of physical activity, physical fitness and body composition

Source: Data from Beets *et al.* (2009).

for young people. More recently, van Sluijs and colleagues (2011) have provided an update of the evidence by reviewing three previous reviews, including van Sluijs *et al.* (2007), and conducted an update on studies up until 2010. In addition to the null findings from van Sluijs *et al.* (2007), Salmon *et al.* (2007) found that only two of seven short-term and one of two long-term family-based interventions showed positive effects on physical activity. Only one of three community-based studies showed positive effects, and this was a weak design. The third review summarised by van Sluijs *et al.* (2011) was a review conducted for NICE in the development of public health guidance for physical activity for young people (NICE Public Health Collaborating Centre – Physical Activity, 2007). For interventions targeted at overweight or obese children, or those at risk for overweight or obesity, it was found that there was evidence from two of four RCTs that family-based physical activity interventions targeting such children can lead to increases in physical activity. Characteristics of successful interventions included being located in the home, and therefore not involving attendance at external sites, and focused on small, specific lifestyle changes (e.g. 2,000 more steps/day). For interventions aimed at non-obese children, there was evidence from four interventions that family-based interventions targeting physical activity can be effective. Two trials failed to show an effect. Successful interventions were located mostly in the home and predominantly involved information packs. Two of the successful interventions involved either mothers and daughters or grandmothers, mothers and daughters exercising together. The same review also looked at community-based interventions. Two studies showed no increases in physical activity in adolescents (NICE Public Health Collaborating Centre – Physical Activity, 2007).

In addition to their review of reviews, van Sluijs *et al.* (2011) conducted their own systematic review by updating evidence from primary studies between 2007 and 2010. Ten new studies were located, with six being family-based and four community-based. Three of the family-based studies showed effects for physical activity, but only one for the community interventions. Overall, van Sluijs *et al.* (2011) concluded that 'the effectiveness of family- and community-based interventions remains uncertain, especially among adolescent populations' (p. 921). Key issues in this field may be the need to better understand different family structures, norms and cultures, such as the role of parents and grandparents. In addition, it seems difficult to generalise from family-based interventions without knowing the environments in which the families are operating. Given that evidence from the correlates of physical activity for young people supports the view that parental support is important, future interventions may want to test this element more closely.

Interventions by settings: active travel

If a child in primary school walks a round trip of one mile to school and back every day of the school year, he or she will accumulate about 200 miles of walking per year. This can be a significant element in the quest to meet national guidelines for physical activity (Stratton *et al.*, 2008). However, over the past few decades parents have increasingly driven their children to school, or the distances from home to school have increased and led to more motorised transport being used. Coupled with parental fears over child safety, rates of active transport for young people remain low in most developed countries.

As part of the process of developing NICE guidance on physical activity for young people, a review was conducted on active travel (NICE Public Health Collaborating Centre – Physical Activity, 2008). Four types of approaches were identified, as shown in Figure 13.7.

It was concluded from five UK studies that cycling promotion projects targeting schoolchildren can lead to large increases in cycling. Successful interventions involved external agencies to facilitate schools to promote and maintain cycling, with the support of parents and the local community.

For 'Safe Routes to Schools' and 'School Travel Plans' there was evidence to suggest that the introduction of school travel plans was not associated with increases in walking and cycling. However, there is evidence showing that a mix of promotional measures, such as curriculum, parental and community promotions (e.g. walk and bike to school days) can increase active transport.

Walking Buses have been promoted for several years now, with parents 'top and tailing' a line of children walking to school. The NICE review found that Walking Buses can increase walking in 5- to 11-year-olds, and reduced car use for children's journeys to and from school.

There is evidence from studies in the UK and Australia that walking promotion schemes can lead to increases in walking to school for primary-age children. These involve promotional materials, incentives and rewards, travel diaries for children and parents, and provision of 'park and walk' areas close to school and restriction of parking outside of schools. Overall, therefore, the NICE review suggests that the use of cycling and walking promotion schemes, and Walking Buses can increase active transport for young people.

A systematic review was conducted by Chillon *et al.* (2011) on interventions promoting active travel to school. From 14 studies they identified the three key elements of school, parents and communities, often used in combination. Nearly all studies reported some increase in physical activity, but this was quite variable. As shown in Figure 13.8, the majority of studies showing some effect reported this to be either trivial or small. The authors said that their conclusions are limited due to the variability in studies and weak research designs used. Nevertheless, some effectiveness was shown, although it remains to be seen if increases in active travel are in addition to other forms of physical activity throughout the day, such as active play for children, or whether it simply acts as a substitute.

Key point: Active travel to school logically holds great promise for increasing physical activity levels in young people. Key strategies involve cycling promotion, walking schemes and Walking Buses.

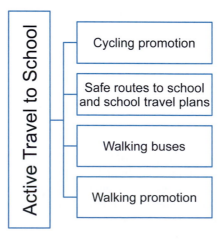

Figure 13.7 Four types of active transport strategies

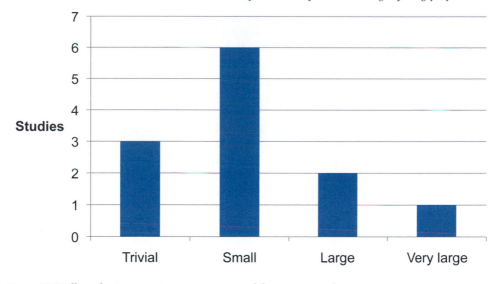

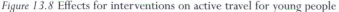

Figure 13.8 Effects for interventions on active travel for young people

Source: Data from Chillon *et al.* (2011).

Interventions using pedometers

Pedometers provide information on the number of steps the wearer has taken. They can provide valuable feedback and 'motivation' at a low cost compared to some more sophisticated new technologies. Using pedometers with young people has been common (Clemes and Biddle, 2013), and has been successful in increasing physical activity in adults (Bravata *et al.*, 2007). Moreover, self-monitoring is seen to be an important strategy enabling behaviour change (Abraham and Michie, 2008).

To see if pedometers promote physical activity in young people, Lubans and colleagues (2009) conducted a systematic review of 14 studies. All but two of these showed increases in physical activity. The majority used the pedometers for self-monitoring and goal-setting, and eight of these 10 studies were effective in behaviour change. Lubans *et al.* concluded that pedometer-based interventions are particularly effective for low active adolescents and most children.

It appears that the pedometer can both self-monitor activity as well as provide feedback and prompting for further gains, often when goal-setting is used. This is where the ubiquitous '10,000-step' target is useful (Brown *et al.*, 2006). Indeed, some have argued that simply wearing a pedometer can create a change in behaviour, and this is referred to as 'reactivity'. While there is evidence for this in adults (Clemes and Parker, 2009), it is less clear for young people (Clemes and Biddle, 2013).

Tudor-Locke and colleagues have suggested that 10,000 steps may not be the correct target for children and adolescents. They reviewed many studies and concluded that 60 minutes of physical activity at moderate to vigorous intensity appeared to be achieved within a total step count per day of 13,000 to 15,000 for boys and 11,000 to 12,000 for girls who were in the primary school age range. For adolescents (both boys and girls), 10,000 to 11,700 was associated with 60 minutes of MVPA (Tudor-Locke *et al.*, 2011). Thus it would appear that children need to aim for more than 10,000 steps per day to achieve the public health recommendations for physical activity.

Key point: Pedometer-based interventions can be effective for increasing physical activity and seem most effective for children and low active adolescents.

Interventions using mass media

Mass media campaigns and messages create diversity of views as to their effectiveness. While such methods are used frequently – after all, we are constantly bombarded with advertising for day-to-day products – many health behaviour mass media campaigns are thought to be too broad and lacking in sufficient 'power' to really change behaviour. It is the classic pay-off between wide reach but limited penetration for individual behaviour change. For example, Wakefield and co-workers (2010) concluded from their review that mass media campaigns can produce positive changes in health behaviours across large populations, although physical activity was not assessed in their research synthesis. They suggested that such outcomes are reliant on the 'availability of required services and products, availability of community-based programmes, and policies that support behaviour change' (p. 1261).

Perhaps the most extensive mass media campaign aimed at promoting physical activity in young people was the VERB campaign in the USA (see Cavill and Maibach, 2008; Collins and Wechsler, 2008). Launched in 2002, VERB – with its strap line 'it's what you do!' – was based on social marketing principles and aimed at 9- to 13-year-olds. Messages were designed to be 'fun, cool and socially appealing' and had TV advertising slots on channels popular with the targeted age group (Huhman *et al.*, 2008).

Campaign awareness was good, with at least some recall being at 74 per cent. Levels of recall were also associated with free-time physical activity levels in the first year of the campaign, as shown in Figure 13.9. The graph shows the median number of weekly free-time physical activity sessions engaged in by boys and girls differing in their levels of campaign

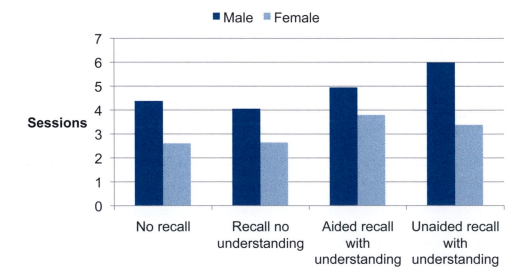

Figure 13.9 Free-time physical activity sessions per week according to level of VERB campaign recall
Source: Data from Huhman *et al.* (2005).

message recall. It is clear that those with better recall were more active. Of course, one explanation could be that more active children, and those more interested in physical activity, may seek out or better engage with such messages anyway (Huhman *et al.*, 2008); nevertheless, the results were encouraging. Those who evaluated the campaign also stated that other strategies are required to complement the mass media approach, including changes in schools and transport environments (Huhman *et al.*, 2005). Two-year follow-up data also showed good effects for the campaign (Huhman *et al.*, 2007).

Chapter summary

In this chapter, we have looked at the evidence concerning interventions designed to increase physical activity in children and adolescents. Readers are referred to Chapter 12 for more information on the nature and design of interventions. The area of behaviour change is a crucial one for physical activity psychology and ultimately, it may be argued, it is the most important area for our field. Naturally, interventions will use various approaches, and not just rely on psychology alone.

From our review of the evidence, largely using systematic reviews, we conclude the following:

1. Overall, interventions designed to increase physical activity in young people have had limited success. The best evidence is for multi-component and 'school plus family or community environment' interventions for adolescents.
2. Self-efficacy is a mediator of successful behaviour change.
3. Intervention for girls seems to work best when it targets girls-only settings and uses multi-component approaches.
4. Schools are a common setting for interventions but have shown patchy success. Short-term behaviour change is possible using physical education curricula changes and printed support materials.
5. Changing playground markings and creating activity zones can be highly effective in increasing physical activity, especially for boys.
6. After-school interventions have shown mixed success in increasing levels of physical activity and may appeal only to a limited range of individuals.
7. Interventions involving families and communities have shown some, but inconsistent, success. Home-based strategies involving focused goals or information packs hold promise.
8. Active travel is a logical area for promotion, with evidence showing success for cycling promotion initiatives, walking schemes and Walking Buses.
9. Pedometers have been successful in increasing levels of physical activity, particularly in children and low active adolescents.
10. Mass media campaigns can have wide reach, and an extensive campaign in the USA was successful.

References

Abraham, C. and Michie, S. (2008). A taxonomy of behavior change techniques used in interventions. *Health Psychology, 27*(3), 379–387.

Atkin, A.J., Gorely, T., Biddle, S.J.H., Cavill, N. and Foster, C. (2011). Interventions to promote physical activity in young people conducted in the hours immediately after school: A systematic review. *International Journal of Behavioural Medicine, 18*, 176–187.

Baranowski, T., Anderson, C. and Carmack, C. (1998). Mediating variable framework in physical activity interventions: How are we doing? How might we do better? *American Journal of Preventive Medicine, 15*(4), 266–297.

Beets, M.W., Beighle, A., Erwin, H.E. and Huberty, J.L. (2009). After-school program impact on physical activity and fitness: A meta-analysis. *American Journal of Preventive Medicine, 36*(6), 527–537.

Biddle, S.J.H., Braithwaite, R. and Pearson, N. (2014). The effectiveness of interventions to increase physical activity among young girls: A meta-analysis. *Preventive Medicine, 62*, 119–131. doi: 10.1016/j.ypmed.2014.02.009.

Bravata, D.M., Smith-Spangler, C., Sundaram, V., Gienger, A.L., Lin, N., Lewis, R. and Sirard, J.R. (2007). Using pedometers to increase physical activity and improve health: A systematic review. *JAMA, 298*(19), 2296–2304. doi: 10.1001/jama.298.19.2296.

Brown, W.J., Mummery, K., Eakin, E. and Schofield, G. (2006). 10,000 steps Rockhampton: Evaluation of a whole community approach to improving population levels of physical activity. *Journal of Physical Activity and Health, 3*, 1–14.

Camacho-Miñano, M.J., LaVoi, N.M. and Barr-Anderson, D.J. (2011). Interventions to promote physical activity among young and adolescent girls: A systematic review. *Health Education Research, 26*(6), 1025–1049. doi: 10.1093/her/cyr040.

Cavill, N. and Maibach, E.W. (2008). VERB: Demonstrating a viable national option for promoting physical activity among our children. *American Journal of Preventive Medicine, 34*(6, Supplement 1), S173–S174.

Chillon, P., Evenson, K., Vaughn, A. and Ward, D. (2011). A systematic review of interventions for promoting active transportation to school. *International Journal of Behavioral Nutrition and Physical Activity, 8*(1), 10. doi: 10.1186/1479-5868-8-10.

Clemes, S.A. and Biddle, S.J.H. (2013). The use of pedometers for monitoring physical activity in children and adolescents: measurement considerations. *Journal of Physical Activity and Health, 10*, 249–262.

Clemes, S.A. and Parker, R.A.A. (2009). Increasing our understanding of reactivity to pedometers in adults. *Medicine and Science in Sports and Exercise, 41*, 674–680. doi: 10.1249/mss.0b013e31818cae32.

Collins, J.L. and Wechsler, H. (2008). The VERB Campaign. *American Journal of Preventive Medicine, 34*(6, Supplement 1), S171–S172.

Crutzen, R. (2010). Adding effect sizes to a systematic review on interventions for promoting physical activity among European teenagers. *International Journal of Behavioral Nutrition and Physical Activity, 7*(1), 29. doi: 10.1186/1479-5868-7-29.

De Meester, F., van Lenthe, F., Spittaels, H., Lien, N. and De Bourdeaudhuij, I. (2009). Interventions for promoting physical activity among European teenagers: A systematic review. *International Journal of Behavioral Nutrition and Physical Activity, 6*(1), 82. doi: 10.1186/1479-5868-6-82.

Dobbins, M., DeCorby, K., Robeson, P., Husson, H. and Tirilis, D. (2009). School-based physical activity programs for promoting physical activity and fitness in children and adolescents aged 6–18. *Cochrane Database of Systematic Reviews, 4*, http://mrw.interscience.wiley.com/cochrane/clsysrev/articles/CD007651/pdf_fs.html.

Dobbins, M., Husson, H., DeCorby, K. and LaRocca, R.L. (2013). School-based physical activity programs for promoting physical activity and fitness in children and adolescents aged 6 to 18. *Cochrane Database of Systematic Reviews, 2*, Art. No.: CD007651. doi: 007610.001002/14651858.CD14007651.pub14651852.

Dzewaltowski, D.A. (2008). Community out-of-school physical activity promotion. In S.J.H. Biddle and A.L. Smith (eds), *Youth Physical Activity and Sedentary Behavior: Challenges and solutions* (pp. 377–401). Champaign, IL: Human Kinetics.

Huhman, M.E., Potter, L.D., Wong, F.L., Banspach, S.W., Duke, J.C. and Heitzler, C.D. (2005). Effects of mass media campaign to increase physical activity among children: Year-1 results of the VERB campaign. *Pediatrics, 116*, e277–e284.

Huhman, M.E., Potter, L.D., Duke, J.C., Judkins, D.R., Heitzler, C.D. and Wong, F.L. (2007). Evaluation of a national physical activity intervention for children: VERB Campaign, 2002–2004. *American Journal of Preventive Medicine, 32*(1), 38–43.

Huhman, M.E., Bauman, A.E. and Bowles, H.R. (2008). Initial outcomes of the VERB campaign: Tweens' awareness and understanding of campaign messages. *American Journal of Preventive Medicine, 34*(6, Supplement), S241–S248. doi: 10.1016/j.amepre.2008.03.006.

Jago, R. and Baranowski, T. (2004). Non-curricular approaches for increasing physical activity in youth: A review. *Preventive Medicine, 39*(1), 157–163.

Kriemler, S., Meyer, U., Martin, E., van Sluijs, E.M.F., Andersen, L.B. and Martin, B.W. (2011). Effect of school-based interventions on physical activity and fitness in children and adolescents: A review of reviews and systematic update. *British Journal of Sports Medicine, 45*, 923–930. doi: 10.1136/bjsports-2011-090186.

Lubans, D.R., Foster, C. and Biddle, S.J.H. (2008). A review of mediators of behavior in interventions to promote physical activity among children and adolescents. *Preventive Medicine, 47*, 463–470.

Lubans, D.R., Morgan, P.J. and Tudor-Locke, C. (2009). A systematic review of studies using pedometers to promote physical activity among youth. *Preventive Medicine, 48*(4), 307–315. doi: 10.1016/j.ypmed.2009.02.014.

NICE Public Health Collaborating Centre – Physical Activity. (2007). *Promoting Physical Activity for Children: Review 7 – Family and community interventions*. London: NICE: http://www.nice.org.uk/guidance/PH17.

———. (2008). *Promoting Physical Activity for Children: Review 5 – Children and active travel*. London: NICE: http://www.nice.org.uk/guidance/PH17.

Pate, R.R. and O'Neill, J.R. (2009). After-school interventions to increase physical activity among youth. *British Journal of Sports Medicine, 43*, 14–18.

Pearson, N.L., Braithwaite, R. and Biddle, S.J.H. (2014). The effectiveness of interventions to increase physical activity among adolescent girls: A meta-analysis. Academic Pediatrics, Online. doi: http://dx.doi.org/10.1016/j.acap.2014.08.009.

Ridgers, N.D., Stratton, G., Fairclough, S.J. and Twisk, J.W.R. (2007). Long-term effects of a playground markings and physical structures on children's recess physical activity levels. *Preventive Medicine, 44*(5), 393–397.

Saelens, B.E. and Kerr, J. (2008). The family. In S.J.H. Biddle and A.L. Smith (eds), *Youth Physical Activity and Sedentary Behavior: Challenges and solutions* (pp. 267–294). Champaign, IL: Human Kinetics.

Salmon, J., Booth, M.L., Phongsavan, P., Murphy, N. and Timperio, A. (2007). Promoting physical activity participation among children and adolescents. *Epidemiologic Reviews, 29*, 144–159.

Stokols, D. (1992). Establishing and maintaining healthy environments: Toward a social ecology of health promotion. *American Psychologist, 47*, 6–22.

Stone, E.J., McKenzie, T.L., Welk, G.J. and Booth, M.L. (1998). Effects of physical activity interventions in youth: Review and synthesis. *American Journal of Preventive Medicine, 15*, 298–315.

Stratton, G. (2000). Promoting children's physical activity in primary schools: An intervention study using playground markings. *Ergonomics, 43*, 1538–1546.

Stratton, G. and Leonard, J. (2002). The effects of playground markings on the energy expenditure of 5–7 year-old school children. *Pediatric Exercise Science, 14*, 170–180.

Stratton, G., Fairclough, S.J. and Ridgers, N.D. (2008). Physical activity levels during the school day. In A.L. Smith and S.J.H. Biddle (eds), *Youth Physical Activity and Sedentary Behavior: Challenges and solutions* (pp. 321–350). Champaign, IL: Human Kinetics.

Townsend, N., Bhatnagar, P., Wickramasinghe, K., Scarborough, P., Foster, C. and Rayner, M. (2012). *Physical Activity Statistics 2012*. London: British Heart Foundation.

Tudor-Locke, C., Craig, C.L., Beets, M.W., Belton, S., Cardon, G.M., Duncan, S. and Blair, S.N. (2011). How many steps/day are enough? For children and adolescents. *International Journal of Behavioral Nutrition Phys Act, 8*, 78. doi: 10.1186/1479-5868-8-78.

van Sluijs, E.M.F., McMinn, A.M. and Griffin, S.J. (2007). Effectiveness of interventions to promote physical activity in children and adolescents: Systematic review of controlled trials. *British Medical Journal, 335*, 703–707.

van Sluijs, E.M.F., Kriemler, S. and McMinn, A.M. (2011). The effect of family and community interventions on young people's physical activity levels: A review of reviews and updated systematic review. *British Journal of Sports Medicine, 45*, 914–922. doi: 10.1136/bjsports-2011-090187.

Wakefield, M.A., Loken, B. and Hornik, R.C. (2010). Use of mass media campaigns to change health behaviour. *Lancet, 376*, 1261–1271. doi: 10.1016/S0140-6736(10)60809-4.

14 Physical activity interventions for adults and older adults

You are never too old!

Purpose of the chapter

There has been global concern about the physical activity levels of adults and older adults. As has been pointed out in Chapter 1, the high prevalence of physical inactivity has far-reaching health, economic and social implications. Despite the widespread interest in the problems of physical inactivity, rates remain high and indeed in high-income countries there is evidence that they continue to increase (Hallal *et al.*, 2012). Interventions to promote physical activity in adults and older adults are required to reverse this trend.

In this chapter, we address the evidence for how effective interventions have been in increasing physical activity in adults and older adults. Specifically, this chapter will aim to:

- summarise the evidence concerning the effectiveness of physical activity interventions for adults and older adults;
- give examples of studies and strategies that have promoted physical activity to adults or older adults in a variety of settings (e.g. worksites and primary health care);
- focus on interventions that have promoted walking and cycling;
- discuss the use of pedometers as a tool to promote physical activity;
- describe the evidence for different mediated approaches to physical activity intervention;
- describe the evidence for physical activity interventions in ethnic minorities and socially disadvantaged groups.

Interventions in organisations

The importance of promoting physical activity through organisations is widely recognised. The advantages of such 'captive audiences' make these appealing settings for intervention. Although there are many organisational settings where physical activity can be, and sometimes is, promoted, such as prisons and churches, the two settings in which systematic work can be located for adults are the workplace and primary health care.

The workplace offers a potentially strong avenue for the delivery of interventions to promote physical activity. It has been estimated that most adults spend about a quarter of their time at their place of work during their working lives (Department of Health, 1993). If physical activity can be built into work time, this could help overcome the commonly cited barrier for physical activity of lack of time (Dugdill *et al.*, 2008). Similarly, the workplace has the advantage of targeting large numbers of adults and, at least for larger companies, may have an infrastructure to support health promotion initiatives. These may include medical support and sport/exercise facilities. Furthermore, workplaces are encouraged to play a role in the promotion of health and well-being within working adults (Department of Health, 2008; World Health Organization (WHO)/World Economic Forum, 2008).

The primary health care (PHC) setting has become popular for the testing of physical activity interventions. There are several good reasons why PHC should address physical activity promotion, including the following:

- PHC has become increasingly oriented towards prevention; therefore physical activity can more easily be promoted alongside other health behaviours, such as smoking cessation and dietary modification.
- The PHC team has regular contact with large numbers of people who could benefit from increases in physical activity. It is estimated that in Great Britain, adults on average make at least four visits to their GP each year, and this increases with age (see Office of Health Economics at http://www.ohe.org/).
- GPs (family physician; 'General Practitioner') are thought to be particularly influential in changing attitudes and behaviours, since they are often viewed as credible sources of information.

Primary care, therefore, seems an appropriate setting in which to target physical activity behaviour change. Physical activity can be promoted in this setting in different ways, including delivery of advice through brief interventions, provision of written materials, and exercise referral schemes.

Promoting physical activity in workplace settings

Public health policy now emphasises the role employers can play in promoting health and well-being among working-age adults (National Institute for Health and Clinical Excellence, 2008; Scottish Government, 2014; World Health Organization (WHO)/World Economic Forum, 2008). For example, a key delivery theme in the physical activity implementation plan for Scotland is physical activity promotion through the workplace setting, with a goal of having employers making it easier for people to be more physically active as part of their everyday working lives (Scottish Government, 2014). Some of the major benefits claimed for workplace health promotion programmes include improved work performance and lower absenteeism (Proper and van Mechelen, 2007), reduced medical costs (Baicker *et al.*, 2010), improved staff morale, and a reduction in the incidence of industrial injuries (American Institute for Preventive Medicine, 2008). In addition, workplace physical activity programmes have been shown to have significant effects on health outcomes, particularly blood lipids, anthropometric measures and diabetes risk, with some evidence for effects on quality-of-life indices and mood (Conn *et al.*, 2009).

Several systematic reviews and meta-analyses have reviewed the evidence for the effectiveness of physical activity promotion interventions at work. An early meta-analysis by Dishman *et al.* (1998) suggested that worksite interventions had little effect on physical activity levels or fitness. However, it was suggested that the lack of effectiveness should be interpreted with caution, as the majority of studies available at that time were of poor quality.

In a systematic narrative review of the effectiveness of workplace physical activity interventions across Europe, Australia, New Zealand and Canada, it was reported that the effectiveness of stair-walking interventions was limited and short-lived. However, the reviewers concluded that workplace walking interventions using pedometers could lead to increases in daily step counts (Dugdill *et al.*, 2008). It was also reported that workplace counselling positively influenced physical activity behaviour. Dugdill *et al.* concluded that there was growing evidence that workplace physical activity interventions can positively influence physical activity behaviour.

Malik *et al.* (2013) systematically reviewed the evidence for three types of worksite physical activity interventions:

1. Physical activity/exercise interventions (e.g. active travel, stair walking, exercise classes).
2. Counselling/support interventions (e.g. telephone counselling or coaching, motivational interviewing, peer support).
3. Health-promotion messages/information interventions (e.g. health checks or screening, delivery of health messages by email, posters, internet, multi-component interventions).

They reported that while all of these workplace approaches showed potential for increasing physical activity there was wide variability both in the quality of the studies and in the outcomes reported. They concluded that there remains a need for further well-designed studies to evaluate the effectiveness of worksite physical activity interventions.

Two recent meta-analyses provide quantitative evidence for the effect of worksite physical activity programmes. Meta-analysis increases the likelihood (power) of detecting a real effect if it exists, as many studies are too small to detect small effects, but when combined within a meta-analysis there is a higher chance of detecting this effect.

Abraham and Graham-Rowe (2009) assessed the effectiveness of worksite interventions to enhance physical activity. Results are depicted in Figure 14.1 and show that overall worksite interventions had small, positive effects on self-reported physical activity (d = 0.23) and fitness (d = 0.15). Some of the worksite interventions promoted general lifestyle change and others focused specifically on physical activity, and these latter interventions showed significantly greater changes in both self-reported physical activity and fitness. In addition, interventions that were focused on promoting walking (with or without a pedometer) were

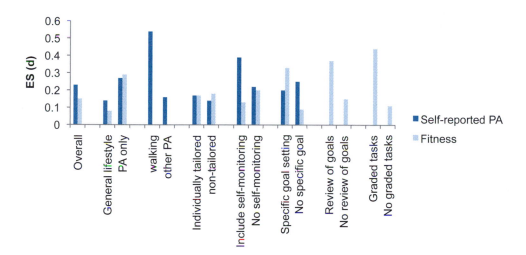

Figure 14.1 Selected results from a meta-analysis of worksite interventions

Source: Abraham and Graham-Rowe (2009).

more effective in increasing self-reported physical activity than those promoting other forms of physical activity. Interventions providing individually tailored information or instructions were not found to be more effective than those without. The inclusion of self-monitoring as a BCT appeared to improve self-reported physical activity but not fitness, suggesting that self-monitoring promotes greater awareness and hence reporting of physical activity, but not necessarily significant gains in fitness. There was evidence that specific goal-setting, goal review techniques and inclusion of graded tasks may enhance fitness gains. Similar results for physical activity behaviour (d = 0.21) were reported in a meta-analysis by Conn *et al.* (2009), although these authors found a larger, moderate effect size for fitness changes (d = 0.57). Conn and colleagues also noted that there were indications that some of the physical activity programmes improved work attendance, job satisfaction and job stress; however, these need further investigation as few studies have assessed these.

While there is some evidence that worksite physical activity interventions are effective in changing physical activity behaviour and fitness it is also useful to look at who engages with these programmes and whether programme characteristics influence participation levels. This information provides evidence about the reach of programmes and has implications for the generalisability of results. Robroek *et al.* (2009) conducted a systematic review of worksite health promotion programmes aimed at physical activity and/or nutrition. They reported that initial participation levels were low, ranging from 10 to 64 per cent with a median of 33 per cent. Low participation rates hamper external validity and will result in low cost-effectiveness. Females were more likely to participate than males in educational and multi-component programmes, but there was no difference in interventions that provided access to fitness centres. No other demographic or health status-related determinants were observed. Several programme characteristics were shown to influence initial participation. Higher initial participation was observed in programmes that offered incentives, were multi-component and which focused on multiple behaviours and not just physical activity. The authors noted that over 80 per cent of the studies identified did not provide any information about non-participants and therefore could not be included in the review. This oversight in reporting needs to be addressed, as this information is essential for the evaluation of reach and thus the public health impact of interventions (see RE-AIM in Chapter 12).

> Key point: There is some evidence that worksite physical activity programmes can lead to increases in physical activity and fitness. However, participation rates are often low, particularly in men.

Worksite example

A good example of a worksite PA intervention is the 'Walk In to Work Out' trial that we conducted in Glasgow (Mutrie *et al.*, 2002). We provided a group of participants who were recruited from workplaces with a 'Walk In to Work Out' pack, which contained written interactive materials based on the Transtheoretical Model of behaviour change (see Chapter 11), local information about distances and routes, and safety information. The control group received the pack six months later. The intervention group was almost twice as likely to increase walking to work as was the control group at six months. As shown in Figure 14.2, the contemplators – that is, those who had been considering active commuting at the beginning of the trial – added more minutes per week to their walking than the preparers. Preparers

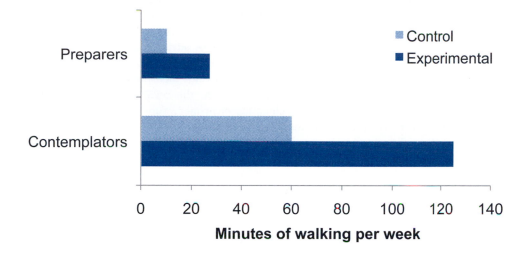

Figure 14.2 Results of the 'Walk In to Work Out' trial

Source: Mutrie *et al.* (2002).

started from a position of already achieving some walking to work and, as may be seen, the intervention was very successful in increasing walking for this group in comparison to the preparers in the control group.

The intervention was not successful at increasing cycling. There were no influences on the results for the variables of distance travelled to work, gender or age. A quarter of the intervention group, who received the pack at baseline, were regularly actively commuting at the 12-month follow-up. These materials were updated and reproduced both in Scotland and England and are now available from Healthy Working Lives (http://www. healthyworkinglives.com/).

Promoting physical activity in primary health care settings

Primary health care (PHC) has become a popular context for the testing of physical activity interventions, with exercise referral schemes (see later) developing rapidly in the UK in the 1990s (Fox *et al.*, 1997). The PHC setting offers the opportunity to counsel people who are not achieving the minimum levels of physical activity and help them become more active. Physical activity can be promoted in PHC in different ways, including delivery of advice, referral to exercise schemes, provision of information through leaflets, etc. (Orrow *et al.*, 2012). We will review evidence for the effectiveness of these different approaches.

Effectiveness of interventions

Early reviews of interventions aimed at PHC or related settings reported that most studies showed some form of improvement in physical activity; however, the effects were small and somewhat inconsistent (Riddoch *et al.*, 1998). Long-term effects were more likely with continuing intervention and multiple intervention components such as supervised exercise, provision of equipment and behavioural approaches (Simons-Morton *et al.*, 1998). A further systematic review of evidence for the effectiveness of clinician counselling to promote physical activity (Eden *et al.*, 2002) found nine trials. The review reports that two studies showed statistically significant improvements in physical activity attributed to physician counselling and three further studies showed an effect if the advice was given under certain conditions, such as with a written prescription or a written goal. There was an interesting gender difference noted in one study where women but not men increased activity levels following counselling and phone call support. However, the review concluded that the available evidence about whether or not clinicians in primary care settings can promote increased physical activity in their patients is inconclusive.

PHC exercise referral schemes are common in the UK and some other European countries. In these schemes a GP or member of the primary health team identifies and refers an individual to a third-party service (e.g. a sports or leisure centre) which typically provides a 10- to 12-week exercise programme, often tailored to the needs of the individual. Pavey and colleagues (2011) conducted a meta-analysis of eight RCTs of exercise referral schemes. The trials mainly recruited inactive, middle-aged white adults with no medical diagnosis but at least one cardiovascular risk factor. The main referrer was the GP. Exercise sessions were usually between 30 and 60 minutes in length and took place twice a week. Participants were encouraged to exercise at either a moderate intensity or individually tailored intensity. Duration of study follow-up ranged from two to 12 months. The meta-analysis showed only weak evidence of success. There was a 16 per cent increase in the likelihood of achieving 90 to 150 minutes of at least moderate physical activity per week, in the short term, as a result of an exercise referral scheme relative to a usual care group (Pavey *et al.*, 2011). No differences were observed between exercise referral schemes compared with alternative physical activity interventions. Pavey and colleagues were critical of the assumption that 10 to 12 weeks of an exercise referral scheme would lead to long-term changes in physical activity behaviour. Similarly, in a meta-analysis only examining PHC interventions with at least 12 months follow-up, Orrow *et al.* (2012) found no significant effect for exercise referral schemes on self-reported physical activity at 12 months. Further trials of exercise referral schemes with different formats (e.g. not facility based and individually tailored), longer follow-up and objective outcome measures are needed to determine whether they are an efficient use of resources. These findings show that the method of physical activity promotion is critical. More investment is needed to test ways of helping patients who require more physical activity to become more active. Currently, typical exercise referral schemes are not very successful at doing this.

An alternative to exercise referral schemes is advice or counselling from primary care practitioners. Orrow and colleagues (2012) conducted a systematic review and meta-analysis of these interventions. They only included RCTs with at least 12 months of follow-up. They identified 15 trials with a total of over 8,500 participants aged 17 to 92 years. Most of the interventions included written materials and two or more sessions of advice or counselling delivered face-to-face. Supplementary advice or counselling was provided in some interventions by telephone. Results showed a small to medium improvement in self-reported physical activity at 12 months (OR = 1.42), although no effect was found for cardiorespiratory fitness. These findings suggest that patients may have undertaken more varied forms of physical activity than typically offered through structured exercise referral, given that the referral schemes have not had much success.

In a commissioned review for the National Institute for Health and Clinical Excellence (NICE) in the UK, Campbell *et al.* (2012) reviewed the evidence for brief advice in primary care. Brief advice was defined as less than 30 minutes in duration, or delivered in one session (allowing for research follow-up only as additional contact). Twenty-one trials, including 12 RCTs, four cluster RCTs and five non-randomised controlled trials, were included in the review. Results suggest a statistically significant increase in self-reported physical activity associated with brief advice interventions compared with usual care controls. Very brief interventions (delivered in less than five minutes) were not effective. There was no clear benefit from the addition of further interventions to support brief advice on physical activity outcomes. For example, there did not appear to be additional benefit from combining brief advice with extra components such as further behavioural counselling, vouchers or written motivational material.

Campbell and colleagues (2012) applied the behaviour change taxonomy (Michie *et al.*, 2009; see also Chapter 12) to identify the most common behaviour change techniques (BCTs) used in the brief advice interventions reviewed. Five BCTs were used in over 50 per cent of the studies: prompt intention formation, provide information on consequences, general information on behaviour–health link, use of follow-up prompts, and prompt specific goal-setting.

Campbell and colleagues (2012) also reviewed 46 studies that looked at the barriers and facilitators of brief advice in PHC. Characteristics of the practitioner influenced how likely they were to provide advice. For example, factors such as how the practitioner perceives the patient and their role, the practitioner's confidence and knowledge with respect to physical activity and providing advice, their own activity levels, and belief in the effectiveness of physical activity advice all seemed to influence how likely they were to provide advice. Structural factors (e.g. lack of time, conflicting priorities, lack of incentives and other support) also influenced how likely practitioners were to provide advice. Perceived characteristics of the patient (e.g. overweight, or perceived motivation) affected a practitioners' decision to discuss or prescribe physical activity. In addition, patient characteristics may also influence the outcomes. For example, patient willingness to comply with the advice may be influenced by their current physical activity levels, their recall and understanding of the advice, and their belief that the advice applies to them and would make a difference. Furthermore, results showed that patients were more receptive of the advice if they were aware of physical activity guidelines and recommendations. A feasibility study of including brief advice and brief interventions for physical activity in routine primary care practice is currently underway in Scotland. Details of this pathway and resources for practitioners, including a useful screening tool, may be found at http://www.healthscotland.com/uploads/documents/20387-PractitionerGuide.pdf.

Guidance issued in 2006 from the National Institute for Health and Clinical Excellence cast some doubt on the continuation of exercise referral schemes (National Institute for Health and Clinical Excellence, 2006). The guidance recommended that there was insufficient evidence about the effectiveness of exercise referral schemes and further suggested that people should only be referred to schemes that are part of a robust evaluation. This may have resulted in premature withdrawal of funding for such schemes before the evidence base had been allowed to grow. This guidance for exercise referral schemes is currently being updated. However, the same 2006 guidance, and an update focused specifically on brief advice (National Institute for Health and Clinical Excellence, 2013), endorsed the use of brief interventions and gave a clear role for primary care in physical activity promotion. The 2013 guidance is more detailed than the earlier advice and recommends the following:

- Primary care practitioners, whose remit includes offering lifestyle advice, should identify adults who are not currently meeting the UK physical activity guidelines using a validated tool to assess physical activity levels. This could be done as part of a consultation, or while the person is waiting.

- For those who are insufficiently active a brief advice intervention should be delivered. This advice should be tailored to the person's motivations and goals, current physical activity and ability levels, and take account of preferences, barriers and health status. It should also include information on local opportunities for physical activity.
- The practitioner should consider giving a written outline of the advice and goals that were discussed.
- Follow-up should occur. This would include a review of what physical activity someone has been doing, and progress towards goals or meeting recommendations.

Example study from primary health care

Project PACE (Physician-based Assessment and Counselling for Exercise) was a large-scale trial of promoting physical activity in primary care (Patrick *et al.*, 1994). PACE was informed by small-scale trials of training physicians to counsel patients to increase physical activity. Project PACE used the Transtheoretical Model (see Chapter 11) to design short interventions that were delivered by family physicians. The project intervention consisted of the GP assessing initial activity levels as well as physical and psychological readiness for exercise and providing brief (three- to five-minute) counselling with each patient. The counselling focused on benefits and barriers to increasing activity, self-efficacy and gaining social support for increasing activity. The strategies differed depending on the stage of exercise behaviour of each patient and in this sense the intervention is described as stage-matched. For example, based on the current physical activity and readiness, the counselling followed one of three protocols:

- *Protocol 1*: 'Getting out of your chair' – designed for those at a low level of readiness and addresses benefits and barriers of moderate-level physical activity.
- *Protocol 2*: 'Planning the first step' – designed for those contemplating and 'ready' for exercise and involves both behavioural and exercise guidance for the adoption of physical activity.
- *Protocol 3*: 'Keeping the PACE' – designed for those who are already active, this intervention involves reinforcement as well as maintenance and relapse prevention strategies and advice.

Physicians themselves found the PACE tools acceptable (Long *et al.*, 1996) and a randomised controlled trial showed that the PACE interventions did increase physical activity, particularly walking (Calfas *et al.*, 1996). In addition, Calfas and colleagues (1997) have shown that the intervention does influence the processes of change (i.e. strategies used for behaviour change). This suggests that there is a good theoretical structure to the intervention tools, although further refinements would enhance validity.

Motivational Interviewing

Health professionals can assist people in changing their behaviour through appropriate methods of advice and counselling. One approach that has received a great deal of interest in health behaviour change is that of 'motivational interviewing' (MI). This is a 'client-centred counselling style for eliciting behaviour change by helping clients to explore and resolve ambivalence' (Rollnick and Miller, 1995, p. 326). Ambivalence is the conflict clients experience when considering the costs and benefits of taking action. For example, in considering the adoption of physical activity, an inactive person may express the view that 'exercise will be good for helping me lose weight', but also believe that 'exercise is time consuming and hard work' (see Breckon (2002) for an application of MI to exercise).

Rollnick and Miller (1995) outline what they see as the 'spirit' of MI and offer seven key points:

- Motivation for behaviour change needs to come from the client rather than be imposed by the counsellor.
- Articulation and resolution of ambivalence must come from the client rather than from the counsellor.
- The counsellor is directive in helping the client identify, examine and resolve ambivalence.
- Direct persuasion is not an effective method for resolving ambivalence.
- The counselling style is often one of quiet elicitation and opposite to direct persuasion and aggressive confrontation.
- The readiness of the client for change is not seen in terms of personality characteristics but rather as a 'fluctuating product of interpersonal interaction' (p. 327). For example, resistance to change, in MI, is a sign that the counsellor needs to modify their strategies.
- The client–counsellor relationship is one of partnership.

Rollnick and colleagues (1999) suggest that behaviour change counselling needs to centre on the three key issues of:

- *Importance*: Why should I change? Is it worthwhile?
- *Confidence*: Can I change? How will I cope if ...?
- *Readiness*: Should I do it now? What about other issues?

Readiness is likely to be strongly associated with the importance attached to change and the confidence (self-efficacy) one has to make changes. This is a very promising approach that should be applied to physical activity research using robust intervention designs in order to determine the efficacy of this behaviour change approach. In the meantime, all involved in physical activity counselling should develop these skills. As Rollnick suggested, 'Enhancing motivation and encouraging change is a complex task that demands skilful consulting and practitioners might benefit from refining their existing skills, particularly in the use of a guiding style' (Rollnick *et al.*, 2005, p. 963).

Rubak *et al.* (2005) conducted a systematic review and meta-analysis of randomised controlled trials that employed MI in a variety of health areas. When looking at the reported data from RCTs focused on physical activity/weight loss, 80 per cent of studies showed an effect for MI. Across the variety of health behaviours reviewed, the median duration of an individual counselling encounter was approximately 60 minutes. The majority of studies (81%) using encounters of 60 minutes showed a positive effect while only 64 per cent of studies using encounters of fewer than 20 minutes showed an effect. Likewise, studies in which participants received more than five sessions were more likely to show an effect (87% of studies with >5 encounters vs. 40% of studies with one encounter). The authors concluded that MI is a method that has potential for facilitating health behaviour change, and outperforms traditional advice giving.

Key point: Motivational interviewing is a counselling style that holds much promise for changing physical activity levels.

Community approaches

The interventions we have considered thus far have typically targeted individuals in specific settings, such as worksites or PHC. Although these interventions may have a significant effect on the lifestyle and health of some groups, they are likely to be local and somewhat restricted. For physical activity to have a significant effect on public health, interventions aimed at communities and mass populations must also be used. Community-wide interventions operate at multiple levels of the ecological framework (see Chapter 1) and include changes to policies and environments, but also individual-level activities such as health screening (Baker et al., 2011).

An early systematic review concluded that there was strong evidence that the use of large-scale, high-visibility, multi-strand community-wide campaigns that used a range of methods was effective in increasing physical activity (Kahn et al., 2002). The community-wide campaigns reviewed tended to address a range of risk factors and not only physical activity. They had strong communication and education elements and were directed at wide-ranging audiences. They were also likely to involve social support activities across a range of settings. The review considered these activities as a combined package and did not separate out different effect sizes for the different interventions. The review included 10 studies with the interventions ranging from six weeks to six months in duration. The median net increase in the proportion of people being active was 4.2 per cent (range -2.9% to 9.4%) and two of the 10 studies showed median net increase in energy expenditure of 16.3 per cent (range 7.6% to 21.4%). The studies were conducted in the USA or Europe and included both rural and urban areas and all socio-economic groups. Kahn et al. (2002) indicated that such interventions are likely to be effective across diverse settings and groups but that those interventions should be adapted to specific target populations.

Additional information about community interventions from the Kahn et al. review concluded that there was strong evidence that strengthening local support networks through buddy systems, walking groups and exercise contacts increased physical activity. The review of interventions that increased physical activity through improved social support in the community considered nine papers. These studies typically involved recruiting groups of people to support each other via phone calls, discussion groups considering strategies to overcome barriers, and buddying systems.

The effect sizes from five interventions showed median net increases in time spent being physically active of 44.2 per cent (Interquartile range of 19.9% to 45.6%). The evidence showed median net increases in frequency of exercise of 19.6 per cent (IQR of 14.6% to 57.6%) and median net increases in aerobic capacity of 4.7 per cent (IQR 3.3% to 6.1%). Highly structured and less formal support appeared to be equally effective. One study showed that more frequent support improved effectiveness. Again these interventions were effective across a range of countries and settings.

Hillsdon et al. (2003) conducted a review of reviews on physical activity interventions in adults. They synthesised evidence from two existing reviews. Based on this synthesis they concluded that community-based interventions which target the individual result in short- to medium-term change in physical activity. Longer term change was associated with interventions which were based on behaviour change theory and which taught behavioural skills. Interventions were more effective when they promoted moderate intensity physical activity, particularly walking, or activities that were not based in a facility. In addition, it was suggested that contact with an exercise specialist can help sustain change. The effective interventions tended to include written materials sent via the post that provide education and guidance on starting and maintaining an exercise programme, self-monitoring via logbooks and ongoing support via the telephone.

The most recent synthesis of evidence for community interventions comes from a Cochrane review by Baker *et al.* (2011). This review focused on community-wide interventions which included at least two broad strategies to increase the physical activity of the whole population. Studies also had to have a minimum six-month follow-up from the start of the intervention. After applying the inclusion criteria 25 studies were included, of which 19 were set in high-income countries. There was considerable variation in the size of the populations targeted (from <1,000 participants in two small villages to almost two million across a large region). There was also considerable variation in the interventions used; however, the majority included a component of building partnerships with local governments of non-government organisations (88%), some form of individual counselling (72%), mass media campaigns (68%), or other communication strategies (76%). Across the 25 studies results were inconsistent. In studies reporting physical activity measured as the attainment of a pre-defined amount, three out of eight studies showed an increase in physical activity, but in two of these effectiveness varied by sex (one was only effective in males, and the other only in females). Three studies used a measure of leisure-time physical activity, and three used a measure of leisure-time physical inactivity. None showed any significant change. Five studies used a measure of physical inactivity, but only one showed some evidence for a significant reduction in the proportion of people classified as inactive. In the seven studies using continuous measures of physical activity there was some evidence of effectiveness in five of the studies. The inconsistency in results may be largely due to serious methodological issues within the studies; for example, none of the studies were identified as having a low risk of bias and 15 were considered at high risk, and the remaining 10 studies were unclear. In contrast to both Kahn *et al.* (2002) and Hillsdon *et al.* (2003), Baker *et al.* concluded that the evidence does not demonstrate that multi-component community-wide interventions are effective for promoting physical activity.

Community-wide interventions thus pose a dilemma. Results for effectiveness are inconsistent, yet such interventions remain potentially the most effective way of making a significant impact on public health. Much of the inconsistency may relate to the non-trivial challenges associated with managing the content, implementation and evaluation of such large-scale and complex interventions. We should not be put off by these challenges and there is a need for further, well-designed studies with better and more frequent measures of physical activity, and attention to the allocation of intervention and control communities (Baker *et al.*, 2011).

Mass media

Mass media campaigns have been used to try to facilitate health behaviour change within large populations (Wakefield *et al.*, 2010; see Chapter 13). Such campaigns use television, radio, outdoor media (e.g. billboards and posters), and print media to disseminate the health or behaviour message. Exposure to the messaging is generally passive. An advantage of mass media campaigns is that a well-defined message can be repeatedly disseminated to a large audience, at a relatively low cost per head (Wakefield *et al.*, 2010). However, such campaigns are not without limitations – audience exposure to the message may not meet expectations, changes in the way individuals engage with media may limit exposure and, although people receive the message, they may lack the resources to actually be able to change. Despite these limitations, physical activity-promoting mass media campaigns have emerged as a promising public health practice (Heath *et al.*, 2012). In a review of mass media campaigns across a variety of health behaviours, Wakefield *et al.* reported that campaigns with mass media components aimed at physical activity yielded short-term increases in physical activity, mainly in highly motivated individuals.

Stronger evidence comes from a meta-analysis on the effect of mass media campaigns on physical activity in adults (Abioye *et al.*, 2013). Nine studies were included, and all the campaigns were conducted in high-income countries. The campaigns lasted from eight weeks to three years, and were conducted on local, regional or national levels. Four studies reported effects on reducing sedentary behaviour, and the pooled relative risk was 1.15. However, this reduced to non-significance when a low-quality study was excluded. Three studies reported effects on achieving sufficient walking (150 minutes per week), and pooled results showed that mass media campaigns increased the likelihood of sufficient walking by 53 per cent. Four studies reported the effects on achieving sufficient physical activity, but no significant effect was observed (pooled RR = 1.02). The authors concluded that mass media campaigns may improve sufficient walking but may not reduce sedentary lifestyles or encourage participants to achieve government recommendations for physical activity.

The evidence for the effectiveness of mass media campaigns for promoting physical activity in adults is mixed. But perhaps we are expecting too much from these campaigns and perhaps their greatest use is to raise awareness rather than change behaviour. For example, in an evaluation of the 'Active for Life' mass media campaign in England in the 1990s, it was shown that knowledge of physical activity guidelines increased following the campaign but physical activity levels showed no change (Hillsdon *et al.*, 2001).

Mediated approaches

Physical activity interventions may be delivered in different ways. Mediated (non-face-to-face) intervention delivery modalities, such as print, telephone and internet, offer the potential to reach large numbers of people at lower cost and more efficiently than traditional face-to-face approaches. They can also provide the repeated contacts that appear necessary to promote behaviour change (Goode *et al.*, 2012). In this section we will review the evidence for physical activity interventions employing these different delivery modalities.

Print

Print media provide a cost-effective way of conveying information to participants in interventions. In an early review of print-based programmes, Marcus *et al.* (1998) reported that they were effective in a range of settings, and led to at least short-term increases in physical activity. The print materials were used in different ways, including dissemination of general information, supplying additional support after counselling and as a means of providing follow-up. Print materials focused on lifestyle activity were more effective than those which promoted structured exercise.

Many early, or first-generation, computer-tailored interventions provided the feedback via printed documentation, although with changes in technology there has been a move away from this (see computer-tailored section). Short *et al.* (2011) suggest that there are several advantages to printed feedback that mean it should continue to be considered. First, printed feedback may have wider reach and acceptability, particularly among those with low access to the internet. Second, personal letters may have greater novelty than the ubiquitous email, and this novelty may lead to greater processing of the information. Third, if participants' preferences for mode of communication are to be taken into account, we need to acknowledge that some people prefer print. In addition, Short *et al.* report that there is some evidence that distance-based interventions are more effective when more than one delivery mode is employed.

To examine the effectiveness of tailored print interventions, Short *et al.* conducted a systematic review. They identified 12 interventions and most focused on promoting moderate to vigorous physical activity. The majority of the interventions were informed by the Transtheoretical Model (see Chapter 11) in conjunction with at least one other theory. The tailoring was based on psychosocial variables (such as barriers and self-efficacy), with some studies also tailoring based on behavioural, demographic and environmental characteristics. The authors of the review concluded that there was preliminary evidence that tailored print interventions were effective in promoting physical activity in adults (seven out of 12 of the interventions reported positive effects). Studies that included multiple contacts were more efficacious than single contact studies, suggesting that more intensive interventions, which can also provide feedback on progress, are better. However, it was not possible to determine the optimum number or time frame in which to provide the contacts. It is likely that the optimum intervention intensity is dependent on participant characteristics, with self-referred, healthy, adults perhaps requiring less contact than sedentary or 'at-risk' individuals.

Telephone

Telephone delivery remains one of the most accessible mediated approaches to intervention (Goode *et al.*, 2012). It is most often used in conjunction with other components such as printed material, pedometers, or initial face-to-face individual or group meetings. The telephone support may follow the principles of motivational interviewing or other counselling/advice approaches. The participants may be called by a real person or alternatively they may be asked to call or be called by an automated system where they 'speak with a computer' (King *et al.*, 2008). The most recent systematic review of telephone-based physical activity interventions found strong evidence for the effectiveness of telephone approaches for producing initiation of physical activity behaviour but only modest evidence for maintenance of behaviour change (Goode *et al.*, 2012). This finding was consistent with an earlier systematic review which reported positive findings in 69 per cent of physical activity studies (Eakin *et al.*, 2007). Completion of a higher number of calls and interventions of longer duration (>12 months) were associated with greater increases in physical activity. Goode *et al.* (2012) suggested that the evidence for telephone delivered interventions is so strong that further RCTs are not needed, and efforts should focus on how to integrate telephone-delivered interventions into health care and health delivery systems. Goode *et al.* reviewed two large-scale dissemination studies in older adults (Hooker *et al.*, 2005; Wilcox *et al.*, 2008), both of which showed pre-post intervention effects consistent with those observed in the original RCTs and that these changes were sustained even after a period of no contact. Although these were uncontrolled studies, they were methodologically sound, and are important for demonstrating the feasibility of translating this approach into practice.

Internet

With widespread access to the internet in many countries it is being increasingly employed as a mode for the delivery of physical activity interventions. One advantage of the internet is that individuals can access large amounts of information at a time convenient to themselves. In an early systematic review of internet-based physical activity interventions including 10 studies, it was concluded that there is indicative evidence that this approach is more effective than a wait list control (van den Berg *et al.*, 2007). In the first meta-analysis of this area, Davies *et al.* (2012) provided stronger evidence for effectiveness. The internet was the main form of delivery in the 32 studies reviewed, with web pages and/or email being used for the delivery and exchange of information. The results are depicted in Figure 14.3. The estimated effect size across the 32 included studies was small but significant (d = 0.14), indicating that internet-delivered physical activity interventions were more effective at changing behaviour than comparison conditions.

Greater effect sizes were observed in studies that targeted inactive individuals compared to those that did not screen participants for physical activity at baseline. No age or gender effects were observed. A variety of intervention components (e.g. goal-setting, self-monitoring, theoretical base) were examined as possible moderators, but only one was significant. Interventions that included educational components were more effective than those that did not. The authors concluded that while the overall effect was small, it was comparable to other intervention approaches and, given the potential reach of internet interventions, such small changes may have large effects at the population level. Furthermore, the authors argue that the public health impact may be even greater as interventions targeting inactive individuals showed the largest effect.

Computer-tailored interventions

Computer-tailored interventions employ computerised expert systems to generate feedback and advice based on information that the participant 'feeds' into the system. Algorithms are used to produce feedback automatically from a database, and this feedback is individualised

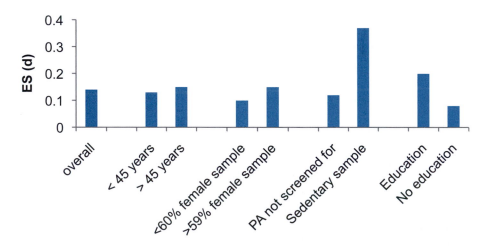

Figure 14.3 Selected results from a meta-analysis of internet-based physical activity interventions

Source: Davies *et al.* (2012).

and specific to the person based on their unique characteristics. Early, first-generation, computer-tailored interventions delivered feedback via print material. Second-generation computer-tailored interventions delivered feedback through websites and email. Third-generation interventions are emerging which employ mobile devices and may improve real-time feedback (King *et al.*, 2008).

In a meta-analysis focused on computer-tailored interventions, regardless of whether the feedback was delivered via print, telephone, or computer terminal, a small, significant, positive effect for physical activity behaviour (Hedges' g effect size = 0.16) was reported (Krebs *et al.*, 2010). The moderator analysis, which included studies focused on a variety of health behaviours, demonstrated that the effect size increased for each additional contact but there were no differences for gender, age, ethnicity or feedback delivery mode. Intervention effects declined after the intervention ended and innovative strategies are needed to maintain the observed changes.

In a review that only included second- or third-generation computer-tailored interventions, 10 of the 16 interventions found reported significant effects on physical activity or weight-reduction outcomes (Neville *et al.*, 2009). The evidence, though, is inconsistent and more work is required. Although these interventions have the potential to reach large numbers of people, there is limited evidence for whether any behaviour changes are sustained in the long term and whether they will generalise beyond the self-selected groups who have typically enrolled in the interventions.

> Key point: Mediated approaches have the potential to reach large numbers of people. Matching the approach to the target audience and individual preferences is likely to be important.

Specific behaviours

In this section we address interventions for adults that have used specific behaviours, including walking, pedometers, stair climbing and cycling.

Walking

Walking is an easily accessible form of physical activity that is popular, familiar, convenient and free (Ogilvie *et al.*, 2007). Requiring no specialised equipment it may be performed at home, at work and during leisure time, and is an activity that can be sustained across the life span. When performed at a moderate pace (~5km/hour), walking meets the definition of moderate intensity physical activity (Ainsworth *et al.*, 2000). In addition, healthy but inactive individuals who take up a programme of regular, brisk walking see improvements in $VO_{2\,max}$ and decreases in body weight, BMI, percentage body fat and resting diastolic blood pressure (Murphy *et al.*, 2007). Indeed, walking has been described as a near-perfect exercise (Morris and Hardman, 1997) and it is now an important component of national and international physical activity strategies (Global Advocacy Council for Physical Activity International Society for Physical Activity and Health, 2010; Scottish Government, 2014) and public health guidance (e.g. National Institute for Health and Clinical Excellence, 2012). The key issue is whether it is possible to successfully promote walking.

Ogilvie *et al.* (2007) conducted a systematic review of the effect of any type of walking intervention on how much people walk. Their review included 19 randomised controlled trials and 29 non-randomised controlled trials. Twenty-seven of these studies focused on walking in general and 21 focused on walking as a mode of transport. Ogilvie *et al.* reported clear evidence for an increase in walking behaviour, at least in the short term, among participants in interventions tailored to individual needs, targeted at the most sedentary individuals, and delivered either at the level of the individual or household or to groups. Strategies used included the following:

- brief advice;
- supported use of pedometers;
- telecommunications;
- individualised marketing.

The evidence for interventions delivered through worksites or the community was less convincing. The most effective intervention led to increases in walking of up to 30 to 60 minutes per week which would make a substantial contribution to increasing the physical activity levels among inactive individuals.

The promotion of walking groups, as a means to increase physical activity levels, has become increasingly popular. For example, a key delivery agent for the Scottish Physical Activity Strategy is the Walking for Health project delivered by Paths for All (http://www.pathsforall.org.uk/). The aim of Walking for Health is to increase the awareness of the benefits of being physically active as well as encourage more people to become active and stay active through walking. Through the project Paths for All have helped establish 200 community walks and 200 workplace-based walks. A similar initiative, the Walking for Health Initiative, operates in England (http://www.walkingforhealth.org.uk/). Kassavou *et al.* (2013) conducted a meta-analysis focused solely on interventions that promote walking in groups, defined as interventions where participants walk together in organised walking groups. This is a more specific focus than Ogilvie *et al.* (2007), who included under the same heading interventions where groups were formed and people walked together, and interventions delivered to groups but where the actual walking was done away from the group setting. Kassavou *et al.* (2013) included 19 studies in their meta-analysis and the results are shown in Figure 14.4. Overall, they reported a moderate effect size, demonstrating that interventions to promote walking in groups are effective at increasing physical activity. This effect size attenuated slightly when only high-quality studies were considered. Studies reporting long-term outcomes (>6 months), or that targeted both genders, or that targeted older adults (60+ years), had larger effect sizes. Interventions delivered by a layperson had similar effect sizes to those delivered by professionals.

> Key point: Walking in groups may be a pragmatic solution to reach larger numbers of people for the promotion of physical activity.

USING PEDOMETERS

Pedometers are currently being widely employed as a means to promote walking in children (see Chapter 13) and adults. Pedometers are small devices, usually worn on the waistband over the hip, that count the steps walked per day, and provide a simple and relatively inexpensive way for individuals to self-monitor their stepping-based physical activity. Most

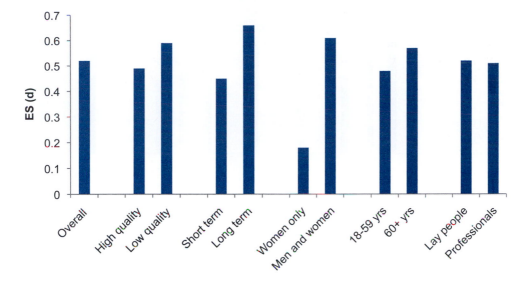

Figure 14.4 Selected results from a meta-analysis of interventions focused on walking in groups

Source: Kassavou *et al.* (2013).

modern phones can also provide pedometers in appropriate 'apps' and more sophisticated pedometers may now be worn in the pocket or even round the neck. A key issue, however, is: can they motivate people to walk more?

In a meta-analysis looking at pedometer use and physical activity in RCTs involving adults, Bravata *et al.* (2007) reported an increase of 2,004 steps per day more in the intervention group compared to the controls. In observational studies pedometer users increased their steps by 2,183 per day over baseline. Intervention effectiveness was increased when participants set a daily step goal, and in fact, pedometer use without a step goal did not result in improvement in physical activity. Furthermore, requiring participants to keep a diary of their daily steps was associated with significant increases in steps, but pedometer use without a diary was not associated with change. Pedometer interventions in worksites did not appear to be effective with only those in other settings predicting change in steps. Intervention duration and the inclusion of physical activity counselling were not predictors of increases in steps.

Another meta-analysis of 32 studies, including some with children, showed a moderate and positive effect size of 0.68 in favour of the pedometer intervention over controls, indicating that pedometers are an effective tool to increase physical activity (Kang *et al.*, 2009). The results are depicted in Figure 14.5. Moderator analyses suggest that the effects of pedometer use were similar across different age groups and intervention lengths. There was evidence that the effects were greater in projects with only female participants, followed by mixed-sex groups, then male-only studies, but this should be interpreted with caution because of the limited number of studies with male-only groups. Studies that set participants the goal of 10,000 steps/day had the largest effect, followed by those that set individualised goals and those using other types of strategies. Interventions that simply required participants to log their step counts had the lowest effect; however, this is still a moderate-sized effect.

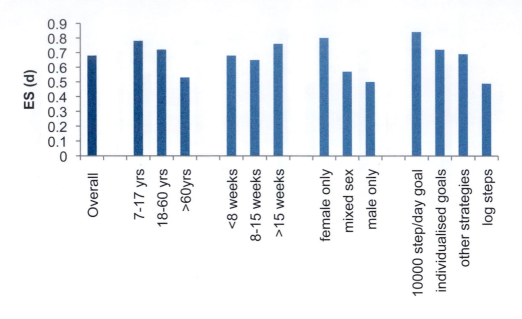

Figure 14.5 Selected results from a meta-analysis of pedometer-based physical activity interventions
Source: Kang *et al.* (2009).

A subsequent systematic review examined pedometer interventions in the workplace for increasing physical activity (Freak-Poli *et al.*, 2013). Four relevant studies were found. Intervention duration was between three and six months, and outcomes were assessed immediately after the intervention had finished. Three studies compared the pedometer intervention to a minimally active control group, but only one observed a significant increase in steps. The fourth programme compared the pedometer intervention to an alternative physical activity programme, but it was not possible to distinguish improvements associated with either programme. The authors concluded that there is insufficient evidence to assess the effectiveness of worksite pedometer interventions, and further well-designed studies are required.

After reviewing evidence-based physical activity from around the world, Heath and colleagues noted that pedometers had the highest effect size (d = 0.68) of a variety of promotional approaches (Heath *et al.*, 2012). Despite this promising outcome we suggest that the next wave of pedometer research must continue to use robust designs, incorporate objective measurement of physical activity other than walking that might be prompted by walking projects, include measures of how the environment facilitates or hinders walking and continue to follow up participants for as long as the research funding will allow. More needs to be known about the motivational effects of pedometer use, including reactivity (Clemes and Parker, 2009) and self-monitoring effects. However, pedometers are ideal self-monitoring devices, and as we suggested in Chapter 12, self-monitoring is a key behaviour change technique. So our conclusion is that pedometers are very useful devices, when used with appropriate goals, to help people self-monitor and change their walking behaviour (see also NICE guidance for walking and cycling: National Institute for Health and Clinical Excellence, 2012).

STAIR CLIMBING

Stair climbing is a specific walking activity that that can be integrated into daily life (Nocon *et al.*, 2010) and even a low volume of stair climbing can lead to positive effects on cardiorespiratory fitness (Kennedy *et al.*, 2007). A common approach to the promotion of stair climbing is the use of point-of-choice prompts. These are informational or motivational posters or banners placed near stairs, lifts (elevators) and escalators that encourage individuals to use the stairs. Nocon *et al.* (2010) conducted a systematic review to assess the effectiveness of this approach. They identified 25 studies which were primarily conducted in public transport stations (train, bus and airport), shopping malls or office buildings. Differences in effectiveness were observed between prompts used in lifts compared with escalator settings. When the prompts were placed near escalators 28 out of 32 studies showed a modest, but significant, increase in stair climbing, although the size of effect varied considerably between studies. Only three out of 10 studies of prompts near elevators showed a significant increase. Most studies reported no difference in response to the prompts between men and women. The authors concluded that point-of-decision prompts increase the rate of stair climbing, especially in escalator settings. Given the variability in size of effects, future research should focus on identifying the most suitable types of point-of-choice prompts for different settings. Soler *et al.* (2010) and Heath *et al.* (2012) reached similar conclusions in their reviews.

Webb *et al.* (2011) looked specifically at the effect of stair-climbing interventions in shopping malls. Six similar studies which used poster or banner point-of-decision prompts were combined and analysed using logistic regression. Stair climbing was shown to increase when the prompts were in place (OR = 2.09). Effects were slightly greater among women compared to men, and in adults under 60 compared to adults over 60. The authors concluded that simple poster/banner prompts can be a useful tool to encourage stair climbing in shopping mall settings.

WALKING INTERVENTION EXAMPLE

'Football Fans in Training' (FFIT) is an innovative programme developed to help men who are football (soccer) fans adopt a healthier lifestyle and lose weight. The programme was developed in Scotland and piloted on two Scottish Premier League Clubs (Gray *et al.*, 2013). The programme involves men attending 12 weekly sessions at their football club and receiving education and practical information from club coaches about how to change their lifestyle and lose weight. The programme was specifically designed for men and described as 'gender sensitised'. Nanette Mutrie has been involved since the outset as the physical activity expert in this multi-disciplinary research team.

A key element of the programme was that in week one coaches taught men how to use a pedometer to monitor their everyday step counts. A suggested set of targets for increasing steps was offered and based on evidence from studies on walking by Mutrie and colleagues (Baker *et al.*, 2008; Fitzsimons *et al.*, 2012). Other sessions focused on changing food portion size, thinking about alcohol, and working through established behaviour change techniques on all aspects of lifestyle. At each session the educational element was completed in an informal atmosphere and the coach and fans enjoyed humorous 'banter' (chat). Also at each session a new aspect of physical activity or exercise was introduced. This might have involved football skills or circuits or strength training. Coaches were trained to pay particular attention to the varying skill and fitness levels and ensure that everyone worked at their own levels.

The pilot study showed promising results in terms of weight loss and physical activity increases. The sessions were evaluated and refined in light of the comments from the participants and coaches. The full details of how we developed the programme may be found elsewhere (Gray *et al.*, 2013). Our pilot study dispelled any ideas that walking would not appeal to men. A qualitative study, with 27 telephone interviews, provided strong evidence that men enjoyed the walking and that the pedometer provided them with an ideal self-monitoring tool (Hunt *et al.*, 2013). The main findings were as follows:

- The pedometer-based part of FFIT was widely accepted.
- The pedometers were a valued technology for motivation, self-monitoring and goal-setting.
- The use of the pedometer quickly became routine in the men's daily lives.

The following quotes from three different men provide the flavour of the views expressed by the participants:

- 'It's given me a good kick up the backside … every day after I've had my shower and got dressed, the first thing that I do is put my pedometer on … it's made me consciously go out of my way to walk more.'
- 'Really good … It's an amazing wee device. … Before you maybe thought you'd been staying active but when you look at your pedometer you realise you hadnae' ['hadnae' – Scottish dialect for 'hadn't'].
- 'I love that part of it but I never go out without my (pedometer). It really is amazing. I wear it every day and record it every day. … That's tangible, something you can touch and see … I think everybody was highly delighted wi' the pedometer.'

With the benefit of funding from the National Institute for Health Research, a fully defined randomised controlled trial with over 700 football fans from all the Scottish Premier League Clubs then took place. The full study showed very similar results to the pilot. The intervention group, in comparison to the control group, lost more weight, reduced waist circumference, increased physical activity levels, changed eating habits, reduced blood pressure, and improved mood, self-esteem and quality of life (Hunt *et al.*, 2013). It was also established that delivering FFIT was cost-effective and funding is now being sought to make FFIT a programme that continues to be delivered in Scotland.

We are also in the process of evaluating this approach for other European countries (http://eurofitfp7.eu), for women fans, for rugby fans, and for prisoners in secure institutions. It really does appear that reaching into the population of sports fans provides an effective and cost-effective means of helping people change lifestyles and become more active. This could have real public health significance if it can cascade to more leagues with large numbers of fans in many parts of the world.

Cycling

Cycling, like walking, offers an active alternative to car use for short journeys (Yang *et al.*, 2010). Cycling to work has been associated with increased cardiorespiratory fitness (De Geus *et al.*, 2009) and with significant reductions in mortality even after adjustment for leisure-time physical activity (Andersen *et al.*, 2000). However, cycling levels are declining in many places and interventions are needed to reverse this decline.

Yang *et al.* (2010) systematically reviewed controlled studies focused on interventions to promote cycling. The intervention approaches reviewed included intensive support for individuals (e.g. three individual meetings with a doctor, physical activity prescriptions and the use of a free bike), improvements in the infrastructure for cycling, and multi-level community packages (e.g. media campaigns, personalised travel planning, cycle repair and cycle training services, and improvements in infrastructure). Interventions that were specifically aimed at promoting cycling were found to be associated with increases in cycling. Those interventions that promoted 'environmentally friendly' modes of transport reported small but consistent increases in cycling. However, these findings should be viewed with caution, as many of the studies were of low quality and did not report whether changes were statistically significant. Furthermore, it is unclear whether the changes observed reflect new cyclists or more cycling by existing cyclists, and the impact of changes in cycling on overall physical activity levels was not assessed. More research, with better measures, is required.

Behaviour change techniques for promoting walking and cycling

A variety of intervention approaches have been taken for the promotion of walking and cycling, and some of the inconsistency in findings may be due to differences in the behaviour change techniques employed. Bird *et al.* (2013) used the Abraham and Michie (2008) taxonomy of BCTs to explore which techniques appear to be associated with changes in walking and cycling behaviour. The studies included in the review were compiled from the Ogilvie *et al.* and Yang *et al.* systematic reviews, plus subsequent publications identified through a database search. Forty-six distinct interventions were reviewed, and were grouped into those that showed significant results (n = 21), those that showed non-significant results (n = 12) and those that did not report statistical significance (n = 13). For interventions showing statistical significance the most frequently identified BCTs were 'prompt self-monitoring of behaviour' and 'prompt intention formation' (both coded in 68 per cent of interventions). Two other BCTs, 'provide instruction' and 'prompt specific goal-setting' were coded within more than 50 per cent of the interventions. The authors concluded that although there was no evidence for a particular combination of BCTs associated with changes in walking and cycling, the 'prompt self-monitoring of behaviour' and 'prompt intention formation' techniques should be included in the design of future interventions. The authors also noted that many of the interventions with statistically non-significant results frequently included 'provide opportunities for social comparison', which may create a focus on ego rather than task orientation (see Chapter 9).

Interventions for different populations

In this final main section of the chapter, we will address intervention issues for older adults and selected other population groups.

Older adults

Older adults are a key target group for physical activity intervention due to the large proportion who are inactive (Nelson *et al.*, 2007). For example, UK data show that self-reported physical activity declines significantly with age in both men and women. When looking at objective data from England, only 5 per cent of men – and no women – older than 65 years meet government recommendations (Townsend *et al.*, 2012). To address these low levels, many interventions have been established to facilitate physical activity among older adults. In this section we will review evidence for the effectiveness of these interventions.

Conn *et al.* (2002) conducted a meta-analysis of interventions with participants with a mean age of 60 years or older. Forty-three studies with over 33,000 participants were included. Results are presented in Figure 14.6. An overall effect size of d = 0.26 was reported, indicating that the interventions had a small positive effect on physical activity behaviour. Larger effect sizes were found for patient populations, suggesting a window of opportunity for these individuals. Moderator analysis supported the inclusion of self-monitoring, but not health education. There were no differences in effect sizes between interventions that did or did not include cognitive modification, social modelling or social support. However, in a follow-up review just examining RCTs, Conn *et al.* (2003) reported that the links between individual intervention components and effectiveness were not clear.

The findings of Conn *et al.* (2002) suggested that interventions were more effective when they made specific physical activity intensity recommendations (moderate vs. low intensity), focused exclusively on physical activity rather than on multiple behaviours, and when intervention delivery was to groups rather than to individuals. Interventions with more intensive contact with participants (defined in minutes across the whole programme) had higher effect sizes.

To determine which interventions are most effective in initiating and maintaining physical activity behaviour change in the older adult, a review was undertaken by van der Bij *et al.* (2002). They analysed 38 randomised control trials reporting on 57 physical activity interventions. These were grouped as home-based (n = 9), group-based (n = 38) or education/counselling (n = 10). In the home-based interventions participants were given an exercise prescription and asked to exercise at home according to this prescription. Most prescriptions required participation in at least three moderate intensity exercise sessions per week.

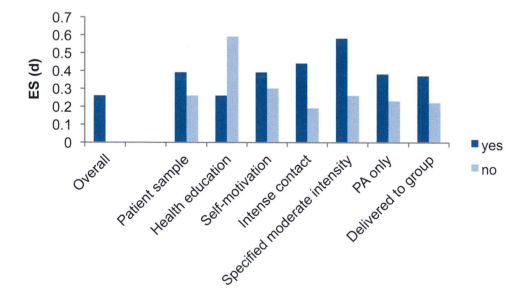

Figure 14.6 Selected results from a meta-analysis of physical activity interventions in older adults
Source: Conn *et al.* (2002).

Behavioural strategies for reinforcement (e.g. telephone calls, rewards or feedback) were included for the home-based interventions. The group-based interventions requested that individuals attend supervised group-based moderate to high intensity exercise programmes, usually three times per week. Some of these interventions also included behavioural strategies such as telephone call or mail reminders or rewards. The education/counselling interventions usually took place in a primary health care setting and involved some sort of health risk appraisal and then counselling on exercise and health with participants being encouraged to engage in regular physical activity. All the education interventions included behavioural strategies, such as follow-up visits, telephone support, goal-setting, feedback, behavioural contracting or vouchers. Participation rates in the short term (< one year) were high for both the home- (90%) and group-based (84%) interventions. However, these participation levels were not maintained in the long term (≥ one year) in either setting, although the decline in participation appeared lower in group-based interventions.

Results for the education/counselling interventions were more variable and few participants attended all sessions. Despite the low attendance rates short-term results showed a significant increase in physical activity within the intervention group, but these effects were not maintained in the long term. The failure to show long-term effects regardless of intervention strategy suggests that new strategies need to be explored with older adults (Taylor et al., 2004). A limitation of the papers included in the review was that the majority only reported participation rates and did not report changes in actual physical activity levels.

Taken together, the evidence from these reviews suggests that interventions with older adults are effective at producing small positive changes in physical activity. However, more work is needed to develop interventions that are effective in promoting larger changes, and to identify the effective behaviour change strategies in this age group (Conn et al., 2002). In addition, many of the interventions used healthy volunteers, and there is a need to explore interventions with more diverse samples, particularly with respect to functional capability.

Promoting physical activity in older adults: an example

As people grow older they consult their GPs more frequently (Eakin et al., 2000), and therefore an effective approach might be to deliver the intervention through primary care. Mutrie and colleagues piloted the idea that it might be appropriate to use the nurse in a general practice to promote activity for older adults who were registered with the primary health care practice (Macmillan et al., 2011).

The 'West End Walkers 65+' randomised controlled trial aimed to examine the feasibility of delivering a pedometer-based walking intervention to adults aged 65 years and above through a primary care setting and to determine the efficacy of this pilot. The intervention consisted of a 12-week pedometer-based graduated walking programme and physical activity consultations. Participants were randomised into an immediate intervention group (immediate group) or a 12-week waiting list control group (delayed group) who then received the intervention. The primary outcome measure was pedometer step counts. Secondary outcome measures of sedentary time and physical activity (time spent lying/sitting, standing or walking; activPAL monitor), mood (Positive and Negative Affect Schedule), functional ability (Perceived Motor-Efficacy Scale for Older Adults), quality of life (Short-Form (36) Health Survey version 2) and loneliness (UCLA Loneliness Scale) were assessed.

The pilot study showed that it was feasible to attract older adults to a physical activity intervention with 66 per cent of the over-65s registered with the practice responding and 90 per cent of those randomised completing the study. Qualitative data suggested that the pedometer and nurse were helpful to the intervention. Step counts showed a significant increase from baseline to week 12 for the intervention group while the control group showed no change. Between weeks 12 and 24, increased step counts were maintained in the intervention group, and were shown for the control group after receiving the intervention. The intervention was associated with improved quality of life and reduced sedentary time (Mutrie et al., 2012). This approach clearly has potential to reach older adults and a full-scale trial is now needed to determine if this approach is efficacious and cost-effective.

Physical activity intervention in other groups of adults

Health inequalities exist across the socio-economic spectrum and within ethnic minority groups (Department of Health, 2011). These health inequalities are reflected in health behaviours such as physical activity (Townsend et al., 2012). To address these inequalities, and avoid a widening of the gap, there may be benefit in targeting interventions specifically at these groups. But is there evidence that such approaches would lead to behaviour change?

Several systematic reviews have examined the effectiveness of physical activity interventions in socially disadvantaged groups. The first review focused on physical activity interventions in socio-economically disadvantaged communities (Cleland et al., 2012a). Fifteen interventions with adults were identified, the majority of which took place in the USA. The intervention approach in three studies targeted individuals and employed either counselling or exercise vouchers plus either a fitness assessment or exercise consultation. Results were inconsistent. The remaining 12 interventions were group-based, and eight targeted only women. Six of these studies showed small to moderate effects, four showed no effects and two provided insufficient detail to determine their effect. The authors concluded that group-based interventions targeting socially disadvantaged adults were effective for increasing physical activity. Most of the interventions were multi-component and included counselling, physical activity, education, social support and relevant incentives (e.g. gym membership, exercise vouchers).

A further systematic review and meta-analysis focused on the effectiveness of interventions to increase physical activity in socially disadvantaged women (Cleland et al., 2012b). This review included 19 studies. Mode of delivery was a key factor in determining intervention effectiveness. Specifically, group-based interventions were more effective than individual-based interventions. Group-based interventions could include group education, practical sessions or both, and could be facilitated by a trained educator, health worker or practitioner. The number of behaviour change techniques employed did not impact on intervention effectiveness and it was not possible to identify which were more effective than others. Consistent with these findings for the relative effectiveness of group-based interventions in socially disadvantaged groups, Campbell et al. (2012) reported that brief advice (which would be individual) in primary health care was less effective among socially disadvantaged groups.

Several reviews have examined interventions within different ethnic minority groups. Ickes and Sharma (2012) found that 72 per cent of the interventions included in their review of interventions in Hispanic adults reported an improvement in physical activity. Community-based interventions were the most prevalent and these likely match the sense of community that has been reported to be important within Hispanic culture. Incorporating community collaborations within the design of the intervention was seen in many of the interventions as important for improving the reach and buy-in to the programmes. There was some evidence that interventions which included staff from the same ethnic group improved recruitment and retention. For a good discussion on culturally appropriate research in physical activity, see Martinez et al. (2008).

Whitt-Glover and Kumanyika (2009) found that while 23 out of 29 studies with African-American adults showed significant within-group changes in physical activity, only 10 of the studies reported significant differences relative to a comparison group. Effectiveness was associated with the use of objective measures of physical activity, and the inclusion of specific goal-setting and structured physical activity or exercise sessions. The majority of studies indicated some attempt to adapt the programme to African-American culture (e.g. through type of music or dance used), but only three studies specifically evaluated the impact of these adaptions, and no significant differences were found between culturally adapted and unadapted programmes.

A further review focused on physical activity interventions with American Indian and Alaska native populations in the USA and Canada (Teufel-Shone *et al.*, 2009). This review included both child and adult studies, with the results presented together. Forty-one per cent of the interventions reported significant changes in health, behaviour or knowledge. Sustainability of programmes was threatened if outside partners took on too many of the leadership responsibilities and if the evaluation and intervention methods were perceived as intrusive or could not be maintained by local personnel.

Collectively, these reviews suggest that interventions targeted at specific populations are effective at facilitating physical activity behaviour change. More work is needed to understand to what extent interventions need 'cultural' adaptation to each group (Martinez *et al.*, 2008). Engaging with the target group at all stages of intervention design, implementation and evaluation is likely to positively influence the outcomes of the intervention.

Chapter summary

In this chapter, we have looked at the evidence concerning interventions to increase physical activity in adults and older adults. Several settings, populations and intervention approaches were reviewed using a combination of systematic reviews and meta-analyses. Given the complexity of physical activity behaviour change it is unlikely that any single approach will be best and a combination of behaviour change techniques and intervention approaches will be needed. Based on our review, we conclude the following:

1. Overall, interventions designed to increase physical activity in adults have a small, but positive, effect on physical activity.
2. There is some evidence that worksite physical activity interventions can lead to increases in physical activity and fitness. There remains a need for further well-designed studies.
3. Primary health care has a clear role in physical activity promotion and this may be best achieved through brief advice rather than exercise referral schemes.
4. The evidence for community-wide interventions is inconsistent.
5. There is mixed evidence for the effect of mass media approaches on physical activity, but they may play an important role in raising awareness.
6. There is evidence for the effectiveness of mediated approaches and these have the potential to reach large numbers of people at relatively low cost. However, further work is needed to establish the most effective way of using these approaches.
7. Walking is an easily accessible form of physical activity, and there is clear evidence of effectiveness for interventions promoting walking. Walking in groups may be a pragmatic solution to reach larger numbers of people.
8. Pedometers are an effective intervention tool.

9. Interventions with older adults are effective in producing small positive changes in physical activity. There is a need for further work with more diverse samples of older adults.

References

Abioye, A., Hajifathalian, K. and Danaei, G. (2013). Do mass media campaigns improve physical activity? A systematic review and meta-analysis. *Archives of Public Health, 71*, 20.

Abraham, C. and Graham-Rowe, E. (2009). Are worksite interventions effective in increasing physical activity? A systematic review and meta-analysis. *Health Psychology Review, 3*(1), 108–144.

Abraham, C. and Michie, S. (2008). A taxonomy of behavior change techniques used in interventions. *Health Psychology, 27*(3), 379–387.

Ainsworth, B., Haskell, W., Whitt, M., Irwin, M., Swartz, A., Strath, S. and Leon, A. (2000). Compendium of physical activities: An update of activity codes and MET intensities. *Medicine and Science in Sports and Exercise, 32*, s498–s516.

American Institute for Preventive Medicine. (2008). The Health and Economic Implications of Worksite Wellness Programs: Wellness White Paper. Retrieved 26 May 2014 from http://www.qigonginstitute.org/html/papers/Wellness_WhitePaper.pdf.

Andersen, L., Schnohr, P., Schroll, M. and Hein, H. (2000). All-cause mortality associated with physical activity during leisure time, work, sports, and cycling to work. *Archives of Internal Medicine, 160*, 1621–1628.

Baicker, K., Cutler, D. and Song, Z. (2010). Workplace wellness programs can generate savings. *Health Affairs, 29*(2), doi: 10.1377/hlthaff.2009.1626.

Baker, G., Gray, S., Wright, A., Fitzsimons, C., Nimmo, M., Lowry, R. and the Scottish Physical Activity Research Collaboration. (2008). The effect of a pedometer-based community walking intervention 'Walking for Wellbeing in the West' on physical activity levels and health outcomes: A 12-week randomized controlled trial. *International Journal of Behavioral Nutrition and Physical Activity, 5*(1), 44–49.

Baker, P., Francis, D., Soares, J., Weightman, A. and Foster, C. (2011). Community wide interventions for increasing physical activity (review). *Cochrane Database of Systematic Reviews, 4*. Art. No.: CD008366. doi: 10.1002/14651858.CD008366.pub2.

Bird, E., Baker, G., Mutrie, N., Ogilvie, D., Sahlqvist, S. and Powell, J. (2013). Behavior change techniques used to promote walking and cycling: A systematic review. *Health Psychology,* Advance online publication. doi: 10.1037/a0032078.

Bravata, D., Smith-Spangler, C., Sundaram, V., Gienger, A., Lin, N., Lewis, R. and Sirard, J. (2007). Using pedometers to increase physical activity and improve health: A systematic review. *Journal of the American Medical Association, 298*(19), 2296–2304.

Breckon, J. (2002). Motivational interviewing and exercise preparation. In D. Lavallee and I. Cockerill (eds), *Counselling in Sport and Exercise Contexts* (pp. 48–60). Leicester: Sport and Exercise Psychology Section of the British Psychological Society.

Calfas, K., Long, B., Sallis, J., Wooten, W., Pratt, M. and Patrick, K. (1996). A controlled trial of physical counseling to promote the adoption of physical activity. *Preventive Medicine, 25*, 225–233.

Calfas, K., Sallis, J., Oldenburg, B. and Ffrench, M. (1997). Mediators of change in physical activity following an intervention in primary care: PACE. *Preventive Medicine, 26*, 297–304.

Campbell, F., Blank, L., Messina, J., Day, M., Buckley Woods, H., Payne, N. and Armitage, C. (2012). Physical activity: Brief advice for adults in primary care (National Institute for Health and Clinical Excellence Public Health Intervention Guidance), from http://www.nice.org.uk.

Cleland, C., Tully, M., Kee, F. and Cupples, M. (2012a). The effectiveness of physical activity interventions in socio-economically disadvantaged communities: A systematic review. *Preventive Medicine, 54*, 371–380.

Cleland, V., Granados, A., Crawford, D., Winzenberg, T. and Ball, K. (2012b). Effectiveness of interventions to promote physical activity among socioeconomically disadvantaged women: A systematic review and meta-analysis. *Obesity Reviews, 14*, 197–212.

Clemes, S.A. and Parker, R.A.A. (2009). Increasing our understanding of reactivity to pedometers in adults. *Medicine and Science in Sports and Exercise, 41*, 674–680. doi: 10.1249/mss.0b013e31818cae32.

Conn, V., Valentine, J. and Cooper, H. (2002). Interventions to increase physical activity among aging adults: A meta-analysis. *Annals of Behavioral Medicine, 24*(3), 190–200.

Conn, V., Minor, M., Burks, K., Rantz, M. and Pomeroy, S. (2003). Integrative review of physical activity intervention research with aging adults. *Journal of the American Geriatrics Society, 51*(8), 1159–1168.

Conn, V., Hafdahl, A., Cooper, P., Brown, L. and Lusk, S. (2009). Meta-analysis of workplace physical activity interventions. *American Journal of Preventive Medicine, 37*(4), 330–339.

Davies, C., Spence, J., Vandelanotte, C., Caperchione, C. and Mummery, W. (2012). Meta-analysis of internet-delivered interventions to increase physical activity levels. *International Journal of Behavioral Nutrition and Physical Activity, 9*, 52.

De Geus, B., Joncheere, J. and Meeusen, R. (2009). Commuter cycling: Effect on physical performance in untrained men and women in Flanders: Minimum dose to improve indexes of fitness. *Scandanavian Journal of Medicine and Science in Sports, 19*, 179–187.

Department of Health. (1993). *The Health of the Nation: A strategy for health for England*. London: HMSO.

———. (2008). *'Working for a Healthier Tomorrow' – Dame Carol Black's review of the health of Britain's working age population*. London: The Author.

———. (2011). *Start Active, Stay Active: A report on physical activity from the four home countries' Chief Medical Officers*. London: Department of Health.

Dishman, R., Oldenburg, B., O'Neal, H. and Shephard, R. (1998). Worksite physical activity interventions. *American Journal of Preventive Medicine, 15*(4), 334–361.

Dugdill, L., Brettle, A., Hulme, C., McCluskey, S. and Long, A. (2008). Workplace physical activity interventions: A systematic review. *International Journal of Workplace Health Management, 1*, 20–40.

Eakin, E., Glasgow, R. and Riley, K. (2000). Review of primary care-based physical activity intervention studies: Effectiveness and implications for practice and future research. *Journal of Family Practice, 49*(2), 158–168.

Eakin, E., Lawler, S., Vandelanotte, C. and Owen, N. (2007). Telephone interventions for physical activity and dietary behavior change: A systematic review. *American Journal of Preventive Medicine, 32*(5), 419–434.

Eden, K., Orleans, C., Mulrow, C., Pender, N. and Teutsch, S. (2002). Does counseling by clinicans improve physical activity? A summary of evidence for the U.S. Preventive Services Task Force. *Annals of Internal Medicine, 137*(3), 208–215.

Fitzsimons, C., Baker, G., Gray, S., Nimmo, M., Mutrie, N. and The Scottish Physical Activity Research Collaboration. (2012). Does physical activity counselling enhance the effects of a pedometer-based intervention over the long-term: 12-month findings from the Walking for Wellbeing in the West study. *BMC Public Health, 12*(1), 206.

Fox, K.R., Biddle, S.J.H., Edmunds, L., Bowler, I. and Killoran, A. (1997). Physical activity promotion through primary health care in England. *British Journal of General Practice, 47*, 367–369.

Freak-Poli, R., Cumpston, M., Peeters, A. and Clemes, S. (2013). Workplace pedometer interventions for increasing physical activity. *Cochrane Database of Systematic Reviews, 4*, Art. No.: CD009209. doi: 10.1002/14651858.CD009209.pub2.

Global Advocacy Council for Physical Activity International Society for Physical Activity and Health. (2010). The Toronto Charter for Physical Activity: A Global Call to Action, from http://64.26.159.200/icpaph/en/toronto_charter.php

Goode, A., Reeves, M. and Eakin, E. (2012). Telephone-delivered interventions for physical activity and dietary behavior change: An updated systematic review. *American Journal of Preventive Medicine, 42*(1), 81–88.

Gray, C., Hunt, K., Mutrie, N., Anderson, A., Leishman, J., Dalgarno, L. and Wyke, S. (2013). Football fans in training: The development and optimization of an intervention delivered through professional sports clubs to help men lose weight, become more active and adopt healthier eating habits. *BMC Public Health, 13*, 232. doi: 210.1186/1471-2458-1113-1232.

Hallal, P., Andersen, L., Bull, F., Guthold, R., Haskell, W. and Ekelund, U. (2012). Global physical activity levels: Surveillance progress, pitfalls, and prospects. *Lancet, 380*, 247–257.

Heath, G., Parra, D., Sarmiento, O., Bo Anderson, L., Owen, N. and Goenka, S. for the Lancet Physical Activity Series Working Group. (2012). Evidence-based intervention in physical activity: lessons from around the world. *Lancet, July*, 45–54.

Hillsdon, M., Cavill, N., Nanchahal, K., Diamond, A. and White, I.R. (2001). National level promotion of physical activity: Results from England's ACTIVE for LIFE campaign. *Journal of Epidemiology and Community Health, 55*, 755–761.

Hillsdon, M., Foster, C., Naidoo, B. and Crombie, H. (2003). *A Review of the Evidence on the Effectiveness of Public Health Interventions for Increasing Physical Activity amongst Adults: A review of reviews*. London: Health Development Agency.

Hooker, S., Seavey, W., Weidmer, C., Harvey, D., Stewart, A., Gillis, D. and King, A. (2005). The California active aging community grant program: Translating science into practive to promote physical activity in older adults. *Annals of Behavioral Medicine, 29*(3), 155–165.

Hunt, K., McCann, C., Gray, C., Mutrie, N. and Wyke, S. (2013). 'You've got to walk before you run': Positive evaluations of a walking program as part of a gender-sensitized, weight-management program delivered to men through professional football clubs. *Health Psychology, 32*(1), 57–65.

Ickes, M. and Sharma, M. (2012). A systematic review of physical activity interventions in Hispanic adults. *Journal of Environmental and Public Health, Article ID 156435*, doi:10.1155/2012/156435.

Kahn, E.B., Ramsey, L.T., Brownson, R.C., Heath, G.W., Howze, E.H., Powell, K.E. and Corso, P. (2002). The effectiveness of interventions to increase physical activity. A systematic review. *American Journal of Preventive Medicine, 22*(4), 73–107.

Kang, M., Marshall, S., Barreira, T. and Lee, J-O. (2009). Effect of pedometer-based physical activity interventions. *Research Quarterly for Exercise and Sport, 90*(3), 648–655.

Kassavou, A., Turner, A. and French, D. (2013). Do interventions to promote walking in groups increase physical activity? A meta-analysis. *International Journal of Behavioral Nutrition and Physical Activity, 10*, 18.

Kennedy, R., Boreham, C., Murphy, M., Young, I. and Mutrie, N. (2007). Evaluating the effects of a low volume stairclimbing programme on measures of health-related fitness in sedentary office workers. *Journal of Sports Sciences and Medicine, 6*(4), 448–454.

King, A.C., Ahn, D.K., Oliveira, B.M., Atienza, A.A., Castro, C.M. and Gardner, C.D. (2008). Promoting physical activity through hand-held computer technology. *American Journal of Preventive Medicine, 34*(2), 138–142.

Krebs, P., Prochaska, J. and Rossi, J. (2010). A meta-analysis of computer-tailored interventions for health behavior change. *Preventive Medicine, 51*, 214–221.

Long, B., Calfas, K., Wooten, W., Sallis, J., Patrick, K., Goldstein, M. and Heath, G. (1996). A multisite field test of the acceptability of physical activity counseling in primary care: Project PACE. *American Journal of Preventive Medicine, 12*(2), 73–81.

Macmillan, F., Fitzsimons, C., Black, K., Granat, M., Grant, M., Grealy, M. and Mutrie, N. (2011). West End Walkers 65+: A randomised controlled trial of a primary care-based walking intervention for older adults: Study rationale and design. *BMC Public Health, 11*, 120. doi: 110.1186/1471-2458-1111-1120.

Malik, S., Blake, H. and Suggs, L. (2013). A systematic review of workplace health promotion interventions for increasing physical activity. *British Journal of Health Psychology, 19*, 149–180.

Marcus, B., Owen, N., Forsyth, L., Cavill, N. and Fridinger, F. (1998). Physical activity interventions using mass media, print media, and information technology. *American Journal of Preventive Medicine, 15*(4), 362–378.

Martinez, S.M., Arredondo, E.M., Ayala, G.X. and Elder, J.P. (2008). Culturally appropriate research and interventions. In A.L. Smith and S.J.H. Biddle (eds), *Youth Physical Activity and Sedentary Behavior: Challenges and solutions* (pp. 453–477). Champaign, IL: Human Kinetics.

Michie, S., Abraham, C., Whittington, C., McAteer, C. and Gupta, S. (2009). Effective techniques in healthy eating and physical activity interventions: A meta-regression. *Health Psychology, 28*(6), 690–701.

Morris, J. and Hardman, A. (1997). Walking to health. *Sports Medicine, 23*, 306–332.

Murphy, M., Nevill, A., Murtagh, E. and Holder, R. (2007). The effect of walking on fitness, fatness and resting blood pressure: A meta-analysis of randomised, controlled trials. *Preventive Medicine, 44*, 377–385.

Mutrie, N., Carney, C., Blamey, A., Crawford, F., Aitchison, T. and Whitelaw, A. (2002). 'Walk in to work out': A randomised controlled trial of self-help intervention to promote active commuting. *Journal of Epidemiology and Community Health, 56*, 407–412.

Mutrie, N., Doolin, O., Fitzsimons, C., Grant, P., Granat, M., Grealy, M. and Skelton, D. (2012). Increasing older adults' walking through primary care: Results of a pilot randomized controlled trial. *Family Practice, 29*(6), 633–642.

National Institute for Health and Clinical Excellence. (2006). Four commonly used methods to increase physical activity: Brief interventions in primary care, exercise referral schemes, pedometers and community based programmes for walking and cycling, from http://www.nice.org.uk/PH2.

———. (2008). Promoting physical activity in the workplace, from http://www.nice.org.uk/PH13.

———. (2012). Walking and cycling: Local measures to promote walking and cycling as forms of travel or recreation, from http://www.guidance.nice.org.uk/ph41.

———. (2013). Physical activity: Brief advice for adults in primary care (NICE public health guidance 44), from http://www.guidance.nice.org.uk/ph44.

Nelson, M., Rejeski, W., Blair, S., Duncan, P., Judge, J., King, A. and Castaneda-Sceppa, C. (2007). Physical activity and public health in older adults: Recommendation from the American College of Sports Medicine and the American Heart Association. *Circulation, 116*(9), 1094–1105.

Neville, L., O'Hara, B. and Milat, A. (2009). Computer-tailored physical activity behavior change interventions targeting adults: A systematic review. *International Journal of Behavioral Nutrition and Physical Activity, 6*, 30.

Nocon, M., Müller-Riemenschneider, F., Nitzschke, K. and Willich, S. (2010). Increasing physical activity with point-of-choice prompts – a systematic review. *Scandinavian Journal of Public Health, 38*(6), 633–638.

Ogilvie, D., Foster, C., Rothnie, H., Cavill, N., Hamilton, V. and Fitzsimons, C. on behaf of SPARColl. (2007). Interventions to promote walking: Systematic review. *British Medical Journal, Online First,* 10.

Orrow, G., Kinmouth, A., Sanderson, S. and Sutton, S. (2012). Effectiveness of physical activity promotion based in primary care: Systematic review and meta-analysis of randomised controlled trials. *British Medical Journal, 344*, e1389 doi:1310.1136/bmj.e1389.

Patrick, K., Sallis, J., Long, B., Calfas, K., Wooten, W. and Heath, G. (1994). PACE: Physician-based assessment and counseling for exercise, background and development. *The Physician and Sportsmedicine, 22*, 245–255.

Pavey, T., Taylor, A., Fox, K., Hillsdon, M., Anokye, N., Campbell, J. and Taylor, R. (2011). Effect of exercise referral schemes in primary care on physical activity and improving health outcomes: Systematic review and meta-analysis. *British Medical Journal, 343*, d6462. doi: 6410.1136/bmj.d6462.

Proper, K. and van Mechelen, W. (2007). *Effectiveness and economic impact of worksite interventions to promote physical activity and healthy diet. Background paper prepared for the WHO/WEF joint event on preventing noncommunicable diseases in the workplace.* Geneva: World Health Organization Press.

Riddoch, C., Puig-Ribera, A. and Cooper, A. (1998). *Effectiveness of Physical Activity Promotion Schemes in Primary Care: A review.* London: Health Education Authority.

Robroek, S., van Lenthe, F., van Empelen, P. and Burdorf, A. (2009). Determinants of participation in worksite health promotion programmes: A systematic review. *International Journal of Behavioral Nutrition and Physical Activity, 6*(26).

Rollnick, S. and Miller, W.R. (1995). What is motivational interviewing? *Behavioural and Cognitive Psychotherapy, 23*, 325–334.

Rollnick, S., Mason, P. and Butler, C. (1999). *Health Behaviour Change: A guide for practitioners.* Edinburgh: Churchill Livingstone.

Rollnick, S., Butler, C.C., McCambridge, J., Kinnersley, P., Elwyn, G. and Resnicow, K. (2005). Consultations about changing behaviour. *British Medical Journal, 331*(7522), 961–963.

Rubak, S., Sandboek, A., Lauitzen, T. and Christensen, B. (2005). Motivational interviewing: A systematic review and meta-analysis. *British Journal of General Practice, April*, 305–312.

Scottish Government. (2014). A more active Scotland: Building a legacy from the Commonwealth Games, from http://www.scotland.gov.uk.

Short, C., James, E., Plotnikoff, R. and Girgis, A. (2011). Efficacy of tailored-print interventions to promote physical activity: A systematic review of randomised trials. *International Journal of Behavioral Nutrition and Physical Activity, 11*(1), 113. doi: 110.1186/1479-5868-1188-1113.

Simons-Morton, D., Calfas, K., Oldenburg, B. and Burton, N. (1998). Effects of interventions in health care settings on physical activity or cardiorespiratory fitness. *American Journal of Preventive Medicine, 15*, 413–430.

Soler, R., Leeks, K., Ramsey Buchanan, L., Brownson, R., Heath, G., Hopkins, D. and the Task Force on Community Preventive Services. (2010). Point-of-decision prompts to increase stair use: A systematic review update. *American Journal of Peventive Medicine, 38*(2S).

Taylor, A., Cable, N., Faulkner, G., Hillsdon, M., Narici, M. and van der Bij, A. (2004). Physical activity and older adults: A review of health benefits and the effectiveness of interventions. *Journal of Sports Sciences, 22*, 703–725.

Teufel-Shone, N., Fitzgerald, C., Teufel-Shone, L. and Gamber, M. (2009). Systematic review of physical activity interventions implemented with American Indian and Alaska native populations in the United States and Canada. *American Journal of Health Promotion, 23*(6), S8–S32.

Townsend, N., Bhatnagar, P., Wickramasinghe, K., Scarborough, P., Foster, C. and Rayner, M. (2012). *Physical Activity Statistics 2012.* London: British Heart Foundation.

van den Berg, M., Schoones, J. and Vilet Vlieland, T. (2007). Internet-based physical activity interventions: A systematic review of the literature. *Journal of Medical Internet Research, 9*(3), e26.

van der Bij, A., Laurant, M. and Wensing, M. (2002). Effectiveness of physical activity interventions for older adults: A review. *American Journal of Preventive Medicine, 22*(2), 129–133.

Wakefield, M., Loken, B. and Hornik, R. (2010). Use of mass media campaigns to change health behaviour. *Lancet, 376*, 1261–1271.

Webb, O., Eves, F. and Kerr, J. (2011). A statistical summary of mall-based stair climbing interventions. *Journal of Physical Activity and Health, 8*, 558–565.

Whitt-Glover, M. and Kumanyika, S. (2009). Systematic review of interventions to increase physical activity and physical fitness in African-Americans. *American Journal of Health Promotion, 23*(6), S33–S56.

Wilcox, S., Dowda, M. and Leviton, L. (2008). Active for life: Final results from the translation of two physical activity programs. *American Journal of Preventive Medicine, 35*(4), 340–351.

World Health Organization (WHO)/World Economic Forum. (2008). *Preventing Noncommunicable Disease in the Workplace through Diet and Physical Activity.* Geneva, Switzerland: The Authors.

Yang, L., Sahlqvist, S., McMinn, A., Griffin, S. and Ogilvie, D. (2010). Interventions to promote cycling: Systematic review. *British Medical Journal, 341*, c5293. doi:5210.1136/bmj.c5293.

15 Physical activity interventions for clinical populations and conditions

Physical activity has a clear role to play in the management and treatment of many chronic diseases. This chapter will review the health benefits associated with participation in regular physical activity, focusing in particular on the psychological effects and issues concerned with adherence among people with diabetes and cancer. We have chosen these two exemplars because diabetes and cancer are, according to the World Health Organization, two of the main chronic diseases (http://www.who.int/mediacentre/factsheets/fs355/en/).

Chronic diseases are also known as non-communicable diseases (NCDs) because they are not passed from person to person and often have risk factors that could be modified. These modifiable factors include increased physical activity, reduced tobacco and alcohol use, and improved diet. NCDs are the main cause of death in all regions of the world except Africa (Lim et al., 2012). The contribution of physical activity and exercise to the management of these chronic disease states is increasingly being recognised.

Initial interest in the role of exercise for clinical populations came from physicians and exercise physiologists. They used exercise tests as part of a medical diagnosis and sought physical improvements and decreased morbidity and mortality for their patients. More recently it has been recognised that longevity is perhaps not the key issue for exercise with these patient groups, but rather quality of life and the ability to function in everyday activities are more salient issues. The American College of Sports Medicine (ACSM) has produced a comprehensive text (now in its third edition) on managing exercise programmes for clinical populations to assist the increasing number of exercise specialists in this area (American College of Sports Medicine, 1997; American College of Sports Medicine with Durstine et al., 2009). Moore (1997, p. 3), in the introductory chapter of the first edition of this text, summarised the short history of the rationale for exercise programmes with clinical populations as follows:

> [I]n the 1980s, research and clinical applications for exercise expanded to populations with a variety of chronic diseases and disabilities, for whom exercise is perhaps more fundamentally related to quality of life rather than quantity of life. Perhaps the greatest potential benefit of exercise is its ability to preserve functional capacity, freedom and independence.

The issue of quality of life has become increasingly important because health economists use measures of quality of life to quantify the benefits of different approaches to treatment. The concept of the quality adjusted life year (QALY) is used to estimate how much it would cost to improve someone's quality of life or extend that person's life with a new treatment. For more information on how the QALY is used to judge the cost-effectiveness of treatments see the National Institute for Health and Care Excellence (NICE) website (http://www. nice.org.uk). Of interest to us is that NICE reviews of physical activity interventions have all shown these interventions to be highly cost-effective.

There are two issues to be considered in discussing the role of physical activity psychology for clinical populations. First, physical activity clearly has a contribution to make to enhancing quality of life for these populations (see Chapter 2). Quality of life could be considered as a broad heading under which various physical and psychological outcomes from exercise programmes could be placed. Quality of life can be measured by life conditions, such as employment status, and, more commonly, by subjective appraisals. Such appraisals may be made using standard 'quality of life' tools such as the SF-36 (Jenkinson *et al.*, 1999) or the EQ-5D (Brooks, 1996), which is the tool often used by health economists to measure cost-effectiveness (http://www.euroqol.org). Assessments may also be made qualitatively because what is important to each person in terms of their perception of their own quality of life will vary. Felce (1997) provided a model of quality of life, which integrated objective and subjective indicators and individual values across a broad range of life domains. These domains include six areas in which quality of life issues emerge: physical, material, social, productive, emotional and civic well-being (Felce, 1997). It is clear that exercise has the potential to influence both objective and subjective indicators in this framework. The framework should assist exercise psychologists to assess the relationship between exercise and quality of life through various techniques, such as standard questionnaires, qualitative interviews and, provided that the psychologists are appropriately trained, through the use of tests of physical function.

The second issue for psychologists to consider is that, if physical activity is to be beneficial to patients, we must be able to keep them involved in activity over the longest time possible. Psychologists clearly have a role to play in understanding the process of adherence and evaluating approaches that will maximise adherence to any given physical activity or exercise plan. The process of keeping people involved in beneficial activity has been under-researched in comparison to the medical outcomes from such activities. In order to promote exercise adherence for people who have a defined medical condition, an understanding of the psycho-logical factors that affect adherence, along with an understanding of the particular challenges to exercise that the various medical conditions create, is required. The prescribed exercise treatment may present problems because people are not confident of their physical abilities, or the medical conditions themselves may present difficulties for the intending exerciser. These two issues of emphasising the psychological benefits (including quality of life) and maximising adherence will be the key points in the following two conditions of diabetes and cancer. Areas for further research will also be highlighted.

> Key point: Quality of life and long-term adherence to physical activity are key aspects for considering the beneficial effects of physical activity for populations with chronic conditions.

Diabetes

Diabetes is a growing global public health problem. The global prevalence of diabetes in 2013 was 382 million. It is estimated by 2035 that this number will rise to 592 million. In the UK, over three million people have diabetes (International Diabetes Federation, 2013).

There are two main types of diabetes. Type 1 diabetes often develops before the age of 40. In Type 1 diabetes the beta cells of the pancreas stop making insulin (hormone-regulating blood glucose) and blood glucose levels become high. The condition develops quickly and is treated with daily insulin injections in addition to healthy lifestyle participation. Type 2 diabetes has typically occurred in people over the age of 40, although the prevalence of a younger age of onset is rising (Wilmot *et al.*, 2010).

Type 2 is the most common form of diabetes, representing 85 to 90 per cent of the diabetes population. Development of Type 2 diabetes is more gradual, involving the inability of the body to produce and utilise insulin properly. Again, the resultant effect is high blood glucose levels. Treatment is healthy lifestyle alone or in combination with oral medication and/or insulin injection. In both Type 1 and Type 2 diabetes, high blood sugar levels cause substantial complications within the body and can lead to blindness, amputation, kidney failure and cardiovascular disease. The deteriorating nature of diabetes impacts upon patients' long-term quality of life and places a huge economic burden on the health service. This section discusses physical activity in relation to both Type 1 and Type 2 diabetes.

People who have either Type 1 (insulin dependent, IDDM) or Type 2 (non-insulin dependent, NIDDM) diabetes are usually advised to exercise as part of their treatment, along with medication, modification of diet and monitoring of glucose levels. The American College of Sports Medicine (Colberg *et al.*, 2010), the American Diabetes Association (American Diabetes Association, 2003) and the International Society for Paediatric and Adolescent Diabetes (ISPAD) (Robertson *et al.*, 2008) have published a comprehensive set of guidelines concerning physical activity, exercise and diabetes. These are a valuable resource for anyone working with people with either Type 1 or Type 2 diabetes. In the guidelines, the physiological and biochemical benefits of physical activity are described, in addition to guidelines on preparing for exercise and exercise prescription. Interestingly, limited information is provided on the psychological effects of physical activity or on the important issue of exercise adherence.

> Key point: The American College of Sports Medicine (ACSM), the American Diabetes Association (ADA) and the International Society for Paediatric and Adolescent Diabetes (ISPAD) provide excellent up-to-date guidelines on exercise and diabetes.

Leading an active lifestyle is also important for the prevention of Type 2 diabetes. Clinical trials (Diabetes Prevention Program Research Group, 2002; Tuomilehto *et al.*, 2001), which include physical activity as an integral part of lifestyle intervention, suggest that the onset of Type 2 diabetes can be prevented or delayed with successful intervention. In these studies, progression from impaired glucose tolerance to Type 2 diabetes was decreased by between 31 per cent and 63 per cent compared to control conditions. This is important information for people at risk of developing Type 2 diabetes, particularly those with impaired glucose tolerance. In addition, in view of the strong genetic link towards developing Type 2 diabetes, it is also important to educate those with Type 2 diabetes of these findings because they can play an important role in encouraging family members to lead a more physically active lifestyle that can prevent or delay the development of Type 2 diabetes.

> Key point: Leading an active lifestyle is important for the prevention of Type 2 diabetes.

Psychological effects of physical activity for people with diabetes

The psychological effects of facing a lifetime of dealing with diabetes, and the consequent emotional and social adjustments, are very well documented by health psychologists, as is the need for patient education about treatment (Dunn, 1993). Diabetes has generally been associated with a poorer quality of life and well-being. Several studies have reported higher levels of depression (Gavard, 1993) and anxiety (Barglow et al., 1984) in people with diabetes and it has been suggested that these states could be associated with poorer diabetes control (Barglow et al., 1984). Given the wealth of literature on these psychological issues in diabetes, and the standard recommendation that physical activity should be part of the treatment, it is surprising that neither the psychological benefits of physical activity for people with diabetes nor patient education in appropriate exercise have received much attention from researchers, although this is changing with more trials involving physical activity (Yates et al., 2008, 2009).

In a two-year observational study, Stewart et al. demonstrated how higher levels of physical activity are associated with overall better psychological functioning and well-being in adults with both Type 1 and Type 2 diabetes (Stewart et al., 1994). Glasgow and colleagues (1997) investigated the association between quality of life and the demographic, medical and self-management characteristics of 2,800 people with diabetes. Results revealed participation in physical activity to be the only significant self-management behaviour predictive of enhanced quality of life. A small number of studies have investigated the effect of physical activity on quality of life in people with Type 2 diabetes. Tessier and colleagues (2000) assessed the effect of supervised aerobic and resistance exercise in 45 elderly people with Type 2 diabetes. At 16-week follow-up no significant changes were recorded in quality of life. Ligtenberg et al. (1998) recorded significant improvements in quality of life in 51 elderly people with Type 2 diabetes after six weeks of supervised exercise training three times a week for one hour. At the end of the supervised exercise period participants were advised to continue training at home without supervision. A follow-up was conducted 14 weeks after the supervised exercise period. At this follow-up, although VO_2 max remained significantly higher than the control group, quality of life scores returned to baseline level.

Research using both individualised and group lifestyle consultation has reported favourable effects on quality of life after successful intervention over periods up to one year (Kirk et al., 2001; Pischke et al., 2006). Pischke et al. (2006) compared the effectiveness over three and 12 months of a lifestyle intervention (including group meetings for diet and exercise education and activity) for people with coronary artery disease with and without diabetes mellitus. Self-reported quality of life was poorer in those with diabetes at all time points. However, all the participants, including those with diabetes, improved their quality of life at both three and 12 months post intervention.

Our systematic review of physical activity interventions for youth with Type 1 diabetes, published in 2013, identified only three studies which included a measure of quality of life as an outcome (Macmillan et al., 2013). Of these three studies only one reported a positive effect, with the others reporting no change. Heyman and colleagues (2007) reported improved scores in the 'satisfaction with diabetes' subscale on the Diabetes Quality of Life question-naire. This was in an intervention group of adolescents with Type 1 diabetes who received a one-year, twice-weekly combined aerobic and strength training exercise programme. Limitations in methodologies, including small sample size and lack of unsupervised physical activity interventions, may account for the overall lack of significant effect reported in quality of life within physical activity interventions for youth with Type 1 diabetes.

Key point: Despite people with diabetes often reporting poorer quality of life, only limited cross-sectional and intervention research has explored the effect of physical activity participation. The small number of studies generally report positive effects.

Physical activity behaviour, barriers and motivations

There has been limited research into the barriers and motivations to physical activity among people with diabetes (see also Chapter 7). Thomas *et al.* (2004) reported that the most significant barriers to physical activity participation from a sample of 408 people with diabetes aged 20 to 84 years were as follows:

- perceived difficulty
- tiredness
- good television viewing
- access to facilities
- lack of time.

A recent qualitative study involving 25 people with Type 2 diabetes identified medical complications, lack of support, and work and family commitments as further barriers (Kirk *et al.*, 2008). Motivations towards physical activity cited were to improve health (particularly blood glucose and weight), remain independent, to have social contact, a sense of achievement, and reduced tiredness. A large-scale survey (n = 1,030) of motivations and barriers to physical activity among people with Type 1 diabetes (Marsden, 1996) suggested that fear of a hypoglycaemic event was not seen as a major barrier. Instead, and similar to non-diabetic populations, time constraints were listed as the major barrier. Motivations for physical activity were to avoid future diabetic complications and to improve physical health.

In a survey of over 23,000 US adults aged 18 years and above with diabetes, Morrato *et al.* (2003) identified that 39 per cent of adults with diabetes self-reported themselves to be physically active (participating in moderate or vigorous activity ≥30 minutes, three times a week) compared to 58 per cent of adults without diabetes. In addition, the majority of diabetic respondents (55%) reported zero minutes of weekly physical activity. Marsden's work also revealed that less than one-third of people with Type 1 diabetes took regular exercise, but that at least another third were contemplating starting or were doing some exercise on an irregular basis (Marsden, 1996). This work highlights the need for exercise education to be part of the diabetes care process.

Research investigating correlates of physical activity has identified the following variables as associated with more physical activity in adults with diabetes: male gender, younger age, more education and higher income, lower level of perceived disability, and greater perceived health benefit and performance expectations (Hays and Clark, 1999). For intervention delivery, Ferrand *et al.* (2008) reported that women with Type 2 diabetes were more likely than men to emphasise the importance of emotional and social support during physical activity behaviour change and the inclusion of group meetings. In contrast, male participants emphasised the importance of knowledge acquisition for disease control. Moreover, female participants indicated the importance of the sense of well-being and the positive body image related to regular physical activity, and male participants underlined the strength of the relationship between physical activity and health-promoting behaviours. To date, little research has explored correlates of physical activity participation in youth with Type 1 diabetes.

> Key point: Levels of physical activity participation for people with diabetes are generally lower than for people without diabetes. Being male, younger, with higher education level and income are associated with higher levels of participation.

Promoting physical activity in diabetes care

There is a clear need for further professional training in physical activity promotion for the diabetes care team. People with Type 2 diabetes report receiving the least amount of support, education and encouragement for physical activity compared to any other aspect of diabetes management. Ary *et al.* (1986) demonstrated that although 75 per cent of people with diabetes were told to exercise, only about 20 per cent received written instructions and advice. In comparison 73 per cent were given written instructions and advice about diet. Health professionals are confused about how to promote physical activity to people with diabetes. Marsden (1996) reported that health professionals admit to putting physical activity promotion last on the agenda in diabetes management largely because they do not understand how to promote physical activity or have the knowledge of the possible value that physical activity could have for their patients. Perhaps it is not surprising that the majority of people with diabetes are inactive and that attempts to become more active are often met with failure (Krug *et al.*, 1991). A study of knowledge and attitude towards physical activity among children with Type 1 diabetes also underlines the need for further education for people with diabetes, family members and professionals because the researchers (Rickabaugh and Saltarelli, 1999) found some serious gaps in knowledge about Type 1 diabetes and exercise among children and their parents and physical education (PE) teachers. Rickabaugh and Saltarelli recommended that PE teachers in particular needed pre-service training on the management of physical activity and exercise for Type 1 diabetes.

> Key point: There is a need for further professional training in physical activity promotion for health professionals and others (e.g. teachers) involved in the care of people with diabetes.

The need to take into account individual motivations and barriers, and the lack of advice regarding physical activity and exercise for this patient group, suggests that people with both Type 1 or Type 2 diabetes could benefit from physical activity consultations. Indeed, an increasing amount of research has reported on the success of physical activity consultation interventions in people with diabetes. We have published guidelines on conducting this type of intervention in people with Type 2 diabetes along with a detailed review of evidence of how effective physical activity consultation has been (Kirk *et al.*, 2007). Figure 15.1 illustrates an example pro forma for the full physical activity consultation process. This is the pro forma used within the randomised control trial by Kirk *et al.* (2004) in which the effectiveness of physical activity consultation was investigated against standard care. In this study we demonstrated the effectiveness of physical activity consultation for promotion of physical activity in people with Type 2 diabetes over six and 12 months (Kirk *et al.*, 2004).

Figure 15.1 Physical activity consultation content with examples

Source: Kirk *et al.* (2004a, 2004b, 2007).

1. Assessing stage of change

Regular physical activity can be defined as either:
- Accumulating at least 30 minutes of moderate intensity physical activity 5 days of the week.
- Participating in three 20-minute continuous sessions of vigorous exercise a week.
- Or a combination of moderate and vigorous sessions.

1: Not thinking about doing more physical activity
2: Starting to think about doing more physical activity
3: Being physically active occasionally, but not regularly
4: Being regularly physically active for less than six months
5: Being regularly physically active for longer than six months

2. Explain what physical activity is and intensity level

Explain different forms of physical activity: *active living (e.g. walking, taking the stairs); exercise (e.g. swimming, exercise class); sport (e.g. football, hockey)*

3. Why be more active?

Detail benefits of physical activity for individual.

4. Decision balance

Go through pros and cons of increasing physical activity.

Pros and cons of becoming more active

Your pros of becoming more active	Your cons of becoming more active
1. Better diabetes control	1. Interfere with other commitments
2. Weight management	2. Cost
3. Feel fitter	

5. Overcoming barriers

Discuss ways of overcoming barriers to becoming more active.

Barriers	Ways to overcome barriers
1. Might have a hypo	1. Educate patient about risk of hypo and how to prevent and treat
2. Feel sore after exercise	2. Discuss suitable activities which will not cause soreness
3. No one to exercise with	3. Establish support buddy for exercise or suggest an appropriate exercise class

6. Evaluate current physical activity level

7. Go through current guidelines and discuss discrepancy between guidelines and individual's level of physical activity

8. Identifying opportunities

Activities you might consider
1. Walking
2. Swimming
3. Dancing

Planning what to do and where and when it will take place. Make first-week goals within reach from where they are now. Two to three days with new activities is a good way to start. Think of taking at least four weeks to build up to the 30 minutes on most days of the week target.

Day of week	What, when and where	✓ When you achieve
Monday	Go for a walk with a friend in the park at lunchtime	
Tuesday		
Wednesday	Go for a walk with a friend in the park at lunchtime	
Thursday	Go and watch the water exercise class at 6 p.m. at the local leisure centre	
Friday	Go for a walk with husband in the evening after tea	
Saturday	Try out some exercises in the house with some music on after breakfast	
Sunday		

9. Assess and develop self-efficacy (modelling, verbal persuasion, mastery experience, emotional arousal)

10. Develop long-term goals

One month	Three months	Six months
1. Walk back from work (10 minutes) at least three days a week	Increase walking to accumulate at least 40 minutes/day, five times a week	Complete sponsored 4km walk
2.		

11. Finding support

What do they need help with? For example, someone to: be active with you, offer expertise or good advice, motivate you to be active.

Name	What things would you like them to do to help?
Friend	Go out walking with during two lunch breaks
Diabetes nurse	Provided information on appropriate types of activity and monitor success

12. Relapse prevention: Maintaining behaviour change

Triggers or risky situations that may cause a lapse in my physical activity	What can you do to prevent these lapses?
1. Busy at work	1. Try to be more active around the workplace. Go for a walk at lunchtime.
2. Going on holiday	2. Try out new activities on holiday. Walk to explore. Arrange with a friend to do an activity on your return.
3. Illness	3. Once you feel better make a plan to gradually get back to doing more activity.

Participants assigned to the intervention group received a physical activity consultation at baseline and six months, with supporting phone calls one and three months after each consultation. Participants in the control group received the standard, usual care, physical activity/ exercise and diabetes leaflet. In comparison to the control group, participants receiving the physical activity consultation intervention demonstrated consistent improvements in both subjective and objective measures of physical activity levels and positive changes in outcomes of behaviour change. Figure 15.2 illustrates the change in physical activity measured objectively using an accelerometer. From baseline to six and 12 months, average increases of 150 and 130 minutes of moderate to vigorous physical activity were recorded, respectively, by the intervention group.

Favourable effects were also recorded in glycaemic control, cardiorespiratory fitness, blood pressure, total cholesterol, and a small number of quality of life indices, including physical functioning and limitations in usual role activities due to emotional health problems, measured by the SF-36 and perceived anxiety measured by the diabetes well-being questionnaire. Throughout the study period, the control group recorded a decrease in physical activity levels, deterioration in glycaemic control and small (although not significant) deteriorations in quality of life (Kirk *et al.*, 2004a). This finding highlights the point that basic educational exercise and diabetes leaflets, often used in current routine care, are not effective in stimulating physical activity behaviour change in people with Type 2 diabetes.

Di Loreto *et al.* (2003) also demonstrated effective physical activity promotion over two years in people with Type 2 diabetes, using brief physician-based physical activity consultation.

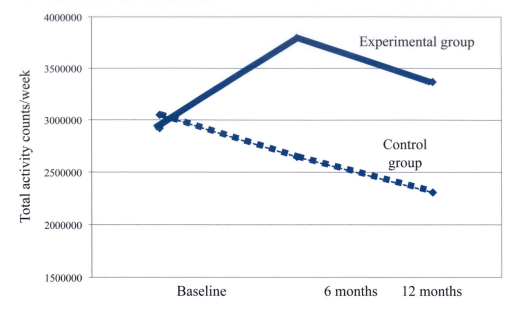

Figure 15.2 Total activity counts/week at baseline, 6 and 12 months by group

Source: Kirk *et al.* (2004a).

The intervention used in this study was individualised and incorporated cognitive behavioural strategies. Each intervention participant received a physical activity consultation at baseline and this was supported with a phone call one month later and appointments at the diabetes outpatient clinic every three months. The control group received usual care in the form of general educational advice. After two years, the intervention group recorded a sevenfold increase in physical activity levels in addition to a significant decrease in BMI and HbA_{1c}. The control group recorded a significant increase in BMI and no significant changes in physical activity levels or $HbA_{1c.}$

> Key point: Physical activity consultation is an intervention with proven success in promoting and maintaining physical activity in people with diabetes. Guidelines are available on how to conduct this intervention.

Marsden and Kirk (2005) have provided an excellent practical guide for undertaking physical activity consultations and constructing exercise and physical activity programmes for people with diabetes (Marsden and Kirk, 2005). The special challenge to people with Type 1 diabetes is to balance insulin control, glucose and physical activity bouts. People with Type 1 diabetes and their families need adequate knowledge of how to do this, including the knowledge that exercise should not be undertaken with high levels (>250 mg/dl) of blood glucose. Blood glucose monitoring should therefore be encouraged before and after exercise. People with Type 2 diabetes may have different challenges that include being overweight and, perhaps, feeling less motivated to deal with their condition, as well as coping with additional health complications. The special challenge in working with overweight individuals is to find activities that do not increase the stress on joints and that avoid potential embarrassment. Swimming may seem like an obvious non-weight-bearing activity, but swimsuits and public swimming pools may be too threatening for many obese people. The active living message, and walking in particular, may prove more realistic for this patient group.

Cancer

Psychologists have recognised for some time that coping with the diagnosis and treatment of cancer may require assistance in the form of psychological interventions (Anderson, 1992). Exercise as part of a treatment regime for cancer patients has the potential to improve both physical (e.g. fatigue, nausea, weight change) and psychological functioning, although it was originally believed that exercise was unlikely to have positive effects on the cancer itself. For example, Simon (1990, p. 586) concluded a discussion of exercise immunity, cancer and infection by stating:

> There is little systematic information dealing with the role of exercise in the functional or psychological rehabilitation of cancer patients. There is little reason to expect that exercise training will help induce remissions in these patients, but there is good reason to expect that exercise may improve their quality of life.

Since 1990, there has been a considerable increase in the knowledge about how physical activity may be of benefit to people who have had a diagnosis of cancer. During cancer treatment and rehabilitation, 'rest is best' was the traditional approach and people with cancer were generally advised to avoid exercise. However, there are several important reasons why people with cancer should be active. Low levels of physical activity in people with cancer result in further deconditioning, and symptoms of fatigue, loss of functional capacity and reductions in quality of life (Courneya and Friedenreich, 1999; Lucia et al., 2003; Stricker et al., 2004). People who are inactive and have cancer may also be at higher risk of secondary tumours (Demark-Wahnefried et al., 2000). A study of breast cancer survivors indicated a 50 per cent risk reduction in mortality among those who are regularly active when compared to those who are inactive (Holmes et al., 2005). Furthermore, physical activity levels tend to reduce following cancer diagnosis and remain low after treatment is completed (Blanchard et al., 2003; Friedenrich and Courneya, 1996). From this low baseline, there is great scope for physical activity interventions to improve the health and well-being of people with cancer.

Key point: There are several important reasons why people with cancer should be active. Low levels of physical activity result in further deconditioning, symptoms of fatigue, loss of functional capacity, reductions in quality of life, and higher risk of secondary tumours.

An early systematic review of 33 controlled trials showed moderate support for physical activity improving physical function, and no evidence of any adverse effects, but there were insufficient studies of good quality to make clear conclusions about quality of life outcomes (Stevinson et al., 2004). The most recent systematic review, conducted to the high standards of the Cochrane Library, found 40 studies of survivors of various cancers and concluded that there was now sufficient evidence to show that physical activity can have a positive impact on health-related quality of life (Mishra *et al.*, 2012). The authors of this review note that there is a need for further research about how to sustain these positive benefits over time.

The contribution of Kerry Courneya

Kerry Courneya and his colleagues in Canada have had a major impact on our knowledge of exercise psychology in relation to cancer. Courneya has contributed to several reviews that indicate the beneficial role (physical, psychological and immunological) exercise can play for people who have had a diagnosis of cancer (Ballard-Barbash *et al.*, 2012; Courneya, 2003; Courneya *et al.*, 2002; Fairey *et al.*, 2002; Schmitz *et al.*, 2005). He has also made a considerable contribution to our understanding of adherence for exercise in people with cancer (Courneya *et al.*, 2004, 2012; Karvinen *et al.*, 2005; Rogers *et al.*, 2006) and shown the importance of the views of cancer care specialists on the role of exercise (Jones *et al.*, 2004). Improving quality of life for people who have had a diagnosis of cancer has been a constant theme in Courneya's work and a good summary of this contribution may be found in Vallance *et al.* (2013).

UK studies

In the United Kingdom there have been several exercise psychology projects related to cancer. Stevinson and Fox (2004) investigated the provision of exercise opportunities for cancer patients within the NHS and found that fewer than 10 per cent of hospitals included exercise in rehabilitation programmes. Despite this, nurses who were surveyed reported willingness to include exercise, but cited lack of expertise and resources as barriers. The same authors presented positive outcomes from a feasibility study on how to include exercise into cancer care in the UK (Stevinson and Fox, 2006).

Daley and colleagues (2004) investigated whether or not aerobic exercise is the key to improvements in quality of life (QoL) for women with breast cancer who had finished their treatment for at least one year. Using a randomised controlled trial design, a total of 108 women who had been treated for breast cancer 12 to 36 months previously were assigned to supervised aerobic exercise therapy (n = 34), exercise placebo (body conditioning; n = 36), or usual care (n = 38). Exercise therapy and exercise placebo sessions took place three times per week for eight weeks. Outcomes included QoL, depression, exercise behaviour and aerobic fitness; outcomes were assessed at baseline and at the eight- and 24-week follow-up. The results showed a significant mean difference of 9.8 units in Functional Assessment of Cancer Therapy – General (the primary outcome) favouring aerobic exercise therapy at eight weeks, relative to usual care. Significant differences that favoured aerobic exercise therapy relative to usual care were recorded for Functional Assessment of Cancer Therapy – Breast, social/family well-being, functional well-being and breast cancer subscale scores at eight-week follow-up. Psychological health outcomes improved modestly for both intervention groups. Daley *et al.* concluded that aerobic exercise therapy had large, clinically meaningful, short-term beneficial effects on QoL in women treated for breast cancer and that this finding cannot be attributable to attention because the placebo group did not report the same kinds of benefits.

A further UK study examined the effects of a lifestyle intervention on body weight and other health outcomes influencing long-term prognosis in overweight women recovering from early-stage (stage I–III) breast cancer (Scott *et al.*, 2013). In this study, 90 women who had been treated three to 18 months previously were randomly assigned to a six-month exercise and hypocaloric healthy eating programme (n = 47) or control group (n = 43). Women in the intervention group received three supervised exercise sessions per week and individualised dietary advice, supplemented by weekly nutrition seminars. A small reduction in body weight in the intervention group (median difference from baseline of -1.09 kg; p = 0.07) was accompanied by significant reductions in waist circumference and saturated fat intake, total cholesterol and resting diastolic blood pressure. Cardiopulmonary fitness and FACT-B quality of life also showed significant improvements in this intervention group. These findings suggest that an individualised exercise and hypocaloric healthy eating programme can positively impact upon health outcomes that are known to influence long-term prognosis in overweight women recovering from early-stage breast cancer.

We have been studying the effects of group exercise opportunities, taking place in community facilities, on various functional and psychological parameters of women who are undergoing breast cancer therapy. Following a promising pilot study (Campbell *et al.*, 2005), we used a randomised controlled trial design to determine the functional and psychological benefits of a 12-week supervised group exercise programme during treatment for early stage breast cancer with a six-month follow-up. The participants were 203 women of whom 177 completed the six-month follow-up. We excluded those with concurrent unstable cardiac, hypertensive or respiratory disease, cognitive dysfunction, and those who were regular exercisers. The control group received usual care. The intervention was a supervised group exercise programme twice weekly for 12 weeks in addition to usual care. The main outcome measures were: Functional Assessment of Cancer Therapy questionnaire, Beck Depression Inventory, Positive and Negative Affect Scale, body mass index, seven-day recall of physical activity, 12-minute walk test, and assessment of shoulder mobility. The results showed both functional and psychological benefits to the intervention group as follows:

- metres walked in 12 minutes: +129 (83 to 176)
- minutes of moderate intensity activity reported in a week: +182 (75 to 289)
- shoulder mobility: +2.6 (1.6 to 3.7)
- breast cancer-specific quality of life: +2.5 (1.0 to 3.9)
- positive mood: +4.0 (1.8 to 6.3).

In general, these effects were maintained at the six-month follow-up, as may be seen in Figure 15.3 (Mutrie *et al.*, 2007).

Our exercise programmes had the aim of developing independent exercisers and we incorporated elements of our approach to individual physical activity counselling into each exercise class which we had established through our work with diabetic patients – see the earlier section of this chapter (Kirk *et al.*, 2007). Six themes were discussed with all the women attending the classes on a rotational basis. These themes were as follows:

- the health benefits of increasing physical activity
- overcoming barriers
- enhancing self-efficacy
- goal-setting
- finding support
- preventing relapse following supervised programme.

In addition, the women in the control group were given a personal physical activity consultation when the six-month follow-up measures were completed. We were, therefore,

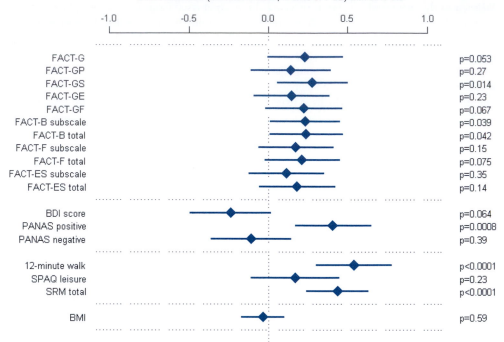

Figure 15.3 Effect estimates (Exercise – Control) with 95% confidence intervals and p-values for outcome variables at the six-month follow-up assessment, expressed in units of one standard deviation (SD) of the outcome distributions, based on mixed effects models adjusting for baseline values, study site, therapy at baseline and age

Source: Mutrie *et al.* (2007).

interested to determine whether adherence levels were improved as a result of using this group format to teach cognitive and behavioural skills that have been shown to help individuals increase activity levels. We were able to follow up all available women five years after this original intervention (Mutrie *et al.*, 2012). Of the 148 women from the original study who agreed to be contacted again, 87 repeated all the original measures at 60 months.

Women in the original intervention group reported more leisure-time physical activity and more positive moods at 60 months than women in the original control group. Irrespective of original group allocation, women who were more active consistently reported lower levels of depression and increased quality of life compared to those who were less active. To our knowledge this is the longest follow-up of any exercise intervention related to cancer survivors. It shows that the experience of the supervised exercise, accompanied by group discussion of evidence-based behaviour change techniques, had a lasting benefit in terms of physical activity adherence and psychological benefit. This evidence suggests that exercise classes for such patients should be provided with the aim of achieving independent exercisers and that group discussion of known behaviour change techniques should be considered as part of this provision.

Key point: Studies from the UK have shown that exercise programmes for women during and after cancer treatment can have benefits for physical and psychological health. Long-lasting effects of increased physical activity five years after the intervention have now been noted.

Barriers to participation

Not all of the women in the study reported above found it easy to continue to be active. Special challenges for exercise for people with cancer include exercising while recovering from intensive treatment such as chemotherapy or muscle weakness. There may also be embarrassment in public facilities because of hair loss due to treatment or fear of what people might think of a mastectomy scar. There has been relatively little attention paid to the barriers that breast cancer survivors may have to remaining active, and so, as part of the five-year follow-up of our original study described above, we undertook qualitative analyses of short exit interviews with the women who provided follow-up data. The data were analysed using inductive thematic analysis.

We noted that there were differences between the original intervention and control groups in terms of their engagement with activity. These differences are noted in Table 15.1 and again reveal the benefits of the approach we used in providing the supervised exercise classes. The findings from the interviews included three main themes and several sub-themes regarding the women's perceived barriers.

1. *Psychological barriers*, such as lack of motivation, fears, dislike of the gym, not being the 'sporty type'. One participant expressed this lack of motivation as follows:

    'I just get bogged into life and I feel I have to deal with that. And then the exercise bit just gets left.'

2. *Physical barriers*, such as the ageing process, cancer treatment and other physical co-morbidities, fatigue and weight gain. For example, a response from one participant about how the process made her feel reveals this barrier:

Table 15.1 Differences in activity engagement between original intervention and control group from qualitative data collected five years after intervention (adapted from Hefferon *et al.*, in press)

Original intervention group	*Original control group*
More aware of importance of exercise to health and well-being	Understood importance but not to same extent as intervention group
More knowledgeable in how to exercise safely	Felt lost as to how to start exercising safely
More self-assured in engagement in different types of activity (weights, classes)	Discussed lower levels of self-efficacy
Integrated exercise into lifestyle	More likely to be at 'Contemplative' stage of change
More likely to be 'Gym go-ers' (44% vs. 2.5%)	More likely to be 'Walkers' (44% vs. 22%)

'Quite lethargic actually and I know that I've put on a bit of weight, I definitely have but I'm definitely going to be addressing that because I really am very uncomfortable with the extra weight and the lack of exercise. I really do feel it, I just feel that I've not got as much energy. Whereas I feel when you're doing regular exercise, you definitely do have more energy for things.'

3.   *Contextual and environmental barriers*, such as employment, traditional female care-giving role, the proximity/access to facilities, seasonality/weather. Many of these issues are similar to those of any woman trying to find time to exercise but here we see the added barrier of recovery from cancer in this response:

'Initially the return to work was very difficult and exhausting, so my social activity if you like, exercise classes and things, dropped off. But that, I think in the main was the struggle to get back to work and then to get back to full-time work, was just so exhausting there was absolutely no room for anything else.'

These findings add support to the current advocacy for the use of activity immediately following diagnosis. However, we also believe that the findings emphasise the need for specially tailored activity programmes in order to overcome potential barriers (Hefferon *et al.*, in press).

The somatopsychic process

We are also interested in how exercise might influence how people feel as they undergo treatment for breast cancer. Psychosomatic principles have suggested for a long time that what we think and feel will have an impact on our physical functioning. When the body's activity affects how we think and feel this should be classed as 'somatopsychic' (Harris, 1973; Hefferon, 2013). In exercise psychology, we explore somatopsychic processes in order to seek answers to why physical activity might help people to feel better. The randomised controlled trial of exercise for breast cancer survivors reported previously in this chapter showed that both psychological and functional benefits were available, thus highlighting the somatopsychic rationale for including exercise in rehabilitation programmes for these cancer patients. Qualitative data provided evidence that the participants viewed the exercise as something that helped them feel better at a time of health challenge (Emslie *et al.*, 2007). For example, one participant in a focus group said: 'You felt better after it … lifted. I just felt generally that my health had improved in that hour. Aye, I think I was on a high possibly!' For some of these women the exercise was associated with a positive change as a result of the trauma of diagnosis and treatment for cancer. This experience has been termed 'post-traumatic growth' and there is a growing literature (especially qualitative) on the possibility of growth after illness (Hefferon *et al.*, 2009). We investigated the possibility of some of the women in our study reporting such post-traumatic growth using interpretative phenomemological analysis. The following quotation from a participant in one of our interviews gives a flavour of our findings that exercise was an element in their experience of growth: 'And I think I have a much better lifestyle now! [Really?] Ya, definitely. That's, that's definite. … So, em, ya, it's definitely changed us now … you know, just happy with what you've got. Contented with what you've got and very grateful for what you have' (Hefferon *et al.*, 2008, 2010).

Key point: Exercise programmes for breast cancer patients may provide the opportunity for experiencing post-traumatic growth.

Chapter summary

Physical activity opportunities should be an integral component of care for people with diabetes or breast cancer. However, many patients are not achieving and/or sustaining the potential benefits because they are failing to adhere to supervised programmes or maintain an active lifestyle after programme completion. The challenge is now to get physical activity advice and support as standard practice and all such provision must include a goal of helping patients become independent exercisers so that the potential for physical activity to improve quality of life for people may be realised. While we have illustrated these issues from two conditions – diabetes and cancer – there will be similar concerns for other special and clinical populations.

We suggest that there is a somatopsychic effect from exercise and that clinicians should promote exercise to help people feel better, and that such benefits will help people adhere to their increased physical activity levels. These somatopsychic effects may be available to many clinical populations and to the general population (Hefferon, 2013).

Acknowledgement

This is an updated and shortened version of the following chapter: Mutrie, N., Kirk, A. and Hughes, A. R. (2011). Adherence and quality of life issues in relation to physical activity: case studies from three clinical populations – coronary heart disease, diabetes and cancer. In A. Morris (ed.), *Sport and Exercise Psychology: To the Cutting Edge*, FIT Technology (pp. 461–481). Sincere thanks and appreciation to Alison Kirk for her willingness to keep the diabetes section up to date.

References

American College of Sports Medicine. (1997). *ACSM's Exercise Management for Persons with Chronic Diseases and Disabilities*. Champaign, IL: Human Kinetics.

American College of Sports Medicine, Durstine, J.L., Moore, G., Painter, P. and Roberts, S. (2009). *ACSM's Exercise Management for Persons with Chronic Diseases and Disabilities*. (3rd edn). Champaign, IL: Human Kinetics.

American Diabetes Association. (2003). Physical activity/exercise and diabetes. *Diabetes Care, 26*, S73–S77.

Anderson, B.L. (1992). Psychological interventions for cancer patients to enhance quality of life. *Journal of Consulting and Clinical Psychology, 60*, 552–558.

Ary, A., Toobert, D., Wilson, W. and Glasgow, R.E. (1986). Patient perspectives on factors contributing to non adherence to diabetes regimen. *Diabetes Care, 9*, 168–172.

Ballard-Barbash, R., Friedenreich, C.M., Courneya, K.S., Siddiqi, S.M., McTiernan, A. and Alfano, C.M. (2012). Physical activity, biomarkers, and disease outcomes in cancer survivors: A systematic review. *Journal of the National Cancer Institute, 104*(11), 815–840. doi: 10.1093/jnci/djs207.

Barglow, P., Hatcher, R., Edidin, D. and Sloan-Rossiter, D. (1984). Stress and metabolic control in diabetes: Psychosomatic evidence and evaluation of methods. *Psychosomatic Medicine, 46*, 127–144.

Blanchard, C.M., Cokkinides V., Courneya, K.S., Nehl, E.J., Stein, K. and Baker, F. (2003). A comparison of physical activity of post-treatment breast cancer survivors and non-cancer controls. [Exercise behaviour]. *Behavioral Medicine, 28*, 140–149.

Brooks, R. (1996). EuroQol: The current state of play. *Health Policy, 37*(1), 53–72.

Campbell, A., Mutrie, N., White, F., McGuire, F. and Kearney, N. (2005). A pilot study of a supervised group exercise programme as a rehabilitation treatment for women with breast cancer receiving adjuvant treatment. *European Journal of Oncology Nursing, 9*(1), 56–63. doi: S1462388904000250 [pii]10.1016/j.ejon.2004.03.007.

Colberg, S.R., Sigal, R.J., Fernhall, B., Regensteiner, J.G., Blissmer, B.J., Rubin, R.R. and American Diabetes Association. (2010). Exercise and Type 2 diabetes: The American College of Sports Medicine and the American Diabetes Association: Joint position statement. *Diabetes Care, 33*(12), e147–167. doi: 10.2337/dc10-9990.

Courneya, K.S. (2003). Exercise in cancer survivors: An overview of research. *Medicine and Science in Sports and Exercise, 35*(11), 1846–1852.

Courneya, K.S. and Friedenreich, C.M. (1999). Physical exercise and quality of life following cancer diagnosis: A literature review. *Annals of Behavioral Medicine, 21*(2), 171–179.

Courneya, K.S., Mackey, J.R. and McKenzie, D.C. (2002). Exercise for breast cancer survivors – Research evidence and clinical guidelines. *Physician and Sportsmedicine, 30*(8), 33–42.

Courneya, K.S., Segal, R.J., Reid, R.D., Jones, L.W., Malone, S.C., Venner, P.M. and Wells, G.A. (2004). Predictors of adherence in a randomized controlled trial of exercise in prostate cancer survivors. *Medicine and Science in Sports and Exercise, 36*(5), S230–S231.

Courneya, K.S., Karvinen, K.H., McNeely, M.L., Campbell, K.L., Brar, S., Woolcott, C.G. and Friedenreich, C.M. (2012). Predictors of adherence to supervised and unsupervised exercise in the Alberta Physical Activity and Breast Cancer Prevention Trial. *Journal of Physical Activity Health, 9*(6), 857–866.

Daley, A.J., Mutrie, N., Crank, H., Coleman, R. and Saxton, J. (2004). Exercise therapy in women who have had breast cancer: Design of the Sheffield women's exercise and well-being project. *Health Education Research, 19*(6), 686–697.

Demark-Wahnefried, W., Peterson, B., McBride, C., Lipkus, I. and Clipp, E. (2000). Current health behaviours and readiness to pursue life-style changes among men and women diagnosed with early stage prostate and breast carcinomas. *Cancer, 88*, 674–684.

Di Loreto, C., Fanelli, C., Lucidi, P., Murdolo, G., Cicco, A., Parlanti, N. and De Feo, P. (2003). Validation of a counselling strategy to promote the adoption and the maintenance of physical activity by Type 2 diabetic subjects. *Diabetes Care, 26*, 404–408.

Diabetes Prevention Program Research Group. (2002). Reduction in the incidence of Type 2 diabetes with lifestyle intervention or metformin. *New England Journal of Medicine, 346*, 396–403.

Dunn, S.W. (1993). Psychological aspects of diabetes in adults. *International Review of Health Psychology, 2*, 175–197.

Emslie, C., Whyte, F., Campbell, A., Mutrie, N., Lee, L., Ritchie, D. and Kearney, N. (2007). 'I wouldn't have been interested in just sitting round a table talking about cancer'; Exploring the experiences of women with breast cancer in a group exercise trial. *Health Education Research, 22* (6), 827–838. doi: 10.1093/her/cyl159.

Fairey, A.S., Courneya, K.S., Field, C.J. and Mackey, J.R. (2002). Physical exercise and immune system function in cancer survivors – A comprehensive review and future directions. *Cancer, 94*(2), 539–551.

Felce, D. (1997). Defining and applying the concept of quality of life. *Journal of Intellectual Disability Research, 41*(Pt. 2), 126–135.

Ferrand, C., Perrin, C. and Nasarre, S. (2008). Motives for regular physical activity in women and men: A qualitative study in French adults with Type 2 diabetes, belonging to a patients' association. *Health and Social Care in the Community, [Epub ahead of print]*.

Friedenrich, C.M. and Courneya, K.S. (1996). Exercise as rehabilitation for cancer patients. *Clinical Journal of Sports Medicine, 6*, 237–244.

Gavard, J. (1993). Prevalence of depression in adults with diabetes: An epidemiological evaluation. *Diabetes Care, 16*, 1167–1178.

Glasgow, R., Ruggiero, L., Eakin, E., Dryfoos, J. and Chobanian, L. (1997). Quality of life and associated characteristics in a large national sample of adults with diabetes. *Diabetes Care, 20*, 562–567.

Harris, D.V. (1973). *Involvement in Sport: A somatopsychic rationale for physical activity*. Philadelphia, PA: Lea & Febiger.

Hays, L. and Clark, D. (1999). Correlates of physical activity in a sample of older adults with Type 2 diabetes. *Diabetes Care, 22*, 706–712.

Hefferon, K. (2013). *Positive Psychology and the Body: The somato-psychic side to flourishing*. Maidenhead, England: Open University Press.

Hefferon, K., Grealy, M. and Mutrie, N. (2008). The perceived influence of an exercise class intervention on the process and outcomes of post-traumatic growth. *Mental Health and Physical Activity, 1*(2), 47–88.

Hefferon, K., Grealy, M. and Mutrie, N. (2009). Post-traumatic growth and life threatening physical illness: A systematic review of the qualitative literature. *British Journal of Health Psychology, 14*, 343–378. doi: 10.1348/135910708X332936.

Hefferon, K., Grealy, M. and Mutrie, N. (2010). Transforming from cocoon to butterfly: The potential role of the body in the process of posttraumatic growth. *Journal of Humanistic Psychology, 50*(2), 224–247. doi:10.1177/0022167809341996. http://dx.doi.org/10.1177/0022167809341996.

Hefferon, K., Murphy, H., McLeod, J., Mutrie, N. and Campbell, A. (in press). Understanding barriers to exercise implementation 5-years post Breast Cancer diagnosis: A large-scale qualitative study. *Health Education Research*.

Heyman, E., Toutain, C., Delamarche, P., Berthon, P., Briard, D., Youssef, H. and Gratas-Delamarche, A. (2007). Exercise training and cardiovascular risk factors in Type 1 diabetic adolescent girls. *Pediatric Exercise Science, 19*(4), 408–419.

Holmes, M.D., Chen, W.Y., Feskanich, D., Kroenke, C.H. and Colditz, G.A. (2005). Physical activity and survival after breast cancer diagnosis. *JAMA, 293*(20), 2479–2486.

International Diabetes Federation. (2013). *IDF Diabetes Atlas* (6th edn). Brussels, Belgium International Diabetes Federation. http://www.idf.org/diabetesatlas.

Jenkinson, C., Stewart-Brown, S., Petersen, S. and Paice, C. (1999). Assessment of the SF-36 version 2 in the United Kingdom. *Journal of Epidemiology and Community Health, 53*(1), 46–50.

Jones, L.W., Courneya, K.S., Peddle, C. and Mackey, J.R. (2004). Oncologists' attitudes towards recommending exercise to cancer patients: A Canadian national survey. *Journal of Clinical Oncology, 22*(14), 763S–763S.

Karvinen, K.H., Courneya, K.S., Campbell, K.L., Pearcey, R.G., Dundas, G. and Tonkin, K.S. (2005). Individual motivational determinants of exercise in endometrial cancer survivors: An application of the theory of planned behavior. *Journal of Sport and Exercise Psychology, 27*, S84.

Kirk, A.F., Higgins, L.A., Hughes, A.R., Fisher, B.M., Mutrie, N., Hillis, S. and MacIntyre, P.D. (2001). A randomized, controlled trial to study the effect of exercise consultation on the promotion of physical activity in people with Type 2 diabetes: A pilot study. *Diabetic Medicine, 18*(11), 877–882.

Kirk, A., Mutrie, N., MacIntyre, P. and Fisher, M. (2004a). Effects of a 12-month physical activity counselling intervention on glycaemic control and on the status of cardiovascular risk factors in people with Type 2 diabetes. *Diabetologia, 47*(5), 821–832.

Kirk, A.F., Mutrie, N., MacIntyre, P.D. and Fisher, M.B. (2004b). Promoting and maintaining physical activity in people with Type 2 diabetes. *American Journal of Preventive Medicine, 27*(4), 289–296.

Kirk, A., Barnett, J. and Mutrie, N. (2007). Physical activity consultation for people with Type 2 diabetes: Evidence and guidelines. *Diabetic Medicine, 24*, 809–816.

Kirk, A., Gannon, M. and Barnett, J. (2008). Patient views of three methods of physical activity promotion for people with Type 2 diabetes. *Diabetic Medicine, 25*, 79.

Krug, L., Haire-Joshu, D. and Heady, S. (1991). Exercise habits and exercise relapse in persons with non-insulin-dependent diabetes mellitus. *The Diabetes Educator, 17*, 185–188.

Ligtenberg, P., Godaert, G., Hillenaar, F. and Hoekstra, J. (1998). Influence of a physical training programme on psychological well-being in elderly Type 2 diabetes patients. *Diabetes Care, 21*, 2196–2197.

Lim, S.S., Vos, T., Flaxman, A.D., Danaei, G., Shibuya, K., Adair-Rohani, H. and Memish, Z.A. (2012). A comparative risk assessment of burden of disease and injury attributable to 67 risk factors and risk factor clusters in 21 regions, 1990–2010: A systematic analysis for the Global Burden of Disease Study 2010. *Lancet, 380*(9859), 2224–2260. doi: 10.1016/S0140-6736(12)61766-8.

Lucia, A., Earnest, C. and Pérez, M. (2003). Cancer-related fatigue: Can exercise physiology assist oncologists. *Lancet Oncology, 4*, 616–625.

Macmillan, F., Kirk, A., Mutrie, N., Matthews, L., Robertson, K. and Saunders, D.H. (2013). A systematic review of physical activity and sedentary behavior intervention studies in youth with Type 1 diabetes: Study characteristics, intervention design, and efficacy. *Pediatric Diabetes*, doi: 10.1111/pedi.12060.

Marsden, E. (1996). *The role of exercise in the well-being of people with insulin dependent diabetes mellitus: Perceptions of patients and health professionals.* Ph.D., University of Glasgow, Glasgow.

Marsden, E. and Kirk, A. (2005). Becoming and staying physically active. In D. Nagi (ed.), *Exercise and Sport in Diabetes* (pp. 161–192). London: Wiley.

Mishra, S., Scherer, R., Geigle, P., Berlanstein, D., Topaloglu, O., Gotay, C. and Snyder, C. (2012). Exercise interventions on health-related quality of life for cancer survivors. *Cochrane Database of Systematic Reviews* (8). doi: 10.1002/14651858.CD007566.pub2.

Moore, G.E. (1997). Introduction. In *ACSM's Exercise Management for Persons with Chronic Diseases and Disabilities* (pp. 3–5). Champaign, IL: Human Kinetics.

Morrato, E., Hill, J. and Wyatt, H. (2003). Physical activity in U.S. adults with diabetes and at risk for developing diabetes. *Diabetes Care, 30*, 203–209.

Mutrie, N., Campbell, A.M., Whyte, F., McConnachie, A., Emslie, C., Lee, L. and Ritchie, D. (2007). Benefits of supervised group exercise programme for women being treated for early stage breast cancer: Pragmatic randomised controlled trial. *British Medical Journal, 334*(7592), 517–520B.

Mutrie, N., Campbell, A., Barry, S., Hefferon, K., McConnachie, A., Ritchie, D. and Tovey, S. (2012). Five-year follow-up of participants in a randomised controlled trial showing benefits from exercise for breast cancer survivors during adjuvant treatment. Are there lasting effects? *Journal of Cancer Survivorship, 6*(4), 420–430. doi: 10.1007/s11764-012-0233-y.

Pischke, C., Weidner, G. and Elliot-Eller, M. (2006). Comparison of coronary risk factors and quality of life in coronary artery disease patients with versus without diabetes mellitus. *American Journal of Cardiology, 97*, 1267–1273.

Rickabaugh, T.E. and Saltarelli, W. (1999). Knowledge and attitudes related to diabetes and exercise guidelines among selected diabetic children, their parents and physical education teachers. *Research Quarterly for Exercise and Sport, 70*, 389–384.

Robertson, K., Adolfsson, P., Riddell, M.C., Scheiner, G. and Hanas, R. (2008). Exercise in children and adolescents with diabetes. *Pediatric Diabetes, 9*(1), 65–77. doi: 10.1111/j.1399-5448.2007.00362.x.

Rogers, L., Courneya, K.S., Verhulst, S., Markwell, S., Lanzotti, V. and Shah, P. (2006). Exercise barrier and task self-efficacy in breast cancer patients during treatment. *Supportive Care in Cancer, 14*(1), 84–90.

Schmitz, K.H., Holtzman, J., Courneya, K.S., Masse, L.C., Duval, S. and Kane, R. (2005). Controlled physical activity trials in cancer survivors: A systematic review and meta-analysis. *Cancer Epidemiology Biomarkers and Prevention, 14*(7), 1588–1595.

Scott, E., Daley, A.J., Doll, H., Woodroofe, N., Coleman, R.E., Mutrie, N. and Saxton, J.M. (2013). Effects of an exercise and hypocaloric healthy eating program on biomarkers associated with long-term prognosis after early-stage breast cancer: A randomized controlled trial. *Cancer Causes Control, 24*(1), 181–191. doi: 10.1007/s10552-012-0104-x.

Simon, H.B. (1990). Discussion: Exercise, immunity, cancer, and infection. In C. Bouchard, R.J. Shephard, T. Stephens, J.R. Sutton and B.D. McPherson (eds), *Exercise, Fitness and Health* (pp. 581–588). Champaign, IL: Human Kinetics.

Stevinson, C. and Fox, K. (2004). Role of exercise for cancer rehabilitation in UK hospitals: A survey of oncology nurses. *European Journal of Cancer Care, 14*, 63–69.

——. (2006). Feasibility study of an exercise programme for cancer care patients. *European Journal of Cancer Care, 15*, 386–396.

Stevinson, C., Lawlor, D. and Fox, K. (2004). Exercise interventions for cancer patients: Systematic review of controlled clinical trials. *Cancer Causes and Control, 15*, 1035–1056.

Stewart, A., Hays, R., Wells, K., Rogers, W., Spritzer, K. and Greenfield, S. (1994). Long-term functioning and well-being outcomes associated with physical activity and exercise in patients with chronic conditions in the medical outcomes study. *Journal of Clinical Epidemiology, 47*, 719–730.

Stricker, C., Drake, D., Hoyer, K. and Mock, V. (2004). Evidence-based practice for fatigue management in adults with cancer: Exercise as an intervention. *Oncology Nursing Forum, 31*(5), 963–976.

Tessier, D., Menard, J. and Fulop, T. (2000). Effects of aerobic physical exercise in elderly with Type 2 diabetes mellitus. *Archives of Gerontological Geriatrics, 31*, 121–132.

Thomas, N., Alder, E. and Leese, G. (2004). Barriers to physical activity in patients with diabetes. *Post Graduate Medicine Journal, 80*, 287–291.

Tuomilehto, J., Lindstrom, J., Eriksson, J., Valle, T., Hamalainen, H. and Ilanne-Parikka, P. (2001). Prevention of Type 2 diabetes mellitus by changes in lifestyle among subjects with impaired glucose tolerance. *New England Journal of Medicine, 344*, 1343–1350.

Vallance, J.K., Culos-Reed, S.N., McKenzie, M. and Courneya, K.S. (2013). Physical activity and psychosocial health among cancer survivors. In P. Ekkekakis (ed.), *Routledge Handbook of Physical Activity and Mental Health* (pp. 518–529). Abingdon, Oxon: Routledge, Taylor & Francis Group.

Wilmot, E.J., Davies, M.J., Yates, T., Benhalima, K., Lawrence, I.G. and Khunti, K. (2010). Type 2 diabetes in younger adults: The emerging UK epidemic. *Postgraduate Medical Journal*, doi:10.1136/pgmj.2010.100917.

Yates, T., Davies, M., Gorely, T., Bull, F. and Khunti, K. (2008). Rationale, design and baseline data from the PREPARE (Pre-diabetes Risk Education and Physical Activity Recommendation and Encouragement) programme study: A randomized controlled trial. *Patient Education and Counselling*, doi:10.1016/j.pec.2008.06.010.

——. (2009). Effectiveness of a pragmatic education program designed to promote walking activity in individuals with impaired glucose tolerance: A randomized controlled trial. *Diabetes Care, 32*, 1404–1410. doi: 10.2337/dc09-0130.

Part V

Sedentary behaviour

16 Psychology of sitting
New kid on the block

Sedentary behaviour is, essentially, 'sitting time'. As defined in Chapter 1 it refers to 'any waking behaviour characterized by an energy expenditure ≤ 1.5 METs while in a sitting or reclining posture' (Sedentary Behaviour Research Network, 2012). Typical examples include TV viewing, computer use, sitting at work or in school, and car travel. Under this definition behaviour performed while standing may be thought of as non-sedentary. It is possible to meet recommended levels of physical activity (e.g. 150 minutes of MVPA per week for adults), and be classified as 'active', but at the same time take part in high levels of sedentary behaviour. That is, the two behaviours may coexist. Furthermore, while the relationship between sedentary behaviour and physical activity in young people has been shown to be negative ($r = -0.108$) in a meta-analysis of 163 studies, the small size of the relationship suggests that these behaviours do not directly displace each other (Pearson et al., 2014). This means that it is important not to refer to those with low levels of physical activity as 'sedentary', as is often the case in the literature. Instead, we should use the term 'inactive'.

Figure 16.1 is a depiction of a continuum of energy expenditure and posture whereby 'light physical activity' (e.g. light ambulation, but not moderate physical activity) falls between sedentary behaviour and MVPA. This helps to see how sedentary behaviour and light PA are likely to easily substitute for each other (i.e. when not sitting there is a good chance you are in light PA, such as standing), but less likely to be in moderate or vigorous PA.

Recognising physical activity and sedentary behaviour as distinct behaviours is important from the point of view of psychology and behaviour change. As they are different behaviours it is likely that they will be influenced by different factors (correlates) and therefore may

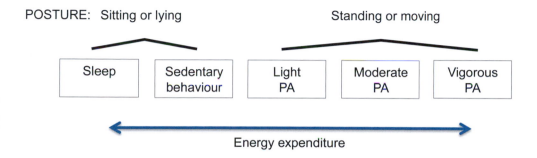

Figure 16.1 A depiction of sedentary behaviour and physical activity along an energy expenditure and posture continuum

require different behaviour change theories, frameworks and intervention approaches to facilitate change.

In this chapter we follow the behavioural epidemiological framework (see Chapter 1) and explore the following key questions with respect to sedentary behaviour:

- What is the relationship between sedentary behaviour and health outcomes in young people and adults?
- How is sedentary behaviour measured?
- What factors influence sedentary behaviour in young people and adults?
- What theories and models help to explain sedentary behaviour?
- What interventions help to change sedentary behaviour in young people and adults?

Sedentary behaviour and health-related outcomes

Young people

There is evidence that young people spend the majority of their leisure time engaged in sedentary behaviours such as television viewing and computer game playing (Rideout *et al.*, 2010) and there is increasing concern that these high levels of sitting are negatively impacting upon the health of young people. A recent systematic review examined the relationship between sedentary behaviour and six health indicators in young people aged 5 to 17 years (Tremblay *et al.*, 2011). The authors reported that sedentary behaviour for more than two hours per day (primarily assessed through TV viewing) was associated with unfavourable body composition, decreased fitness, lowered scores for self-esteem and pro-social behaviour and decreased academic achievement. Weaker evidence was found to suggest that increased sedentary time was associated with increased metabolic and cardiovascular disease risk factors. The authors concluded that there is consistent evidence that increased sedentary time is associated with negative health outcomes in young people, with the majority of studies reporting similar relationships.

The review by Tremblay *et al.* (2011) had broad inclusion criteria and included all eligible studies regardless of design. In contrast, the systematic review of Chinapaw *et al.* (2011) only included prospective studies. These provide a stronger design for examining the relationship between a behaviour and health indicators. Using these stricter inclusion criteria, Chinapaw *et al.* found insufficient evidence for a longitudinal relationship between 'sedentary time' (usually TV time) and body mass index (BMI), blood pressure, blood lipids or bone mass. However, moderate evidence was found for an inverse longitudinal relationship between sedentary time and aerobic fitness. They concluded that the possible detrimental health effects of prolonged or excessive sitting on health indicators in young people needs further study, with stronger designs. They also noted that the relationships may not be strong in young people because some of the health outcomes may not be easily manifested, and thus observable, in young people. Furthermore, small relationships observed during childhood may still be reflected in health problems in adulthood. In addition, children who are high television viewers tend to remain high television viewers, relative to others over time (Biddle *et al.*, 2010), and therefore may be at greater risk of negative health outcomes.

Most of the evidence linking sedentary behaviour to health outcomes has focused on physical health outcomes or indicators. Much less attention has been paid to mental health outcomes. In a brief review, Biddle and Asare (2011) identified nine studies examining the relationship between sedentary behaviour and some measure of mental well-being in children and adolescents. These studies showed consistent, small, negative associations between sedentary behaviour and mental well-being. However, all but one of the studies were cross-sectional and reverse causality is plausible in that those with poorer mental health may choose to be more sedentary (see Chapter 2). In addition, physical activity levels were not controlled for in half the studies. This makes it difficult to untangle the independent effects of sedentary behaviour on mental well-being. Despite these limitations, the authors concluded that high levels of sedentary behaviour are associated with poorer mental health and that sedentary behaviours should be considered alongside physical activity in the study of mental health.

Adults

In a systematic review of prospective studies, Thorp *et al.* (2011) concluded that there was a consistent relationship between self-reported sedentary behaviour and increased risk of all-cause mortality, CVD-related mortality and all-other-causes mortality in men and women, and that this relationship was independent of both physical activity and BMI. A similar finding was reported by Proper *et al.* (2011). In a subsequent meta-analysis, Wilmot *et al.* (2012) reported that those with the greatest sedentary time compared to the lowest had a 90 per cent increase in risk of cardiovascular mortality and a 49 per cent increase in risk of all-cause mortality. Wilmot *et al.* included studies with mixed exposures to sedentary behaviour (e.g. TV viewing, leisure-time sedentary behaviour and sitting) and heterogeneous units and categories (e.g. minutes per day, quartiles of exposure). Chau *et al.* (2013), in a meta-analysis looking only at the association between all-cause mortality and daily total sitting, reported that each hour of daily sitting is associated with an overall 2 per cent increased risk of all-cause mortality. However, this relationship was non-linear, with a 5 per cent increased risk for each one-hour increment for adults sitting >7 hours/day and dose–response modelling suggested a 34 per cent higher mortality risk in adults sitting 10 hours/day, after taking physical activity into account. These authors also calculated an overall weighted population attributable fraction for all-cause mortality for total daily sitting time of 4.9 per cent, after adjustment for physical activity.

When examining chronic disease, Thorp *et al.* and Proper *et al.* both reported a significant positive relationship between sitting time and risk for Type 2 diabetes. This was further supported by Wilmot *et al.*'s meta-analysis which reported that those with the highest sedentary levels had an increase in the risk ratio for Type 2 diabetes of 112 per cent. Consistent evidence has also been found between high levels of sedentary behaviour and site-specific cancers (ovarian, colon and endometrial), although the mediating effect of BMI and physical activity needs further exploration (Thorp *et al.*, 2011). There is limited evidence that a longitudinal relationship exists between sedentary behaviour, weight gain and risk of obesity in adults (Proper *et al.*, 2011; Thorp *et al.*, 2011), but sedentary behaviour during childhood and adolescence is a predictor of obesity in adulthood (Thorp *et al.*, 2011).

There is insufficient evidence to draw conclusions about the longitudinal relationship between sedentary behaviour and individual markers of cardiometabolic health (Thorp *et al.*, 2011). However, Edwardson *et al.*'s (2012) meta-analysis showed that those in the highest sedentary group had a 73 per cent increased risk of metabolic syndrome compared with those in the lowest sedentary group. This remained unchanged when accounting for physical activity, thus suggesting that sedentary behaviour is an independent risk factor. However, sedentary behaviour, mainly in the form of TV viewing, has also been shown to cluster with other deleterious lifestyle practices, such as a poor diet (Pearson and Biddle, 2011), which could act to overestimate the independent effect of sedentary behaviour. For a review of sedentary behaviour and mental health, see Chapter 2.

The majority of the evidence has focused on the link between total sedentary time or individual sedentary behaviours (e.g. TV viewing) and health. However, emerging evidence is suggestive that the nature of sedentary behaviour may also be important. For example, it might be informative to know if periods of sitting are prolonged or whether they take place in a more sporadic form. Healy *et al.* (2008) found that objectively assessed breaks in sedentary time were beneficially associated with waist circumference, BMI, triglycerides and 2-h plasma glucose, and these associations were independent of total sedentary time and MVPA. Similarly, Henson *et al.* (2013), in a study of adults at risk of diabetes, found that breaks in sedentary time were inversely associated with measures of adiposity but not other cardiometabolic outcomes. Increasing the number of breaks from sitting may be important for health.

Older adults

Compared to younger adults, older adults (>60 years) spend a greater proportion of their waking time engaged in sedentary activities (Hallal *et al.*, 2012). Despite this, there has been limited work examining the impact of this behaviour on health outcomes in this age group. In a systematic review of 24 studies, Rezende *et al.* (2014) found evidence for a relationship between sedentary behaviour and all-cause mortality in older adults. There was some evidence for a relationship between sedentary behaviour and metabolic syndrome, cardio-metabolic biomarkers, obesity and waist circumference; however, the quality of the studies reviewed means that these findings should be interpreted with caution. The authors also noted that there was some evidence for a protective effect of some types of sedentary behaviour (e.g. board games, craft activities) on the odds of cognitive impairment or dementia.

> Key point: There is consistent evidence that high levels of sedentary behaviour are associated with negative health outcomes. These findings are stronger in adults, and appear independent of the amount of physical activity participated in.

How is sedentary behaviour measured?

The measurement of sedentary behaviour is important for psychologists, as they need to have a good understanding of the behaviour itself. However, it is also challenging because of the variety of behaviours involved and the often intermittent, habitual and incidental nature of these sedentary behaviours. Currently, there is a lack of consensus on the most appropriate methods of assessing sedentary behaviour (Atkin *et al.*, 2012), but Owen (2012) argues that both objective and self-report measures will be needed. Objective devices allow precision and time-stamped data, but Owen suggests that alongside this there remains a need to charac-terise the nature of sedentary behaviour and sedentary behaviour patterns through the use of high-quality self-report measures.

Psychologists are very familiar with self-report measures of various kinds. Self-reports of sedentary behaviour have been widely used but often lack validity (Atkin *et al.*, 2012; Bryant *et al.*, 2007; Clark *et al.*, 2009). Moreover, few instruments have been assessed for their capacity to identify change in behaviour over time. Many of the self-report methods commonly reported in the literature have focused on TV viewing or other screen-based behaviours. This may be problematic as people find many ways to be sedentary and TV viewing time does not appear to be a good marker of overall sedentary behaviour (Biddle *et al.*, 2009; Sugiyama *et al.*, 2008). This has led to more recent work which has attempted to develop more refined self-report measures which assess multiple sedentary behaviours that might include TV viewing, reading and socialising. In addition, domain-specific behaviours may be assessed, such as sitting at work or at home, or in motorised travel (Clark *et al.*, 2009; Hardy *et al.*, 2007; Marshall *et al.*, 2010). These show promise, but further development and validation work is required. An advantage of self-report over other methods is that self-report allows for the assessment of not just the type of behaviour (e.g. watching TV vs. reading) but also the context (e.g. alone, with family members, etc.). This may be particularly useful for intervention design.

Objective methods, such as accelerometry, are increasingly being used for the assessment of sedentary time. This can overcome the recall limitations of self-report methods and provide an objective assessment of overall levels of sedentary behaviour, and also patterns of sedentary behaviour across a day. However, accelerometry is not without limitations. First, the detection of specific behaviours is not currently possible. Second, there is a lack of consensus as to the most appropriate way to process accelerometer data which limits comparability between studies. For example, commonly used accelerometers, such as the Actigraph, assess movement, and hence sedentary time is inferred from lack of movement. It is not a direct measure of sitting, therefore, whereas some devices, such as the ActivPal, are designed to detect limb angles (e.g. at the thigh), and hence are a more direct measure of sitting. Accelerometers are now being used to assess sedentary time in large-scale surveillance studies (Colley *et al.*, 2011; Matthews *et al.*, 2008).

The best choice of measurement approach will be determined by the specific question to be addressed. However, given the limitations in all existing sedentary measurement technologies it is possible that multiple measurement approaches will be needed. For a comprehensive discussion on the measurement of sedentary behaviour, see Atkin *et al.* (2012).

What factors influence sedentary behaviour in young people and adults?

In order to design effective interventions it is important to first understand the factors related to that behaviour. These are the 'correlates' of behaviour, as described in Chapter 7. Knowledge of correlates allows the identification of target groups that may be at particular risk from a given behaviour, and also allows interventions to better target factors known to cause, or at least influence, sedentary behaviour. The majority of the work examining correlates of sedentary behaviour has focused on young people and TV or screen viewing. There is a need for further systematic research examining the correlates of a broader range of sedentary behaviour and across more diverse population groups.

Young people

Several systematic reviews of the correlates of sedentary behaviour covering different age groups of young people have been published (Cillero and Jago, 2010; Gorely *et al.*, 2004; Hinkley *et al.*, 2010; Uijtdewilligen *et al.*, 2011; van der Horst *et al.*, 2007). The results from these reviews are summarised in Table 16.1. Collectively, the findings from these reviews highlight the significant gaps in our knowledge concerning the influences on sedentary behaviour. All the review authors noted that although many potential correlates have been

Table 16.1 Correlates of sedentary behaviour in young people identified within systematic reviews

Author	Gorely et al. (2004)	Van der Horst et al. (2007)	Van der Horst et al. (2007)	Cillerio and Jago (2010)	Hinkley et al. (2010)	Uitdewilligen et al. (2011)	Uitdewilligen et al. (2011)
Type of review	Systematic	Systematic	Systematic	Systematic	Systematic	Systematic	Systematic
Study design included	Cross-sectional or prospective	Cross-sectional or prospective	Cross-sectional or prospective	Cross-sectional or prospective	Cross-sectional or prospective	Prospective	Prospective
Age group	2–18 years old	4–12 years old	13–18 years olds	<8 years old	3–5 years old	4–12 years	13–18 years
Behaviour	TV/video viewing	TV/video viewing and computer games	TV/video viewing and computer games	Screen viewing	Sedentary behaviour (including overall measures, TV, DVD, gaming, computer use and reading)	Sedentary behaviour	Sedentary behaviour
Correlates							
Positive	Body weight; Snacking; Parent viewing habits; Day of week (weekend); TV in bedroom; Ethnicity (non-white)	Insufficient evidence	Sex (male); Ethnicity (non-white European); BMI; depression	Age; Ethnicity (non-white European); Family TV viewing; Parental viewing; Maternal depression; Parental body mass; Media access	Insufficient evidence	Insufficient evidence	Insufficient evidence
Negative	Parent income; Parent education; Number of parents in household		SES; Parental education	SES; Parental rules and safety	Insufficient evidence	Insufficient evidence	Insufficient evidence

studied, few of these have been investigated frequently enough to be able to draw firm conclusions. It is also evident within the reviews that the correlates of sedentary behaviours other than screen-viewing behaviours have received little attention. This gap needs to be addressed to facilitate the development of effective interventions to reduce the time children and adolescents spend on a wider range of sedentary behaviours. In addition, the findings suggest that the majority of correlates identified have been unmodifiable correlates (moderators) and more work with better designs is required to identify the modifiable correlates (mediators) of sedentary behaviour. The over-reliance on cross-sectional designs is also problematic and there is a need for more high-quality prospective studies to identify the determinants of sedentary behaviours.

Adults

Data on correlates of sedentary behaviour in adults are quite limited and rely largely on self-reported estimates of only a few sedentary behaviours, such as TV viewing. This is particularly limiting given that single behaviours may not be accurate markers of overall sedentary time (Sugiyama *et al.*, 2008) and that there are likely to be different correlates for different behaviours (e.g. transport-related behaviours vs. occupational sitting vs. leisure-time TV viewing or computer use) and potentially for the same behaviour performed in different contexts.

Rhodes *et al.* (2012) presented the findings of a systematic review focused on the correlates of sedentary behaviour in adults. Most of the studies used TV viewing as a measure of sedentary behaviour, were of a cross-sectional design and focused on socio-demographic and behavioural correlates. The review demonstrated that those who watch more TV tend to be less educated, older, unemployed or retired, and have higher BMI. In contrast, computer use was higher among younger, more educated adults, with computer game users more likely to be male. An association was also observed between higher TV viewing and lower leisure-time physical activity. Although psychological correlates have not been widely studied, a sedentary attitude construct (e.g. preference, utility and enjoyment) emerged as a strong positive correlate of all sedentary behaviours. Various theoretical frameworks were used for the study of attitude, including Theory of Planned Behaviour (see Chapter 8).

Depressive symptoms (+) and life satisfaction (−) also emerged as potential correlates. Rhodes *et al.* noted that there are differences in correlates by the type of sedentary behaviour investigated. For example, age and education were correlates of both TV viewing and computer use, but related to these behaviours in opposite directions. This finding supports the notion that it is important to study multiple sedentary behaviours and to avoid generalised assessments of 'screen time' where correlates are concerned. In a narrative review, Owen *et al.* (2011) suggested that TV viewing is associated with lower socio-economic status (SES) and the nature of the built environment. There is a negative association between TV viewing and having a more 'walkable' neighbourhood. In addition, some occupations will involve long periods of sitting. There is a need for more research focused on different sedentary behaviours and contexts, and a broad range of psychological, social and environmental factors.

Key point: The influences on sedentary behaviour in children and adults are not well understood. Few studies differentiate correlates by specific sedentary behaviours.

What theories might be appropriate for sedentary behaviour change?

Physical activity interventions have typically relied on social cognitive theories to either help explain participation in physical activity or inform intervention design. The most common approaches have been Social Cognitive Theory, including the extensive study of self-efficacy, the Theory of Planned Behaviour (TPB) and the Transtheoretical Model (TTM) (Biddle *et al.*, 2007; see also Chapters 8 to 11 for an overview of these and related theories). However, it is questionable to what extent models applied to one health behaviour (i.e. physical activity) transfer optimally to explain other behaviours (i.e. sedentary behaviour), or even the same behaviour performed in a different context (e.g. sedentary behaviour at home vs. sedentary behaviour at work). The demands and characteristics of different behaviours mean that the antecedents and influences are potentially different. For example, Table 16.2 illustrates some of the different behavioural characteristics of physical activity and sedentary behaviour in two contexts (leisure-time TV viewing and office-based desk work). These different characteristics, including different levels of conscious processing, or 'thoughts' and 'planning' about sedentary behaviours, suggest that different theoretical approaches for behaviour change may be needed. However, this suggestion is yet to be tested. In this section we outline two approaches, 'behavioural choice theory' and 'habit'. These may have particular utility for sedentary behaviour change.

Behavioural choice theory

Behavioural choice theory (BCT) is based on behavioural economics and is a theoretical approach that attempts to understand how time and resources are allocated given a choice between two or more alternatives. BCT contends that choosing a specific behaviour, such as watching television, is a function of the accessibility of the behaviour, availability of alternatives, and the reinforcement value ('appeal' or 'enjoyment') of the behaviour. Accessibility relates to the amount of effort (or 'cost') required to engage in a particular behaviour. When

Table 16.2 Possible differentiating qualities between moderate to vigorous structured physical activity (MVPA) and two examples of sedentary behaviours

Quality	MVPA	Sedentary behaviour: TV viewing	Sedentary behaviour: office desk work
Frequency across the day/week	Low; likely to be no more than once per day	High; regular, prolonged bouts of sedentary behaviour likely on a daily basis, particularly in evenings and at weekends	High; regular, sustained, and prolonged bouts of sedentary behaviour during office hours
Daily duration	Short (e.g. 30–60 minutes); <7% of waking day	Long, such as 2–3 hours per day	Very long, such as 6–7 hours a day, with only periodic breaks
Effort	Moderate to high	Low	Low
Conscious processing	Moderate to high; requires planning	Low and habitual	Low (none?) and habitual
Primary behavioural 'drivers'	Mix of individual motivation and goals, and supportive social and physical environment	Habit; social norms; physical environment	Habit; social norms/ job expectations; physical environment

physically active and sedentary options are equally accessible, children tend to select the sedentary option. According to Epstein (1998), the choice of sedentary behaviours is very responsive to 'cost' and effort, and therefore making access more difficult (e.g. keeping video games machines in the box when not being used) may lead to reductions in sedentary behaviour. However, it is important to note that reducing access to highly liked sedentary activities is more likely to lead to shifts in behaviour, but reducing access to less preferred sedentary behaviours is likely to have little effect, as the individuals were less likely to have chosen these behaviours anyway.

Availability of alternatives refers to whether or not there are attractive and positively reinforcing alternative behaviours available. Although people may choose the sedentary option, a different decision may be made if the alternative behaviour(s) are highly desirable (e.g. a trip to the park).

Reinforcement value refers to the appeal of the behaviour. Reinforcement value could be targeted through rewards and praise for choosing alternative behaviours. The notion of choice to obtain the reinforcement is important (Epstein, 1998). If individuals perceive that they are forced into physical activity, and that they have not made a voluntary choice, they may not be motivated in the future (see Chapter 9). It is also important to consider the delay between choosing a behaviour and receiving the reinforcement. When two reinforcers are immediately available people reliably choose the more valuable one. However, when there is a delay in receiving the valuable reinforcer, people may switch to a behaviour with a less valuable, but more immediately available reinforcer. This may be particularly important in sedentary behaviour/physical activity decision-making as the benefits of physical activity are often delayed but the benefits of sedentary alternatives may be immediately experienced (Epstein, 1998).

The task of health behaviour interventions is often to shift the choice from an unhealthy but highly reinforcing behaviour (e.g. sedentary screen-viewing behaviour), to potentially less immediately reinforcing but healthier alternatives (e.g. physical activity). Under the BCT perspective it is considered possible to shift behaviour from sedentary screen viewing, for example, by making non-screen-viewing activities more appealing (reinforcement value) and easy to do (accessible and available) relative to sedentary screen viewing. Epstein and colleagues have used BCT as a framework for the study of sedentary behaviour and physical activity in children (Epstein and Roemmich, 2001). This work has shown that by making alternative active behaviours more accessible, and sedentary pursuits less reinforcing, reductions in sedentary behaviour and increases in physical activity are possible (Epstein and Roemmich, 2001; Epstein *et al.*, 1995).

Habit

In Table 16.2 we suggested that sedentary behaviour may have a significant habitual component. That is, people engage in sedentary behaviour without really thinking about it. For example, a child comes home from school, grabs a biscuit and flops down in front of the TV without actually making a conscious decision that this was what they wanted to do. This suggests that psychologists may need to consider theories allied to notions of 'habit' and less conscious processing when investigating ubiquitous sedentary behaviours. This contrasts with the theories typically used to explain physical activity, some of which have been outlined in this book (see Chapters 8 to 11). These are based on notions of conscious decision-making and portray behaviour as the outcome of conscious deliberation (Gardner *et al.*, 2011). For example, the TPB is based on the proposition that individuals make rational decisions as they form behavioural intentions, and these decisions are based on attitudes, subjective norms and perceived behavioural control. However, it is not likely that people 'intend' to sit or not to sit at their work desk, or at their TV set, at least in the sense of deliberate conscious processing or weighing up the pros and cons. They just 'do' – driven towards the behaviour by relatively automatic processing based on habit, social norms and environmental cues.

Dual-process models in social psychology suggest that information processing occurs along a continuum (Moskowitz *et al.*, 1999). At one end, deliberative conscious decision-making occurs, with decisions requiring thought, planning and cognitive effort. The theories used to explain physical activity typically rely on this mode. At the other end, behaviour or decisions are postulated to occur automatically in response to environmental cues, with no effort, volitional control or awareness (Bargh and Chartrand, 1999). The notion of habit falls at this end of the continuum (see Chapter 9).

Habit may be defined as behavioural patterns learned through situation-dependent repetition (Aarts *et al.*, 1997; Gardner *et al.*, 2011). As a new behaviour is performed, a mental association is made between the situation and the behaviour; repetition of this behaviour in the same situation strengthens this association, and makes alternative behaviours less likely (Wood and Neal, 2009). Over time, when the situation is encountered the habitual response occurs automatically (Lally and Gardner, 2011). For example, a child receives a computer game console for their birthday. They play with this game on the couch in the lounge at home. Over time the act of sitting down in the lounge at home becomes sufficient to automatically cue the habitual response of picking up the console and playing games. According to habit theory, in novel contexts behaviour is more likely to be regulated by conscious decisions through intentions, but in familiar contexts behaviour will be much more affected by habit (Gardner *et al.*, 2011). This means that in familiar contexts habits may dominate over intentions to regulate action. Given the high frequency of many sedentary behaviours, such as sitting at a desk at work or sitting in front of the TV at home, it is easy to see how habitual such behaviours become.

Kremers *et al.* (2007) demonstrated that screen-viewing behaviour has a habitual component for many adolescents. As part of a wider study, 383 Dutch adolescents completed questionnaires assessing screen-viewing behaviour and habit strength for screen viewing. Results showed a moderately strong correlation between screen-viewing behaviour and habit strength. This result suggests that habit is worthy of further investigation with respect to sedentary behaviour. Using the same dataset, Kremers and Brug (2008) also showed that intentions were unrelated to behaviour in adolescents with strong habits, and it was suggested that interventions to decrease sedentary behaviour should not just provide information to increase motivation. Indeed, this is similar to Fogg's notion that behaviour change may more readily be achieved by making behaviours easier to perform rather than increasing motivation to perform already challenging behaviours (see http://www.behaviormodel. org/). Reducing sedentary behaviour, therefore, may require disrupting environmental factors that automatically cue habitual behaviours.

As habits are formed through repetition, it is going to require time and repetition to break one habit and replace it with another. Few interventions have been explicitly based on habit formation or habit change, however, Lally and Gardner (2011) make some suggestions for interventions:

1.   Identify the cues for specific behaviours. This will require people to self-monitor their behaviour over time to identify situations in which they perform unwanted habitual behaviour. The cue can then either be avoided or strategies developed so that when the cue occurs, the behavioural response to the cue is something less sedentary.

2.   Implementation intentions may be a useful tool (see Chapter 8). These if-then statements could highlight cues that may result in unwanted behaviour. Using implementation intentions to identify new cue responses may help replace unwanted habits.
3.   Unwanted habits could be broken by restructuring personal environments, or programming new responses to existing environments. Where context change is unfeasible as an intervention strategy, intervening at a point when people are changing the environments in which they live or work is recommended (see the Gorman *et al.* (2013) example in the section on sedentary behaviour interventions in adults). Within existing environments placing reminders in the contexts where unwanted habits are performed can provide a useful reminder to implement an alternative response.

Another popular concept with respect to automatic processes and health behaviour change is 'nudging' (Thaler and Sunstein, 2008), and this too is relevant to sedentary behaviour as well as to physical activity (see Chapter 9). Nudging is when behaviours are encouraged through indirect suggestions and with no incentives offered. It does not involve direct instruction, government policies, legislation or enforcement. The idea is that the best option for people's behaviour is highlighted but the individual has to choose to do it. Thaler and Sunstein (2008, p. 6) define a nudge as follows:

> [A]ny aspect of the choice architecture that alters people's behaviour in a predictable way without forbidding any options or significantly changing their economic incentives. To count as a mere nudge, the intervention must be easy and cheap to avoid. Nudges are not mandates. Putting fruit at eye level counts as a nudge. Banning junk food does not.

Governments like this approach because it is cheap and because they cannot be accused of running a 'nanny' state. Nudging less sedentary behaviour may involve environmental changes, such as removing chairs from some meeting rooms and thereby encouraging standing meetings, or providing standing desks in the workplace. Nudging to encourage less sedentary screen viewing in children may involve environmental changes such as the removal of TV sets from bedrooms.

> Key point: Nudging to encourage less sedentary behaviour could be promising and will likely need to involve environmental changes.

Interventions

Awareness of the potential negative effects of sedentary behaviour has led several countries or organisations to issue public health guidance focused on limiting sedentary behaviour. Table 16.3 provides examples of this guidance for young people. The awareness of the potential for negative health outcomes and the issuing of official guidance to limit sedentary behaviour have led to increasing interest in interventions that try to reduce sedentary behaviour. Much of this work has focused on changing sedentary behaviour in young people, although interventions with adults are also emerging. In young people, many of the interventions have focused on reducing television or screen-based media use, while in adults the focus has been on reducing sitting at work as well as screen-based leisure-time behaviour.

Table 16.3 A sample of sedentary behaviour recommendations for young people

Country / organisation	Recommendation
Canada (Canadian Society for Exercise Physiology, 2012)	Young people should minimise the time spent being sedentary and to limit recreational screen time to no more than two hours per day
Australia (Commonwealth of Australia, 2014)	To reduce health risks, children aged 5–12 years, and adolescents 13–17 years should minimise the time they spend being sedentary every day. To achieve this: • Limit use of electronic media for entertainment (e.g. television, seated electronic games and computer use) to no more than two hours a day – lower levels are associated with reduced health risks. • Break up long periods of sitting as often as possible.
United Kingdom (Department of Health, 2011)	Young people should minimise the amount of time spent being sedentary (sitting) for extended periods.
USA (American Academy of Pediatrics, 2001)	Children should limit total entertainment media time to less than two hours per day.

Young people

As already stated, research on interventions to reduce sedentary behaviour has focused almost exclusively on young people, and there are at least 10 systematic reviews or meta-analyses synthesising some aspect of this work (Biddle *et al.*, 2011, 2013; DeMattia *et al.*, 2007; Kamath *et al.*, 2008; Leung *et al.*, 2012; Luckner *et al.*, 2011; Maniccia *et al.*, 2011; Schmidt *et al.*, 2012; Steeves *et al.*, 2012; Wahi *et al.*, 2011). Many of these systematic reviews have included studies that did not focus explicitly on sedentary behaviour change but may have measured sedentary behaviour as a secondary outcome of a physical activity or weight management intervention.

The majority of the interventions included in these reviews focus on reducing TV or screen media use in 8- to 11-year-old children with few interventions in the early years or adolescence (Maniccia *et al.*, 2011). The interventions have been conducted in schools, homes, community settings and clinics (Biddle *et al.*, 2013). Regardless of the primary setting of the intervention, almost all studies include a home component (Schmidt *et al.*, 2012), and the majority of interventions are delivered to both the child and the parents (Steeves *et al.*, 2012).

The meta-analysis by Biddle *et al.* (2011) only included studies that specifically targeted a reduction in sedentary behaviour. We reported a small, significant and robust effect in favour of the intervention group (Hedges' $g = -0.192$, $p = 0.001$), indicating that it is possible to change sedentary behaviour in young people. Similar-sized effects have been reported in other meta-analyses that focused only on sedentary behaviour interventions for weight management and/or have also included studies that were designed to increase physical activity but have had an assessment of sedentary behaviour as a secondary outcome (e.g. Kamath *et al.*, 2008; Maniccia *et al.*, 2011).

While these are only minor effects, it may be argued that such small changes across a large population could have significant public health implications given the prevalence of screen media use among young people (Biddle *et al.*, 2011; Maniccia *et al.*, 2011). The small effect sizes observed may also reflect real difficulties in changing behaviour with a strong habitual element.

Biddle *et al.* (2013) summarise the findings of the published systematic reviews and meta-analyses by performing a review of 10 reviews. It was concluded that interventions which focused on decreasing sedentary behaviour resulted in a reduction in sedentary behaviour and/or improvements in body composition. However, the long-term effects of these interventions could not be established due to limited data. In addition, few moderators could be identified, with some evidence that behaviour change may be greater in children (younger than 6 years), or when studies measure in-treatment outcomes rather than post-treatment outcomes.

Schmidt *et al.* (2012) and Steeves *et al.* (2012) focused on the intervention strategies employed to reduce screen time among children. Most interventions employed multiple behaviour modification strategies with the most common being goal-setting and self-monitoring, followed by pre-planning, problem-solving and positive reinforcement (Steeves *et al.*, 2012). Although these are the most frequently mentioned techniques it is not clear whether they are the most successful or whether they are causally associated with behaviour change (Biddle *et al.*, 2013).

A number of interventions also included electronic monitoring devices or contingent TV devices to assist behaviour change (Schmidt *et al.*, 2012; Steeves *et al.*, 2012). Electronic monitoring devices allow participants to set a time goal for viewing after which point the television will turn off. Contingent TV devices operate in one of two ways. In the first, a closed-loop system is used which makes TV viewing contingent on a concurrent behaviour such as stationary cycling. The second method employs an open-loop system, in which TV viewing is made contingent on physical activity accumulated at other times, and participants may choose when they use the TV time they have earned. While the inclusion of these devices has considerable effects on reducing TV viewing, with estimated reductions of between 30 and 90 per cent (Steeves *et al.*, 2012), little is known about the long-term effectiveness and sustainability of device use (Schmidt *et al.*, 2012; Steeves *et al.*, 2012). In addition, there are questions over acceptability, as the device may impact upon TV access by all family members and not just the individuals who agreed to the intervention (Schmidt *et al.*, 2012). It may also be argued that using screen viewing as a reward for completing physical activity is counter-intuitive, particularly if a reduction in screen viewing is the goal, and may be especially problematic as there is a risk that using TV as a reward may actually lead to an increased liking for TV (Steeves *et al.*, 2012).

In summary, interventions to reduce sedentary screen use have been shown to have small positive effects, particularly among children. Effective interventions include both behaviour modification techniques and electronic TV control devices or making TV contingent on other behaviours. Future interventions need to build on this work to identify the most effective strategies and to examine the long-term sustainability of behaviour change. In addition, other non-screen sedentary behaviours need to be investigated.

> Key point: Interventions to reduce sedentary screen use in children have been shown to have small positive effects.

Example intervention

Dennison *et al.* (2004) conducted an intervention designed to reduce TV viewing in American pre-school children. Baseline and post-intervention measures were made by parents, and intervention materials comprised educational and informational support to both children and parents. For example, children made 'No TV' signs to take home and place next to the TV, and parents were encouraged to read to their children and provide family meals away from the TV. Seven educational sessions were provided at day-care or pre-school settings. Results showed reductions in TV viewing for the intervention group for weekdays, Saturdays and Sundays, as shown in Figure 16.2. It was reported that the intervention was 'well accepted' by the children as well as by the parents and staff.

Adults

Interventions to reduce sitting behaviour in adults are beginning to emerge, but these are mostly small-scale pilot studies. Earlier interventions that have been suggested to change sedentary behaviour were most often physical activity interventions that assessed sedentary behaviour as a secondary outcome. For example, Chau *et al.* (2010) purported to systematically review interventions to reduce sitting in the workplace. They included six studies in the review and found no evidence for intervention effectiveness as far as sitting was concerned. This finding is perhaps unsurprising given that all of the included studies were designed to increase physical activity and did not have a clear focus on sedentary behaviour reduction. In addition, the studies relied on self-report measures of sedentary or sitting behaviour, of which only one specifically assessed occupational sitting.

    More recent studies have used a variety of approaches to target sedentary behaviour more directly and these provide better evidence on whether changing sitting behaviour is possible and, if so, what are likely to be effective strategies. The majority of these recent studies have

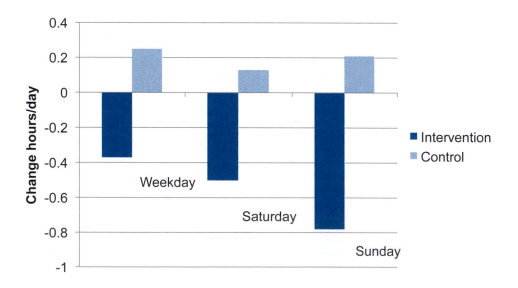

Figure 16.2 Changes in TV viewing from intervention

Source: Dennison *et al.* (2004).

focused on workplaces, and office workplaces in particular. There is a need to broaden the focus and consider other types of worksites or occupations (e.g. drivers), and also other contexts in which sedentary behaviour takes place.

Workplace interventions

In a randomised controlled trial conducted in workplaces in the Netherlands, Verweij *et al.* (2012) examined the effectiveness of a draft occupational guideline aimed at preventing weight gain on employees' physical activity, sedentary behaviour and dietary behaviour. The guideline included evidence-based methods and strategies to prevent weight gain and was designed for use by occupational physicians. Participants were randomised to either a usual care group (control; n = 249 employees with nine occupational physicians) or an intervention group (n = 274 with seven occupational physicians). The intervention was delivered by the occupational physicians associated with the different workplaces who had received behaviour change training suitable for brief consultations in health care settings. Intervention participants received up to five 20- to 30-minute counselling sessions over six months. Participants could choose which target behaviour they would like to discuss (decreasing sedentary behaviour, increasing physical activity or reducing snacking). The counselling sessions covered pros and cons of behaviour change, perceived confidence to change, goal-setting and potential barriers to change. Sedentary behaviour, physical activity and dietary behaviour were all assessed through self-report at baseline and immediately post intervention.

At the end of the six months participants in the intervention group had significantly lower sedentary behaviour at work (-15 vs. -3 minutes/day) and increased fruit intake (+1.5 vs. -0.8 pieces/week). No significant effects were found on physical activity, total or leisure-time sedentary behaviour, or snack intake. The authors concluded that guideline-based care can result in less sedentary behaviour at work and increased fruit consumption, but work is required to increase adherence by the occupational physicians to the guideline and to enhance attendance by participants.

Another approach to reducing sitting time at work has been to employ prompting software on PCs used at work. This type of software may be used as 'pop-up' advice windows at regular intervals reminding users to take a break. In a small-scale randomised trial, employing a convenience sample, Evans *et al.* (2012) investigated the effect of installing prompting software, on the computer used at work (PC), to reduce long, uninterrupted sedentary bouts and total sedentary time at work. There were two groups. The first group (n = 14) received a brief education session on the importance of reducing prolonged sitting at work. The second group (n = 14) received the same education along with software for their computer that reminded them to stand up every 30 minutes. Sitting time was measured objectively using the activPAL device (see earlier) for five days prior to the intervention and for the five days of the intervention. The main outcome measures were the number of bouts of sitting longer than 30 minutes and the total amount of sitting accumulated in bouts longer than 30 minutes.

Results showed that during the intervention period the education-plus prompt group reduced the number and duration of sitting events longer than 30 minutes, and this compared to a lack of change in the education-only group. These are encouraging results; however, the small sample employed, the short duration of the intervention and the lack of long-term follow-up mean that more work is needed before firm conclusions may be drawn.

Another approach receiving substantial attention is the use of standing desks and sit-stand workstations. The latter may be fitted to traditional desks. Sit-stand workstations are height adjustable and may be moved up and down to allow working in either a seated or standing posture. The effect of the introduction of standing desks to workplaces has been investigated in several small-scale studies, with mixed results. Alkhajah *et al.* (2012) conducted a pilot study assessing the short- (one-week) and long-term (three-month) changes in objectively measured sitting time (both workplace and total sitting) in office workers who were assigned to either a sit-stand desk intervention group (n = 18) or to a control group (n = 14; no change to normal desk). Sitting time was measured objectively using the activPAL, and data were collected for one week at baseline, one week after the sit-stand desks were installed, and again after three months. Results showed that compared to the control group the intervention group reduced their workplace sitting by more than two hours per day at both the one-week and three-month follow-up. There were also significant differences between the groups in overall sitting time which favoured the intervention group.

In another study, Gilson *et al.* (2012) investigated the use of standing desks within an open-plan shared office environment. Sedentary behaviour was monitored using the SenseWear pro armband accelerometer for one week. After a baseline assessment week, a pod of four standing desks was fitted into the centre of the office space and the 11 employees involved in the study were briefed on the benefits of reducing sitting and encouraged to use any of the standing desks within the pod to stand and work as often as possible during the week. The participants continued to wear the SenseWear armband throughout this intervention week. There was no overall change in the proportion of time spent in sedentary behaviour during the intervention week. When looking at the data for individual participants, some individuals had made a lot of use of the shared standing workstations and others had made no use at all. Further work is needed to identify reasons that influence the use of the shared desks.

Sit-stand desks were also incorporated within a multi-component intervention to reduce office workers' sitting time (Healy *et al.*, 2013). A single organisation was used and, to prevent contamination, workers on one floor were invited to be in the control group (usual working patterns maintained; n = 22) and those on the other floor to be in the intervention group (n = 22). The intervention comprised organisational, environmental and individual elements, and emphasised three key messages: Stand Up, Sit Less, Move More. In the organisational element the researcher led consultations with worksite representatives during which they brainstormed and selected organisation-specific strategies that were then conveyed to all participants in a workshop. The environmental element involved the installation of sit-stand workstations for the four weeks of the study. Participants were briefed on the use of the stations and also received an information sheet. The individual-level element comprised an initial 30-minute face-to-face consultation with a health coach, and this was followed by three phone calls (one per week). In the initial session, participants received feedback on their baseline activity and standing, and this information was used to construct personally relevant goals around the three key messages of Stand Up (at least once every 30 minutes), Sit Less (by using the workstation), and Move More (by increasing incidental physical activity). These sessions emphasised behaviour change strategies, prompts and problem-solving.

Total sitting time, sitting time accumulated in prolonged bouts (>30 minutes), standing time and stepping time were assessed using the activPAL at baseline and at the end of the intervention (four weeks). Compared to the control there were significant reductions in workplace sitting time in the intervention group, in the order of 125 minutes per eight-hour working day. These changes appeared to be the result of reductions in prolonged bouts of sitting. The sitting was replaced with standing but not stepping. The authors concluded that substantial reductions in sitting time are achievable in the office setting, although larger and longer studies are needed to assess sustainability of the changes and their potential impact on health-related outcomes.

An alternative to standing desks are treadmill desks. These consist of a treadmill that fits under a sit-to-stand table, with room for a desk chair next to the treadmill in case the user wishes to sit. The treadmill is operated at a slow walking speed while the individual works. John *et al.* (2011) investigated whether access to a treadmill desk resulted in changes in sedentary time, physical activity, body composition and cardiovascular and metabolic variables in 12 overweight or obese office workers. After baseline measures, treadmill workstations were installed in the participants' offices. Follow-up measures were taken after three months and again at the end of the intervention (nine months). Participants wore an activPAL for two workdays at each measurement point to assess sitting time and physical activity. Significant increases in standing time, stepping time and total steps were observed, and there was a corresponding decrease in sitting time. Favourable changes in waist and hip circumference and lipid and metabolic profiles were also observed. Some might perceive treadmill desks as quite a challenging intervention and more information is needed regarding how acceptable such a change may be viewed.

The physical environment of many workplaces lends itself to sedentary behaviour, with many sitting and few non-sitting options available. While large, structural changes to buildings to make them more activity-permissive are complex and not always readily available, when they do occur they provide the opportunity to observe what effect whole-of-workplace environmental change may have. Gorman *et al.* (2013) report on a natural experiment looking at changes in standing, stepping and sitting time before and after a move from a conventional workplace (with no standing options in offices or meeting rooms) to an activity-permissive workplace (this was a purpose-built building, including a glass-enclosed staircase, height-adjustable desks, standing option meeting rooms and common areas, centralised printing, and a layout that encouraged movement across floors). Workers, who were from a university research centre, received no information or education about the benefits of sitting less and moving more at work. Almost one-third of the workforce volunteered for the study. ActivPAL data were collected for seven days pre-move and again at an average of four months post-move once workers had acclimatised to their new environment. Post-move there was a significant increase in workplace standing time (18.5 minutes/8-hour working day) which was reflected in a decrease in sitting time (-19.7 minutes/8-hour working day). There were no changes in stepping behaviour. There was considerable variation in the degree of change achieved, and this seemed to be influenced by employment level, with general non-academic staff showing greater change compared to academic staff (faculty) members.

Table 16.4 summarises the preliminary evidence for approaches to reduce sedentary behaviour in adults during office work. This is not a definitive list and it is important that the limitations of this evidence are acknowledged. The evidence comes from a limited number

Table 16.4 Summary of preliminary evidence for approaches that have been trialled in worksites to reduce sitting among employees

	Change in sedentary time
Education only	N
Education plus computer prompt	Y
Standing desk	Y
Shared standing desk	N
Treadmill desk	Y
Building changes	Y
Multi-component	Y

of small-scale studies. Convenience samples have often been employed. The studies were generally of short duration and there is limited evidence for the sustainability of changes and people's willingness to engage with intervention approaches such as standing desks in the long term (see Grunseit *et al.*, 2013). Consideration also needs to be given to social factors and worksite culture that may influence someone's willingness to change the way they work (e.g. not wanting to be the only one standing).

> Key point: Initial studies on reducing sitting time at work are promising but more needs to be known about the acceptability and longevity of changes.

Other intervention contexts

Very few interventions to reduce sedentary behaviour in adults have been undertaken outside of the workplace context, although published protocol papers (e.g. Martin-Borras *et al.*, 2014; Wilmot *et al.*, 2011) suggest that there are ongoing trials which will start to address this gap. One published feasibility study, 'Stand Up For Your Health', has shown favourable results in adults aged 60 years and older (n = 59; Gardiner *et al.*, 2011). In this trial they used a 45-minute face-to-face meeting to assist participants to reduce sitting time and to increase breaks in sitting. The intervention was informed by Social Cognitive Theory and behavioural choice theory, and focused on building self-efficacy (via goal-setting), self-control (via self-monitoring and goal-setting), outcome expectancies (via barriers and benefits), reinforcement (via rewarding behaviour change) and preference (via identifying enjoyable non-sedentary pursuits). During the intervention session participants: (1) reviewed their accelerometer-assessed sedentary time from the previous day; (2) received normative feedback on their self-reported sedentary time, using graphs to compare to an average Australian of a similar age and gender; (3) completed a goal-setting exercise to reduce sedentary time and increase the number of breaks in prolonged sedentary time, and (4) formulated a behaviourally specific action plan. Generic strategies to reduce and break up sedentary time were suggested, and participants identified strategies specific to their circum-stances. The participants were also encouraged to self-monitor their sitting behaviour using a tracker. Sedentary time was derived from the Actigraph accelerometer and defined as <100 counts per minute. At the end of the first week of data collection participants received the intervention and were then monitored for another week. During this post-intervention week there was a small but significant reduction in sedentary time of 3.2 per cent and an increase in the number of breaks from sedentary time. Participants reduced their sedentary time mainly during the day, and increased their breaks in sedentary time in the evening. This intervention is promising but a full randomised trial with a representative sample is required before we can make definitive conclusions about its effectiveness.

Sedentary behaviour change in adults: Summary

While the field of research on interventions to reduce sedentary behaviour in adults is still in its infancy, results from the early pilot studies indicate that reductions in sedentary behaviour are achievable, at least in the short term and in the workplace. Until further more robust intervention evidence is available, possible strategies may need to involve a mixture of individual (goal-setting, self-monitoring, prompts), social (targeted social support, changing norms for standing) and physical environment actions (e.g. modified office design such as standing desks and waste bins away from desks; standing or walking meetings; public prompts and signs).

Chapter summary

Sedentary behaviour is a new area for those who study physical activity and health psychology. The wider field of sedentary behaviour, including epidemiological trends, measurement and health outcomes, is growing rapidly. However, behaviour change, and the psychological issues associated with it, is still in its infancy. From the evidence presented in this chapter, we conclude the following:

- There is growing evidence for a relationship between sedentary behaviour and health outcomes. This is stronger in adults than in young people and has been shown to be independent of MVPA.
- Sedentary behaviour can be measured using objective devices as well as by self-report. The former can capture total time being sedentary as well as the number of breaks in sedentary time. Self-report measures can be useful for assessing different types and contexts of sedentary behaviour.
- Studies on the correlates of sedentary behaviour in young people are still quite limited, with many focusing only on screen time. Few modifiable correlates have been identified. The evidence concerning adults is even less well developed.
- Theories and models have been used to help explain sedentary behaviour but often these have been taken from research on physical activity. It may not be appropriate to use the same approaches.
- Interventions helping to change sedentary behaviour have a longer history for young people than for adults. For young people most studies have been limited to sedentary screen time, while for adults studies are emerging on reducing sitting in the workplace. Initial evidence shows that sedentary behaviour can be reduced, but often changes are small with limited evidence on how long term such changes may be.

References

Aarts, H., Paulussen, T. and Schaalma, H. (1997). Physical exercise habit: On the conceptualization and formation of habitual health behaviours. *Health Education Research, 12*, 363–374.

Alkhajah, T., Reeves, M., Eakin, E., Winkler, E., Owen, N. and Healy, G. (2012). Sit-stand workstations: A pilot intervention to reduce office sitting time. *American Journal of Preventive Medicine, 43*(3), 298–303.

American Academy of Pediatrics. (2001). Policy statement: Children, adolescents and television (RE0043). *Pediatrics, 107*(2), 423–426.

Atkin, A., Gorely, T., Clemes, S., Yates, T., Edwardson, C., Brage, S. and Biddle, S. (2012). Sedentary behaviour: A methods of measurement in epidemiology paper. *International Journal of Epidemiology, 41*, 1460–1471.

Bargh, J. and Chartrand, T. (1999). The unbearable automaticity of being. *American Psychologist, 54*, 462–479.

Biddle, S. and Asare, M. (2011). Physical activity and mental health in children and adolescents: A review of reviews. *British Journal of Sports Medicine, 45*, 886–895.

Biddle, S., Hagger, M., Chatzisarantis, N. and Lippke, S. (2007). Theoretical frameworks in exercise psychology. In G. Tenenbaum and R.C. Eklund (eds), *Handbook of Sport Psychology* (3rd edn, pp. 537–559). Hoboken, NJ: John Wiley.

Biddle, S., Gorely, T. and Marshall, S. (2009). Is television viewing a suitable marker of sedentary behaviour in young people. *Annals of Behavioral Medicine*, Published online 07 October 2009. doi: 10.1007/s12160-12009-19136-12161.

Biddle, S., Pearson, N., Ross, G.M. and Braithwaite, R. (2010). Tracking of sedentary behaviours of young people: A systematic review. *Preventive Medicine, 51*, 345–351.

Biddle, S., O'Connell, S. and Braithwaite, R. (2011). Sedentary behaviour interventions in young people: A meta-analysis. *British Journal of Sports Medicine, 45*, 937–942.

Biddle, S., Pertolini, I. and Pearson, N. (2013). Interventions designed to reduce sedentary behaviours in young people: A review of reviews. *British Journal of Sports Medicine*, Published online first: 17 December 2013. doi: 10.1136/bjsports-2013-093078.

Bryant, M.J., Lucove, J.C., Evenson, K.R. and Marshall, S. (2007). Measurement of television viewing in children and adolescents: A systematic review. *Obesity Reviews: An Official Journal of the International Association for the Study of Obesity, 8*(3), 197–209.

Canadian Society for Exercise Physiology. (2012). *Canadian Physical Activity Guidelines, Canadian Sedentary Behaviour Guidelines*. http://www.csep.ca/guidelines.

Chau, J., van der Ploeg, H., van Uffelen, J., Wong, J., Riphagen, I., Healy, G. and Brown, W. (2010). Are workplace interventions to reduce sitting effective? A systematic review. *Preventive Medicine, 51*, 352–356.

Chau, J., Grunseit, A., Chey, T., Stamatakis, E., Brown, W., Matthews, C. and van der Ploeg, H. (2013). Daily sitting time and all-cause mortality: A meta-analysis. *PLoS ONE, 8*(11), e80000. doi:80010.81371/journal.pone.0080000.

Chinapaw, M., Proper, K., Brug, J., van Mechelen, W. and Singh, A. (2011). Relationship between young peoples' sedentary behaviour and biomedical health indicators: A systematic review of prospective studies. *Obesity Reviews*, doi: 10.1111/j.1467-789X.2011.00865.x.

Cillero, I. and Jago, R. (2010). Systematic review of correlates of screen-viewing among young children. *Preventive Medicine, 51*, 3–10.

Clark, B., Sugiyama, T., Healy, G., Salmon, J., Dunstan, D. and Owen, N. (2009). Validity and reliability of measures of television viewing time and other non-occupational sedentary behaviour of adults: A review. *Obesity Reviews, 10*(1), 7–16.

Colley, R., Garriguet, D., Janssen, I., Craig, C., Clarke, J. and Tremblay, M. (2011). Physical activity of Canadian children and youth: Accelerometer results from the 2007 to 2009 Canadian Health Measures Survey. *Health Reports, 22*, 15–23.

Commonwealth of Australia. (2014). *Make Your Move – Sit less. Be active for life!* Canberra: Commonwealth of Australia. Retrieved from http://www.health.gov.au.

DeMattia, L., Lemont, L. and Meurer, L. (2007). Do interventions to limit sedentary behaviours change behaviour and reduce childhood obesity? A critical review of the literature. *Obesity Reviews, 8*, 69–81.

Dennison, B.A., Russo, T.J., Burdick, P.A. and Jenkins, P.L. (2004). An intervention to reduce television viewing by preschool children. *Archives of Pediatrics and Adolescent Medicine, 158*(2), 170–176.

Department of Health. (2011). *Start Active, Stay Active: A report on physical activity from the four home countries' Chief Medical Officers*. London: Department of Health.

Edwardson, C., Gorely, T., Davies, M., Gray, L., Khunti, K., Wilmot, E. and Biddle, S. (2012). Association of sedentary behaviour with metabolic syndrome: A meta-analysis. *PLoS ONE, 7*(4), e34916.

Epstein, L.H. (1998). Integrating theoretical approaches to promote physical activity. *American Journal of Preventive Medicine, 15*(4), 257–265.

Epstein, L.H. and Roemmich, J.N. (2001). Reducing sedentary behaviour: Role in modifying physical activity. *Exercise and Sport Sciences Reviews, 29*, 103–108.

Epstein, L.H., Saelens, B.E. and O'Brien, J.G. (1995). Effects of reinforcing increases in active behavior versus decreases in sedentary behavior for obese children. *International Journal of Behavioral Medicine, 2*(1), 41–50.

Evans, R., Fawole, H., Sheriff, S., Dall, P., Grant, P. and Ryan, C. (2012). Point-of-choice prompts to reduce sitting time at work: A randomized trial. *American Journal of Preventive Medicine, 43*(3), 293–297.

Gardner, B., de Bruijn, G. and Lally, P. (2011). A systematic review and meta-analysis of applications of the Self-Report Habit Index to nutrition and physical activity behaviours. *Annals of Behavioral Medicine, 42*, 174–187.

Gardiner, P., Eakin, E., Healy, G. and Owen, N. (2011). Feasibility of reducing older adults' sedentary time. *American Journal of Preventive Medicine, 41*(2), 174–177.

Gilson, N.D., Suppini, A., Ryde, G., Brown, H. and Brown, W. (2012). Does the use of standing 'hot' desks change sedentary work time in an open plan office? *Preventive Medicine, 54*, 65–67.

Gorely, T., Marshall, S. and Biddle, S. (2004). Correlates of TV viewing in adolescents. *International Journal of Behavioural Medicine, 11*, 152–163.

Gorman, E., Ashe, M., Dunstan, D., Hanson, H., Madden, K., Winkler, E. and Healy, G. (2013). Does an 'activity-permissive' workplace change office workers' sitting and activity time? *PLoS ONE, 8*(10), e76723. doi:76710.71371/journal.pone.0076723.

Grunseit, A.C., Chau, J.Y-Y., van der Ploeg, H.P. and Bauman, A. (2013). 'Thinking on your feet': A qualitative evaluation of sit-stand desks in an Australian workplace. *BMC Public Health, 13*(1), 365. doi: 10.1186/1471-2458-13-365.

Hallal, P., Andersen, L., Bull, F., Guthold, R., Haskell, W. and Ekelund, U. (2012). Global physical activity levels: Surveillance progress, pitfalls, and prospects. *Lancet, 380*, 247–257.

Hardy, L., Booth, M. and Okely, A. (2007). The reliability of the Adolescent Sedentary Activity Questionnaire (ASAQ). *Preventive Medicine, 45*(1), 71–74.

Healy, G., Dunstan, D., Salmon, J., Cerin, E., Shaw, J., Zimmet, P. and Owen, N. (2008). Breaks in sedentary time: Beneficial associations with metabolic risk. *Diabetes Care, 31*, 661–666.

Healy, G., Eakin, E., LaMontagne, A., Owen, N., Winkler, E., Wiesner, G. and Dunstan, D. (2013). Reducing sitting time in office workers: Short-term efficacy of a multicomponent intervention. *Preventive Medicine, 57*, 43–48.

Henson, J., Yates, T., Biddle, S., Edwardson, C., Khunti, K., Wilmot, E. and Davies, M. (2013). Associations of objectively measured sedentary behaviour and physical activity with markers of cardio-metabolic health. *Diabetologia, 56*(5), 1012–1020. doi: 10.1007/s00125-013-2845-9.

Hinkley, T., Salmon, J., Okley, A. and Trost, S. (2010). Correlates of sedentary behaviours in preschool children: A review. *International Journal of Behavioural Nutrition and Physical Activity, 7*, 66.

John, D., Thompson, D.L., Raynor, H., Bielak, K., Rider, B. and Bassett, D.R. (2011). Treadmill workstations: A worksite physical activity intervention in overweight and obese office workers. *Journal of Physical Activity and Health, 8*, 1034–1043.

Kamath, C.C., Vickers, K.S., Ehrlich, A., McGovern, L., Johnson, J., Singhal, V. and Montori, V.M. (2008). Behavioural interventions to prevent childhood obesity: A systematic review and meta-analyses of randomized trials. *Journal of Clinical Endocrinology and Metabolism, 93*(12), 4606–4615.

Kremers, S.P. and Brug, J. (2008). Habit strength of physical activity and sedentary behavior among children and adolescents. *Pediatric Exercise Science, 20*, 5–17.

Kremers, S.P., van der Horst, K. and Brug, J. (2007). Adolescent screen-viewing behaviour is associated with consumption of sugar-sweetened beverages: The role of habit strength and perceived parental norms. *Appetite, 48*, 345–350.

Lally, P. and Gardner, B. (2011). Promoting habit formation. *Health Psychology Review, 7*(supp. 1), S137–S158.

Leung, M., Agaronov, A., Grytsenko, K. and Yeh, M-C. (2012). Intervening to reduce sedentary behaviours and childhood obesity among school-age youth: A systematic review of randomized trials. *Journal of Obesity, 2012*, 14pp.

Luckner, H., Moss, J. and Gericke, C. (2011). Effectiveness of interventions to promote healthy weight in general populations of children and adults: A meta-analysis. *European Journal of Public Health*, 1–7. doi:10.1093/eurpub/ckr1141.

Maniccia, D., Davison, K., Marshall, S., Manganello, J. and Dennison, B. (2011). A meta-analysis of interventions that target children's screen time for reduction. *Pediatrics, 128*, e193.

Marshall, A.L., Miller, Y.D., Burton, N.W. and Brown, W.J. (2010). Measuring total and domain-specific sitting: A study of reliability and validity. *Medicine and Science in Sports and Exercise, 42*(6), 1094–1102.

Martin-Borras, C., Gine-Garriga, M., Martinez, E., Martin-Cantera, C., Puigdomenech, E., Sola, M. *et al.* (2014). Effectiveness of a primary care-based intervention to reduce sitting time in overweight and obese patients (SEDESTACTIV): A randomized controlled trial; rationale and study design. *BMC Public Health, 14*, 228.

Matthews, C., Chen, K., Freedson, P., Buchowski, M., Beech, B., Pate, R. and Troiano, R. (2008). Amount of time spent in sedentary behaviors in the United States, 2003–2004. *American Journal of Epidemiology, 167*, 875–881.

Moskowitz, G., Skurnik, I. and Galinski, A. (1999). The history of dual-process notions, and the future of preconscious control. In S. Chaiken and Y. Trope (eds), *Dual Process Theories in Social Psychology* (pp. 12–36). New York: Guilford Press.

Owen, N. (2012). Ambulatory monitoring and sedentary behaviour: A population-health perspective. *Physiological Measurement, 33*, 1801–1810.

Owen, N., Sugiyama, T., Eakin, E., Gardiner, P., Tremblay, M. and Sallis, J. (2011). Adults' sedentary behavior: Determinants and interventions. *American Journal of Preventive Medicine, 41*(2), 189–196.

Pearson, N. and Biddle, S. (2011). Sedentary behaviour and dietary intake in children, adolescents and adults: A systematic review. *American Journal of Preventive Medicine, 41*, 178–188.

Pearson, N., Braithwaite, R., Biddle, S., van Sluijs, E. and Atkin, A. (2014). Associations between sedentary behaviour and physical activity in children and adolescents: A meta-analysis. *Obesity Reviews*. doi: 10.1111/obr.12188.

Proper, K.I., Singh, A.S., van Mechelen, W. and Chinapaw, M.J.M. (2011). Sedentary behaviors and health outcomes among adults: A systematic review of prospective studies. *American Journal of Preventive Medicine,, 40*(2), 174–182.

Rezende, L., Rey-Lopez, J., Matsudo, V. and Luiz, O. (2014). Sedentary behavior and health outcomes among older adults: A systematic review. *BMC Public Health, 14*, 333.

Rhodes, R.E., Mark, R.S. and Temmel, C.P. (2012). Adult sedentary behavior: A systematic review. *American Journal of Preventive Medicine, 42*(3), e3–e28.

Rideout, V., Foehr, U. and Roberts, D. (2010). GENERATION M2 media in the lives of 8- to 18-year-olds: A Kaiser Family Foundation Report. Retrieved 30 July 2010 from http://www.kff.org/entmedia/upload/8010.pdf.

Schmidt, M., Haines, J., O'Brien, A., McDonald, J., Price, S., Sherry, B. and Taveras, E. (2012). Systematic review of effective strategies for reducing screen time among young children. *Obesity,* doi: 10.1038/oby2011.348.

Sedentary Behaviour Research Network. (2012). Letter to the Editor: Standardized use of the terms 'sedentary' and 'sedentary behaviours'. *Applied Physiology, Nutrition and Metabolism, 37*, 540–542.

Steeves, J., Thompson, D., Bassett, D., Fitzhugh, E. and Raynor, H. (2012). A review of different behavior modification strategies designed to reduce sedentary screen behaviors in children. *Journal of Obesity, 16*, 16.

Sugiyama, T., Healy, G., Dunstan, D., Salmon, J. and Owen, N. (2008). Is television viewing time a marker of a broader pattern of sedentary behavior? *Annals of Behavioral Medicine, 35*, 245–250.

Thaler, R. and Sunstein, C. (2008). *Nudge: Improving decisions about health, wealth, and happiness.* New Haven, CT: Yale University Press.

Thorp, A., Owen, N., Neuhaus, M. and Dunstan, D. (2011). Sedentary behaviors and subsequent health outcomes in adults: A systematic review of longitudinal studies, 1996–2011. *American Journal of Preventive Medicine, 41*(2), 207–215.

Tremblay, M., LeBlanc, A., Kho, M., Saunders, T., Larouche, R., Colley, R. and Connor Gorber, S. (2011). Systematic review of sedentary behaviour and health indicators in school-aged children and youth. *International Journal of Behavioral Nutrition and Physical Activity, 8*, 98.

Uijtdewilligen, L., Nauta, J., Singh, A., Van Mechelen, W., Twisk, J., Van der Horst, K. and Chinapaw, M. (2011). Determinants of physical activity and sedentary behaviour in young people: A review and quality synthesis of prospective studies. *British Journal of Sports Medicine, 45*, 896–905.

van der Horst, K., Chin A Paw, M., Twisk, J. and Van Mechelen, W. (2007). A brief review on correlates of physical activity and sedentariness in youth. *Medicine and Science in Sports and Exercise, 39*(8), 1241–1250.

Verweij, L.M., Proper, K., Weel, A.N.H., Hulshof, C.T. and van Mechelen, W. (2012). The application of an occupational health guideline reduces sedentary behaviour and increases fruit intake at work: Results from an RCT. *Occupational and Environmental Medicine, 69*, 500–507.

Wahi, G., Parkin, P., Beyene, J., Uleryk, E. and Birken, C. (2011). Effectiveness of interventions aimed at reducing screen time in children: A systematic review and meta-analysis of randomized controlled trials. *Archives of Pediatric and Adolescent Medicine, 165*(11), 979–986.

Wilmot, E., Davies, M., Edwardson, C.T.G., Khunti, K., Nimmo, M. and Biddle, S. (2011). Rationale and study design for a randomised controlled trial to reduce sedentary time in adults at risk of Type 2 diabetes mellitus: Project STAND (Sedentary Time ANd Diabetes). *BMC Public Health, 11*, 908.

Wilmot, E., Edwardson, C., Achana, F., Davies, M., Gorely, T., Gray, L. and Biddle, S. (2012). Sedentary time in adults and the association with diabetes, cardiovascular disease and death: Systematic review and meta-analysis. *Diabetologia, 55*(11), 2895–2905.

Wood, W. and Neal, D.T. (2009). The habitual consumer. *Journal of Consumer Psychology, 19*, 579–592.

Part VI

Conclusions

17 Summary, conclusions and recommendations

All's well that ends!

Those were the days, my friends

The forerunner of this book was published quite a long time ago (Biddle and Mutrie, 1991). Unfortunately, it was produced in hardback only and was available at a very high price. Consequently, its visibility was limited to the extent that another publisher advertised their own book on 'exercise psychology' a year later as the first ever! However, our initial publishers no longer wanted to publish psychology books, and hence we moved to Routledge where we produced the 'first' edition of the current book with them in 2001 (Biddle and Mutrie, 2001). The second edition was published in 2007 (Biddle and Mutrie, 2007), and now here is the third edition. Thus, from initial publication to 2015, it has been almost a quarter of a century.

A great deal has changed during this time in the interconnected worlds of research, physical activity, health and psychology. The field has changed and moved on and, we would like to think, so have we. But what have we learned over this 20-plus-year period and what are the big issues for the future? This chapter will allow us some reflection over the past few years, and especially the past seven years or so since we prepared the last edition of this book. We will do this by posing some key questions and offering some thoughts in response. Each chapter in this book has its own set of conclusions so we do not feel we need to repeat those here, although we will discuss some future directions.

What has progressed?

$r = 0.30$, but so what?

Looking back on the earlier editions of this book it is clear that we wrote a great deal about psychological theory that we thought underpinned involvement in physical activity. Much of this drew on papers that were heavy on theorising or were observational studies correlating one psychological variable with another, usually showing modest strength correlations – the ubiquitous 0.30! If you were lucky, these psychological variables might be associated with intentions and a weak self-reported measure of behaviour, but the latter were in the minority. In other words, we had a great deal of theory to go on but precious little intervention evidence or larger observational studies combining psychological with social and environmental variables. That has now changed, although the field is still guilty of producing a plethora of observational studies with poor behavioural outcome measures. But we do have a great deal more evidence on interventions, and signs that this expansion is continuing.

Less chaos in the brickyard

Moreover, when we first reviewed the evidence, we relied on collating a large number of primary studies and giving it our best shot at summarising the trends. While no textbook can realistically conduct and report a new systematic review for every chapter, it can at least draw on review-level evidence as a way of synthesising the literature and providing a good guide to current trends. This has changed greatly over the past 20 years to the extent that we had almost too many systematic reviews to handle for the current book. For example, in Table 5.2, we have summarised the evidence from 10 systematic reviews concerning the relationship between physical activity and cognitive functioning only in young people. In Chapter 16, we draw on five systematic reviews of correlates of sedentary behaviour and 10 reviews of interventions, also only in young people. The list could go on. There has been an explosion in this type of research, and systematic reviews, including meta-analyses, have often provided much-needed coherence and structure to previous chaos. To use the long-standing analogy of bricks and wall building, we now have a better and more organised 'wall' of knowledge rather than the somewhat chaotic 'brickyard' of yesteryear (Biddle, 2006; Forscher, 1963). That said, we may be in danger of some chaos returning. We have many different systematic reviews on the same topic, as highlighted above. These reviews often use slightly different inclusion criteria and can reach slightly different conclusions. One way to keep this under control is to conduct a review of reviews, and we do have some in our field (e.g. Biddle and Asare, 2011; Biddle *et al.*, 2014; Daley, 2008; Greaves *et al.*, 2011; Kriemler *et al.*, 2011).

   In addition to research synthesis coming to the fore, the field has also recognised that different research designs have their place. Not only has this brought about more variety in methods, including greater recognition and use of qualitative methods, it has also led to the appreciation that not all methods are equal. With behaviour change often being the key objective for psychologists, it is apparent that much greater use of intervention designs is needed and, fortunately, this is now taking place. The identification of correlates of physical activity is all well and good, and necessary (see the behavioural epidemiological framework described in Chapter 1 and the content of Chapter 7), but research cannot stop there. Correlates must inform intervention design and be tested under rigorous experimental conditions with suitable process evaluation.

And I'm feeling good

We know that connections between physical activity, fitness and mental health have been discussed for centuries, and even in the relatively young field of sport and exercise science there is a literature going back many decades. For example, researchers such as Bill Morgan (e.g. Morgan, 1969) were instrumental in the development of this area that is still expanding today (see Ekkekakis, 2013).

   The area of physical activity and mental health has developed on several fronts. First, while research continues to explore links between physical activity and discrete elements of mental health, such as depression, it has now expanded to address special populations, such as women with breast cancer, adults with schizophrenia, those with sleep problems, and links to helping with problem behaviours (e.g. smoking cessation). In addition, researchers are more aware that mental health responses to physical activity are not just outcomes in their own right, but are also linked to how people feel about continuing their active lifestyles. In other words, they have a motivational influence. Moreover, expansion is evident in the area of cognitive functioning. Physical activity is being increasingly recognised as an important element for children's school learning and for older adults' mental function and independence. These are powerful arguments in support of the role of physical activity in the promotion of good mental health and prevention of poor mental health.

Rollin' and tumblin'

Even with greater use of experimental designs, other things are changing. Researchers are increasingly seeking greater 'impact' for their work. They need to know what works and why. In addition, they want to 'roll out' practical behaviour change solutions. It is interesting to see the emergence of 'implementation' and 'translational' journals such as *Implementation Science* and *Translational Behavioral Medicine*. While there is obviously a place for more basic science on physical activity, we are essentially interested in getting more people more active and less sedentary. This requires translation of research and rolling out behaviour change solutions, preferably at low cost.

Too many interventions in physical activity are either not working well or we do not know why they have limited effectiveness. Greater use of comprehensive process evaluation is required (see Chapter 12). In this respect, researchers need to broaden their outlook beyond the emphasis on psychology in this book, and this is another noteworthy trend which we have observed. Physical activity behaviour change is not just 'exercise psychology'. A good intervention will certainly require appropriate choice of psychological/behavioural theory, with elements mapped on to behaviour change techniques, but successful interventions may also require good measurement tools, including those for certain biomarkers, as well as for assessing the primary outcomes of physical activity and sedentary behaviour. All of this requires multi-disciplinary research teams leaving their 'ology' baggage at the door as they enter! Some academics find that hard to do. One may argue that we have moved in our different editions of this book from just psychology to a greater focus on psychology embedded within a wider behavioural epidemiological framework. Interestingly, both Stuart and Nanette have moved from professorial positions with psychology in the title to positions that focus more on physical activity for health.

Are you sitting comfortably?

Those familiar with earlier editions of this book may notice one very significant difference between then and now: sedentary behaviour. There has been an explosion of research investigating 'sitting time' alongside moderate to vigorous physical activity. This focus on sedentary behaviour has not necessarily had much connection with psychology per se, although there are numerous examples of behaviour change interventions with elements of psychology included (see Chapter 16). What this shift has done is to highlight a continuum of energy expenditure and posture – from sleep to vigorous physical activity – and not just a focus on MVPA (see Figure 16.1). As this field develops, more integration between environmental changes, such as standing desks, and psychological strategies, such as self-monitoring with prompts, will be evident as we seek better ways of reducing excessive sitting alongside ways of increasing MVPA. Perhaps the next edition of this book will include sedentary behaviour in the title!

Context is king

Another change which we detect from the many years of involvement in this field is the shift towards a more public (population) health approach, even when using individualistic psychology principles. There is now a much greater emphasis not just on the person, but on the context in which the individual operates. This means that psychology has had to embrace a wider public health approach and ask how its principles may be applied successfully across a wide range of contexts and populations. While many of the theoretical approaches covered in this book have been developed from a more individualistic slant, they may still be applied across larger populations. For example, self-efficacy is known to be an important construct in the initiation and maintenance of physical activity, and it was developed from experiences in individual counselling (see Chapter 10). Yet the same construct may be applied in a public health approach through mass media messages and community-wide strategies.

   Ultimately, psychology is about individual behaviour, and indeed any behaviour change strategy will ultimately involve the individual. But we are essentially interested in making the greatest difference with the widest population reach. This requires a dual approach through understanding the behaviour and context. The behaviour may be walking (high reach) or high intensity exercise (low reach) (see the RE-AIM framework in Chapter 12). Whatever the behaviour, we need to better understand what it is, how people feel about it, what contexts it takes place in, and how it can be promoted across different people and contexts. If the behaviour is not adopted by large numbers, it is not a successful public health strategy. We are getting better at addressing these issues and moving beyond narrowly defined psychological constructs and models (but see comment later in the next section), although more needs to be done. As psychologists, we certainly need to see the 'bigger picture'.

Think about it … or not

There seems to be a greater recognition of some health behaviours being driven by non-conscious processing – health by stealth! While physical activity is likely to require conscious planning, sedentary behaviour is clearly influenced by habit and information processing at a subconscious level. We always reinforce this concept to our students in a lecture class. We ask how many entered the lecture theatre, stopped to think whether they should stand or sit, and then made their choice about sitting or not. It's fairly obvious that no one really does this – it's an automatic process to sit, driven by social convention and context as well as by physical environment (i.e. a seated lecture theatre). Indeed, most students sit in the same seat week after week. While it is recognised that less conscious, more automatic processing goes on, more needs to be known about this across different contexts of physical activity, and how this may be used to change behaviour, such as through nudge-type strategies (see Chapters 9 and 16).

What has not progressed?

In theory …

Psychologists interested in physical activity and health have been particularly enthusiastic about the use of theory and the range of theories used. We still subscribe to the view that behaviour change needs to use theory appropriately, but it is also clear that the field remains narrow in its use of particular theories. This is best illustrated by the ubiquitous use of the Theory of Planned Behaviour (TPB). We have argued in Chapter 8 why we believe an understanding of this theory is important, but equally we can see that it may have been overplayed and, in the view of some, may be in need of 'retirement' (Sniehotta *et al.*, 2014). However, it may also be to do with the way we test some theories. With the TPB, a great deal of emphasis has been placed on predicting intentions rather than behaviour. Where behaviour has been assessed, it is either too general a construct (e.g. 'physical activity' rather than certain types of physical activity), or it is assessed poorly through a weak self-report instrument.

It was in 2004 that one of us (Stuart) said in his keynote lecture at the annual conference of the British Association of Sport and Exercise Sciences that we have placed too much emphasis on the 'left' side elements of models such as the TPB and not enough on *predicting actual behaviour* – the right side (see Figure 8.3 if you are not sure what we mean by this). This is certainly true of much of the research on physical activity motivation where motivational constructs have usually been linked with outcomes such as enjoyment, need satisfaction and effort rather than actual behaviour. Moreover, we still know little about translating good intentions into behaviour. Better integration of elements across theories may be needed (Hagger and Chatzisarantis, 2014).

Perhaps a more important issue is to do with the theories we do *not* use in physical activity research. Physical activity studies are highly likely to utilise one of only a handful of theories: social cognitive theory, TPB, the Transtheoretical Model and self-determination theory. Maybe we are also guilty of this and, of course, these theories are summarised in this book because that is where the evidence has been accumulated. Interestingly, we suggest that other approaches may be more appropriate for the study of sedentary behaviour (see Chapter 16). It was also in the 2004 BASES keynote lecture where this issue was raised. It was suggested that greater attention be paid to social and environmental theories, as well as theories of policy, and not just those focusing on individual psychology (see Bartholomew *et al.*, 2001). Little seems to have changed in this regard even though the field is now embracing nudge-type approaches (Thaler and Sunstein, 2008; Wise, 2011), and approaches based on lower levels of conscious processing, as well as social and environmental frameworks.

It seems to work, but how?

Another area where rather little progress seems to have taken place is in identifying the mechanisms accounting for the mental health outcomes of physical activity. We have been unable to say a great deal more in this version of the book compared with the previous two editions. We believe that breakthroughs are likely to be made, and maybe soon, especially regarding neuroscience explanations. It is ironic that the popular media have picked up on the potential role of endorphins for many years, yet scientists see endorphin release as being just one of several neurobiological mechanisms at play. Determining the mechanisms for the psychological benefits of physical activity is perhaps the greatest challenge for exercise scientists trying to illuminate the relationship between physical activity and mental health. It is clear that the answer to this complex question will not be found in exercise laboratories alone. We must collaborate with colleagues in neuroscience and psychological medicine to expand our knowledge.

In short, we are confident in saying that there are significant mental health benefits from physical activity, but we still do not really know why.

Different strokes for different folks

There seems to have been a lack of progress in understanding the extent to which different types of physical activity are affected by different correlates. If we believe that modifiable correlates provide the 'active ingredients' for behaviour change, why have we been so slow in looking at different correlates for different types of physical activity? One of the few examples where this has been done is Edwardson and Gorely's (2010) systematic review of parental correlates of youth physical activity. Instead of synthesising the correlates of 'physical activity', they reviewed studies by types and intensities of physical activity. This makes sense and should help future interventions to be more targeted and successful. The same may be said for sedentary behaviour. We should not expect the correlates of sitting for evening TV to be the same as for sitting at work.

What is missing?

It's really about the long term

As we say in Chapter 11 with reference to the natural history model, we know more about starting physical activity involvement than we do about maintaining such involvement. Similarly, interventions showing effective behaviour change often do not assess or demonstrate long-term maintenance. Ultimately it is continued involvement in physical activity that will provide public and personal health benefits. The health benefits cannot be stored up. We need to help people get started and maintain their involvement. Yet we seem unable to make much of a contribution to knowledge on this. Of course the issue is a tough one to address, and maybe funding agencies are too conservative to 'risk' investing long term.

Measure where, not just what

We have already alluded to the premise that 'context is king'. However, while we have made considerable progress in assessing how much physical activity we undertake (e.g. with objective monitoring tools), we are still missing good measures of the context in which physical activity takes place. It is argued that such measures will be self-reported, such as saying where the behaviour took place, who the person was with, etc. However, progress is needed in combining the quantification of objective outcome measures with simultaneous context data. For example, radio frequency identification (RFID) tags could be used to link an individual with an environmental context such that location may be coupled with other behavioural data. While the intrusive nature of such measures may be an issue, the principle of linking behavioural frequency with temporal and environmental context remains an important one to investigate in the future. New technologies should help a great deal here.

The work using geographic information systems (GIS) and position systems (GPS) are now being seen in physical activity research. This is clearly an advance, but more work is required. GPS, for example, has the key role of providing context/location data, but could also be used for motivational purposes, such as through GPS running and cycling apps on smart phones. We need to know more about how people use and interact with such devices.

Similarly, wearable cameras have been used recently to capture multiple images of the context where different behaviours are taking place (Doherty et al., 2013). More work is needed on this to see if such detailed context data can help us better understand how to change behaviour.

Wish you were here

While some population groups have better representation in the physical activity literature (e.g. older adults), there is still a great deal of imbalance. Sadly, we must confess to having reinforced some of this in the current book, although we guess our defence is that we are merely reporting what is available. Research commonly deals with age and gender differences, but not much is known about ethnic differences in physical activity, and particularly the associated correlates and behaviour change approaches. Similarly, mention of groups with disabilities is still quite sparse, yet it is known that adults with disabilities are much more likely to be inactive compared with those without disabilities (Carroll *et al.*, 2014).

It's more than what happens between the ears

It may be said that the current zeitgeist in psychology is cognitive. That is to say, we are in a school of thought in which what we think and feel (all from the neck up, as it were) is the predominant theory of psychology. In others times other schools had their moments, such as behaviourism or psychoanalysis (see Weiner, 1980). If cognitive psychology is the zeitgeist, where does that leave experiences and feelings from the body or the opportunity to learn from physical experience? Even positive psychology, which may be one of the newest schools of thought in psychology, could be accused of having a 'neck-up' focus on flourishing (Peterson, 2013). Martin Seligman talks of building strength as one of the key principles of positive psychology (Seligman, 2002). But gaining physical strength or capacity is not often mentioned (see Hefferon (2013) for the exception). Even in a book entitled *Psychology of Physical Activity* we have highlighted theories which are mostly cognitive. What is missing is an alternative theoretical approach in which what we experience from physical activity and what we might learn through more structured approaches, such as physical education, is appropriately acknowledged. Of course, the brain still processes all of that, but taking account of the body is currently lacking in cognitive psychology. The well-known phrase 'mens sana in corpore sano' ('a healthy mind in a healthy body') neatly describes what we have proposed elsewhere in the book as the 'somatopsychic' principle and more attention to this principle is needed. This was first introduced to us by Dorothy V. Harris in the 1970s and 1980s when first Stuart, and then Nanette, studied with Dr Harris at Penn State University. Indeed, Harris used the term somatopsychic in the subtitle of one of her books (Harris, 1973). She wanted to use this term in preference to 'psychosomatic', as it better captured the direction of influence – body to mind.

Future research directions

Having reviewed the evidence as we compiled this new edition of the book we have some suggestions for future research directions. In addition, we will offer future directions for professional practice and policy in later sections. We will present research directions in respect of the four main sections of this book: physical activity and mental health, physical activity correlates and theories, physical activity behaviour change, and sedentary behaviour.

Physical activity and mental health

- While good mental health should be a central goal of physical activity and health programmes in its own right, researchers must devote more time to the integration of affective responses with adherence to physical activity (see Chapter 2). The nature of the physical activity undertaken (i.e. intensity, type, context) will be important in this regard.
- Greater use of longitudinal population studies is needed to show connections between physical activity and mental health. Physical activity and mental health must be adequately measured, with the former assessed using objective monitors.

- More studies are required that explore the relationship between physical activity and mental health for children and adolescents as well as special populations (e.g. certain disabilities).
- Further studies on comparisons of exercise treatment and standard drug treatments are required in mental health, including anxiety, depression and other mental health conditions.
- Multi-disciplinary research is required to determine the mechanisms by which exercise can produce the 'feel-better' or other mental health effects.
- Developments in links between physical activity and cognitive functioning need to address how best the promotion of physical activity can impact upon academic learning for young people and maintained or even enhanced cognitive functioning in older adults. The preventative effect of physical activity on dementia needs further epidemiological evidence.
- Further exploration is needed on the role of sitting time in mental health outcomes, including testing for reverse causality.
- Studies that explore the relationship between physical activity, fitness change and self-esteem are required.
- There is a need for rigorous research evaluating the effectiveness of physical activity on the self-esteem of young people and older adults. This may be achieved through well-designed randomised controlled trials.
- Future research should focus on investigating the psychological effects of physical activity through comparisons of different types of activity (e.g. supervised vs. home-based, aerobic vs. resistance, or flexibility/balance-based activity).

Physical activity correlates and theories

- More needs to be known about how the correlates of physical activity may differ across different intensities and types of activity.
- Physical activity must be adequately measured – including objective assessment – to capture both the amount and context of activity.
- Better integration of aspects across different psychological theories should be considered, including more automatic and conscious processing approaches.
- Research should investigate the role of social, environmental and policy theories alongside theories of psychology.

Physical activity behaviour change

- The factors that contribute to the maintenance of physical activity following supervised programmes, such as those offered in breast cancer rehabilitation, have not been fully explored.
- How best to integrate physical activity promotion into routine clinical care requires further research.
- Researchers must involve potential participants and other stakeholders in all stages of behaviour change research, including design and development.
- We need follow-up data to demonstrate the extent to which the effects of interventions are maintained over time.
- Better use of process evaluations is required to understand successful and unsuccessful behaviour change efforts.

Sedentary behaviour

- More needs to be known about the influences on different sedentary behaviours among different groups and within the same group across different contexts.
- More needs to be known about the acceptability of different strategies and behaviours designed to reduce sitting. In addition, we need to know more about how messages concerning 'less sitting' are interpreted and understood.
- In addition to environmental influences, we need to develop our understanding of social context and influences on sedentary behaviour.
- Progress is required in the development of sedentary behaviour self-monitoring tools.
- Research is needed on sedentary behaviour change, including habit breaking, using a wider range of theories, and not just relying on theories used in physical activity.
- Little is known about the longevity of some behaviour change strategies, such as sit-to-stand stations in office environments.
- We need improvements in measurement of sedentary behaviour to capture the amount, type and context of behaviours.

Future directions for professional practice

- Better links to, and communication with, physical activity groups and 'industry' are required, including the fitness industry, schools, workplaces, community groups, non-government agencies (e.g. 'Paths for All') and governments.
- Greater emphasis on the skills needed to promote physical activity to individuals and groups, and knowledge of appropriate measurement techniques, is needed for accreditation processes for sport and exercise psychologists.
- The professional development for those working in the fitness, health and physical activity industries, and initiatives such as 'Exercise is Medicine', should include more training material on psychology and behaviour change (see Nigg, 2014).

Future directions for policy

- Governments need to avoid placing too much emphasis on 'sport' in efforts to promote population-wide physical activity. In most countries 'sport', defined as suggested in Chapter 1, is a minority activity in population terms.
- More advocacy work is needed at all levels, and including academics alongside other health professionals.
- More national and local walking and cycling strategies are needed that are aimed at increasing physical activity and reducing our reliance on cars (because of pollution, congestion and reducing global oil resources).
- There is a need for government departments to work collaboratively in tackling physical activity, including departments responsible for health, education and transport.
- Academic organisations should consider adopting a strong advocacy role along their research and dissemination roles.
- Governments should adopt the principles of the Toronto Charter and the seven investments that work for promoting physical activity which we described in Chapters 1 and 12. These policies must be resourced at similar levels to the resourcing that was provided for the reduction of smoking levels.
- Objective monitoring of physical activity levels in national surveillance should become the norm.

References

Bartholomew, L.K., Parcel, G.S., Kok, G. and Gottlieb, N.H. (2001). *Intervention Mapping: Designing theory- and evidence-based health promotion programs*. Mountain View, CA: Mayfield.

Biddle, S.J.H. (2006). Research synthesis in sport and exercise psychology: Chaos in the brickyard revisited. *European Journal of Sport Science, 6*(2), 97–102.

Biddle, S.J.H. and Asare, M. (2011). Physical activity and mental health in children and adolescents: A review of reviews. *British Journal of Sports Medicine, 45*, 886–895. doi: 10.1136/bjsports-2011-090185.

Biddle, S.J.H. and Mutrie, N. (1991). *Psychology of Physical Activity and Exercise: A health-related perspective*. London: Springer-Verlag.

——. (2001). *Psychology of Physical Activity: Determinants, well-being and interventions*. London: Routledge.

——. (2008). *Psychology of Physical Activity: Determinants, well-being and interventions* (2nd edn). London: Routledge.

Biddle, S.J.H., Petrolini, I. and Pearson, N. (2014). Interventions designed to reduce sedentary behaviours in young people: A review of reviews. *British Journal of Sports Medicine, 48*, 182–186. doi: 10.1136/bjsports-2013-093078.

Carroll, D.D., Courtney-Long, E.A., Stevens, A.C., Sloan, M.L., Lullo, C., Visser, S.N. and Dorn, J.M. (2014). Vital signs: Disability and physical activity – United States, 2009–2012. *Morbidity and Mortality Weekly Report, 63*(18), 407–413.

Daley, A.J. (2008). Exercise and depression: A review of reviews. *Journal of Clinical Psychology in Medical Settings, 15*, 140–147.

Doherty, A.R., Hodges, S.E., King, A.C., Smeaton, A.F., Berry, E., Moulin, C.J.A. and Foster, C. (2013). Wearable cameras in health. *American Journal of Preventive Medicine, 44*(3), 320–323. doi: 10.1016/j.amepre.2012.11.008.

Edwardson, C.L. and Gorely, T. (2010). Parental influences on different types and intensities of physical activity in youth: A systematic review. *Psychology of Sport and Exercise, 11*(6), 522–535.

Ekkekakis, P. (ed.). (2013). *Routledge Handbook of Physical Activity and Mental Health*. London: Routledge.

Forscher, B.K. (1963). Chaos in the brickyard. *Science, 142*, 35.

Greaves, C., Sheppard, K., Abraham, C., Hardeman, W., Roden, M., Evans, P. and the IMAGE Study Group. (2011). Systematic review of reviews of intervention components associated with increased effectiveness in dietary and physical activity interventions. *BMC Public Health, 11*(1), 119.

Hagger, M.S. and Chatzisarantis, N.L.D. (2014). An integrated behavior change model for physical activity. *Exercise and Sport Sciences Reviews, 42*(2), 62–69. doi: 0091-6331/4202/62-69.

Harris, D.V. (1973). *Involvement in Sport: A somatopsychic rationale for physical activity*. Philadelphia, PA: Lea & Febiger.

Hefferon, K. (2013). *Positive Psychology and the Body: The somato-psychic side to flourishing*. Maidenhead: Open University Press.

Kriemler, S., Meyer, U., Martin, E., van Sluijs, E.M.F., Andersen, L.B. and Martin, B.W. (2011). Effect of school-based interventions on physical activity and fitness in children and adolescents: A review of reviews and systematic update. *British Journal of Sports Medicine, 45*, 923–930. doi: 10.1136/bjsports-2011-090186.

Morgan, W.P. (1969). Physical fitness and emotional health: A review. *American Corrective Therapy Journal, 23*, 124–127.

Nigg, C.R. (ed.). (2014). *ACSM's Behavioral Aspects of Physical Activity and Exercise*. Philadelphia, PA: Lippincott Williams & Wilkins.

Peterson, C. (2013). *Pursuing the Good Life: 100 reflections on positive psychology*. New York: Oxford University Press.

Seligman, M.E.P. (2002). Positive psychology, positive prevention and positive therapy. In C.R. Snyder and S.J. Lopez (eds), *Handbook of Positive Psychology* (pp. 3–9). New York: Oxford University Press.

Sniehotta, F.F., Presseau, J. and Araujo-Soares, V. (2014). Editorial: Time to retire the theory of planned behaviour. *Health Psychology Review, 8*(1), 1–7. doi: 10.1080/17437199.2013.869710.

Thaler, R. and Sunstein, C. (2008). *Nudge: Improving decisions about health, wealth, and happiness.* Newhaven, CT: Yale University Press.

Weiner, B. (1980). *Human Motivation.* New York: Holt, Rinehart & Winston.

Wise, J. (2011). Nudge or fudge? Doctors debate best approach to improve public health. *British Medical Journal, 342*, d580.

Subject index

Page references in *italics* are for figures and a **bold** reference indicates a table.

Author index

Page references in *italics* are for figures and a **bold** reference indicates a table.